Withdrawn
Outdated Material
Hepatitis

WITHDRAWN

ALSO BY ELAINE A. MOORE

*Autoimmune Diseases and
Their Environmental Triggers* (2002)

WITH LISA MOORE

Encyclopedia of Sexually Transmitted Diseases (2005)

*Encyclopedia of Alzheimer's Disease; With Directories
of Research, Treatment and Care Facilities* (2003)

Graves' Disease: A Practical Guide (2001)

ALL FROM MCFARLAND

Hepatitis

Causes, Treatments and Resources

ELAINE A. MOORE

McFarland & Company, Inc., Publishers
Jefferson, North Carolina, and London

Library of Congress Cataloguing-in-Publication Data

Moore, Elaine A., 1948–
    Hepatitis : causes, treatments and resources / Elaine A. Moore.
        p.   cm.
    Includes bibliographical references and index.

    ISBN-13: 978-0-7864-2623-2
    ISBN-10: 7864-2623-3
    (softcover : 50# alkaline paper) ∞

    1. Hepatitis—Popular works.
    I. Title.
    RC848.H42M66 2006
    616.3'623–dc22   2006020688

British Library cataloguing data are available

Cover photograph ©2006 Comstock.

Manufactured in the United States of America

McFarland & Company, Inc., Publishers
  Box 611, Jefferson, North Carolina 28640
    www.mcfarlandpub.com

Table of Contents

Preface

Developing hepatitis can be compared to being struck by a stray ball. For some people, the ball merely grazes the skin and is soon forgotten. For a smaller number of individuals, this acute assault, like acute hepatitis, can have serious ramifications, including death. For most people, symptoms are mild and resolve within a few weeks to a few months. If the ball caused irreparable internal damage or if hepatitis progressed into a chronic condition, tissue damage could persist indefinitely although complications might not be noticed for many years. Whether the hepatitis is acute or chronic, preventive measures are available, injuries may cause no symptoms; treatment options offer benefits; and individual occurrences are unique events capable of permanently resolving or causing a legacy of lingering effects.

Hepatitis, a disease characterized by liver inflammation or injury, is an ancient disorder with both infectious and non-infectious origins. Virtually any assault to the liver can damage the liver's cells and elicit an immune response resulting in inflammation.

The word hepatitis stems from "hepato," derived from the Greek word *hepatikos*, which refers to the liver, and "-itis," a suffix meaning "the fire within," which is used to describe inflammation. The word hepatitis was first coined in 1912 to describe the epidemic viral form of the disease.

However, hepatitis doesn't refer to viral hepatitis alone. Hepatitis is a collective term referring to a broad class of diseases causing liver injury or inflammation. Hepatitis can also be caused by bacteria and toxins, and it can result from metabolic disorders, including obesity and the iron overload disorder hemochromatosis.

The first records of epidemic hepatitis, presumably caused by the hepatitis A virus (HAV), date back to Hippocrates, in his description of an

1

epidemic of jaundice on the Greek island of Thassos in 510 B.C. Since that time there have been numerous hepatitis epidemics reported worldwide, especially during wars, with 10-year cycles of increased prevalence.

Before 1948, all infectious hepatitis was presumed to be caused by one virus referred to as hepatitis A. HAV had, by then, been found in the feces of infected patients and was known to be spread by contaminated food and water. Serum hepatitis had also been identified by 1948, but no one had yet discovered its viral origin.

By 1961, however, scientists realized that other viruses, toxins, parasites and bacteria could all cause hepatitis with most infectious hepatitis presumably caused by HAV. The 1962 *Merck Manual* refers to serum hepatitis as inoculation hepatitis, transfusion hepatitis, viral hepatitis and hepatitis B as a means of distinguishing it from hepatitis caused by HAV [43].

Soon after the discovery of hepatitis B virus (HBV) in 1966, blood tests for it were developed. People with symptoms of infectious hepatitis with negative tests for HAV and HBV were said to have non-A, non-B (NANB) hepatitis. In 1988 the hepatitis C virus was isolated and found to be the primary cause of NANB hepatitis. The discoveries of the hepatitis D, E, F and G viruses soon followed.

In the United States the hepatitis viruses A–D are responsible for most cases of viral hepatitis. However, other viruses, such as cytomegalovirus (CMV), Epstein-Barr virus, varicella and herpes viruses, described in chapter four, can also be responsible.

Hepatitis causes an acute disease that may persist, causing chronic disease. Chronic hepatitis is responsible for the true disease burden of hepatitis. Approximately 1.25 million Americans are chronically infected with HBV, and an estimated 2.7 million Americans are chronically infected with HCV [17]. Blood products used before 1990 account for most of the chronic hepatitis in the U.S. The introduction of blood tests for HBV and HCV has dramatically reduced hepatitis transmission. Today, 61 percent of new HCV cases are caused by intravenous drug use.

The hepatitis A virus (HAV), which causes acute but not chronic illness, affects about 25 percent of the population worldwide, usually children, in whom it seldom causes symptoms. In some undeveloped countries, HAV is endemic. Although the course of HAV tends to be milder than that of HBV and HCV, in the United States HAV causes approximately 100 fatalities related to acute liver failure annually [17].

Besides transmission through blood products, hepatitis viruses can be transmitted via intravenous drug use, hemodialysis, childbirth, organ transplants, contaminated food, unsanitary conditions, occupational exposures, and sexual intercourse. Patients with the clotting factor deficiencies hemophilia and thallasemia, an inherited form of anemia, have the highest risk because they typically receive multiple transfusions or blood products made from hundreds of different donors.

Hepatitis caused by drugs results from more than 1,000 different medications. Alcohol abuse, toxic chemicals, bacteria and parasites can also be responsible. Hepatitis also occurs in several metabolic disorders, including shock (ischemic hepatitis or shock liver); Wilson's disease, a copper storage disease; hemochromatosis, an iron overload disorder; and alpha antitrypsin deficiency. Hepatitis can also occur as an autoimmune liver disorder known as chronic autoimmune hepatitis.

The first three chapters of *Hepatitis: Causes, Treatments and Resources* focus on the history, symptoms, causes and disease course of the various hepatitis disorders. Normal liver function, the immune system response, and the changes in liver function caused by hepatitis and the effects of these changes on general health are also described. Risk factors and special concerns for the prison population, hemodialysis patients, children, and pregnant women are included.

Chapters 4 through 9 describe the infectious causes of hepatitis including hepatitis viruses, bacteria, parasites, cytomegalovirus, herpes viruses, varicella, and Epstein-Barr virus. For each microorganism, the epidemiology, symptoms, diagnosis, and disease course are included.

The non-infectious causes of hepatitis are described in chapters 10 through 12. Chapter 10 describes autoimmune hepatitis, and chapter 11 describes hepatitis caused by drugs, alcohol, and toxins. Chapter 12 describes hepatitis in metabolic disorders, such as Wilson's disease, non-alcoholic fatty liver, alpha 1-antitrypsin deficiency, galactosemia, tyrosinemia, and hemochromatosis.

Chapter 13 describes the advanced stages of hepatitis, including liver failure, cirrhosis, sclerosing hepatitis, and hepatocellular cancer (primary liver cancer). Chapter 14 describes laboratory and imaging tests used to diagnose and assess hepatitis. Chapter 15 describes the cellular changes of hepatitis seen on liver biopsies, and it explains how these changes are used to interpret disease staging, severity and prognosis.

Chapters 16 through 18 focus on treatment and lifestyle influences. Chapter 16 describes conventional treatment, including transplants. Chapter 17 describes alternative treatment options including glandular extracts and herbal medicine. Chapter 18 describes lifestyle influences including diet, exercise and stress reduction techniques.

The book concludes with a comprehensive resource chapter, including government resources, Internet websites, drug assistance programs, organ transplant sources, hotlines, and support groups. The resource chapter is followed by a glossary of terms, a list of references, and an index.

This book is intended to empower and educate patients with hepatitis, including the many people whose hepatitis has no definitive cause. With insight into the nature and course of hepatitis and the diagnostic tests used to diagnose disease and monitor treatment, patients can understand what a diagnosis of hepatitis means and what resources are available for improving their condition and its outcome.

I'd like to take this opportunity to thank everyone who helped with this project, especially my good friend and former co-worker Marvin G. Miller, who created the insightful drawings that accompany this text. Thanks also goes to the educational departments at Abbott Diagnostics and Bayer Healthcare Diagnostics Division for sharing their resources on hepatitis testing. I'm also grateful to the Centers for Disease Prevention and Control in Atlanta, commonly known as the CDC, for their gracious sharing of educational resources. Thanks also to Lisa, Brett and Rick Moore and Diane Foster for their assistance with proofreading and for their general support.

I'd also like to take this opportunity to acknowledge the many dedicated medical technologists and pathologists I've worked with in hospital laboratories in Colorado, Idaho and Ohio during the past three decades, especially the late Dr. Raoul Urich.

Changes in the field of viral hepatitis testing are among the most dramatic seen in the clinical laboratory. Early tests for hepatitis B in the 1970s brought awareness of the window period, a time when patients can be infectious despite having negative test results. With the discovery of HCV and the introduction of viral nucleic acid testing (NAT), the nation's blood supply became safer and the incidence of acute hepatitis infections declined. The goal of laboratory medicine is providing timely and accurate results to aid in the diagnosis and management of disease. The challenge for laboratories in the next few decades will be identifying and developing tests for hepatitis markers that can rapidly assess disease progression and facilitate early treatment.

1

Understanding Hepatitis

A diagnosis of hepatitis can be frightening and confusing. It can also mean different things to different people. Some people may recall an obese or alcoholic friend known to have hepatitis and wonder how this relates to them. Or they might think of a friend who developed hepatitis years after receiving blood transfusions during surgery. Others might immediately consider a relative who abused drugs years ago and now is on the list for a liver transplant. Still others might recall a co-worker who came down with hepatitis after a trip to Mexico or a friend's newborn who was diagnosed with hepatitis shortly after birth. A diagnosis of hepatitis can indeed mean many different things.

Hepatitis is a broad term used to describe a diverse group of related medical conditions, both infectious and non-infectious, that cause liver inflammation and liver disease involving degenerative or necrotic (cell death) alterations of liver cells. In some people hepatitis causes no discernible symptoms. In others, it can cause symptoms ranging from mild fatigue to life-threatening liver failure. Viruses, toxins, therapeutic drugs, vitamin overdoses, parasites and bacteria can all cause hepatitis. In addition, hepatitis can develop as a result of several different metabolic diseases, including obesity and the iron storage disorder hemochromatosis.

This chapter focuses on the nature of hepatitis including its typical causes, disease course, signs, symptoms, stages, associated syndromes, and complications. Readers will also learn about the history of hepatitis, the differences between acute, chronic, and fulminant disorders, the various types of hepatitis and some of the special considerations of hepatitis in neonates and children and in pregnancy.

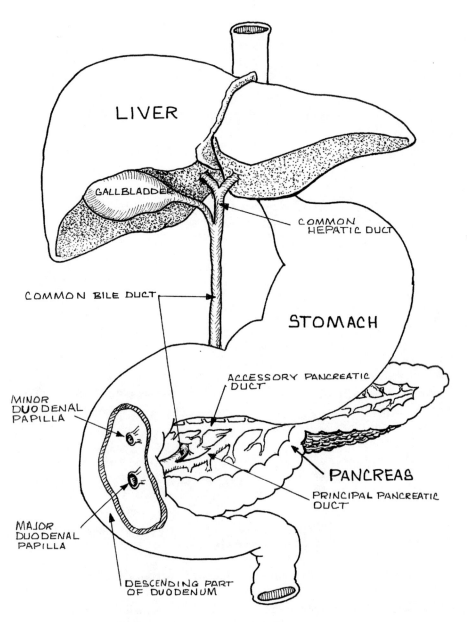

Liver and adjacent organs (Marvin G. Miller).

What Is Hepatitis?

Hepatitis is a disease of liver inflammation and liver cell destruction. The liver is the body's primary metabolic organ, responsible for converting food into energy and medications into effective compounds. Inflammation is one of the immune system's ways of responding to injury and disease.

In inflammation, white blood cells rush to the site of the injury. Here, they work together to produce toxic chemicals that offer protection. These immune substances contribute to cell damage and symptoms in liver disease.

In hepatitis caused by toxins, symptoms and their severity are primarily related to the liver cell damage inflicted by the responsible toxin. In infectious hepatitis the immune system's response to injury or to viral or bacterial invasion causes most symptoms. In either case, the injured liver can no longer carry out its functions efficiently.

Hepatitis typically occurs as an acute disorder of sudden onset lasting several months before resolving. In some cases of hepatitis, if its cause persists or if the damage to the liver is particularly severe, even in the absence of symptoms, hepatitis can cause chronic or long-term illness, with serious symptoms developing decades later.

Causes of acute hepatitis

Approximately 46,000 cases of acute hepatitis are reported in the United States annually. These represent only a fraction of cases. Specialists in the field estimate that only 1 out of every 5–10 cases is diagnosed and reported. The most common cause of acute hepatitis is shock resulting from bleeding, infection, trauma, heat stroke, cardiac problems and related conditions. The liver and the heart work closely together. Damage to either organ affects the other.

Viral hepatitis is another prominent cause of acute hepatitis. The hepatitis A virus (HAV) is the most common cause (50 percent of cases) in the United States although the hepatitis B virus (HBV) accounts for more reported cases. The hepatitis C virus (HCV) accounts for about 15 percent of cases. Toxins are a less common cause of acute hepatitis, but they are the most common cause of fulminant hepatic failure, a severe life-threatening form of hepatitis.

ENZYMES IN ACUTE HEPATITIS

Enzymes are proteins found within the body's cells that are essential for the cell's various functions. Enzymes are catalysts acting in a manner similar to kerosene added to a fire. They ignite chemical reactions and keep them going. Liver enzymes help the liver carry out its many functions such as converting sugar into stored energy. When liver cells are damaged, enzymes leak from the cells and spill out into the blood circulation.

Hepatocytes are the most predominant type of liver cell. That is, most areas of liver tissue are composed of these cells. The hepatocyte cell cytoplasm, which surrounds the cell nucleus, contains several different liver enzymes, primarily alanine aminotransferase (ALT) and aspartate aminotransferase (AST). Hepatocytes contain approximately one and a half to two times as much ALT as AST. These enzymes are also found in other organs, but ALT is primarily found in the liver. Besides being present in liver cells, high amounts of AST are found in the bone.

ENZYMES IN SHOCK HEPATITIS (ISCHEMIC SHOCK)

Shock arising from blood loss, infection, or trauma can damage the liver. The clinical picture is the same in all types of shock. There are rapid, marked increases in AST and ALT which also fall rapidly, indicating a rapid massive necrosis (cell death). The prothrombin time, which measures a clotting factor produced in the liver, rises very quickly and to very high levels although there is only a minimal increase in levels of bilirubin, a bile pigment found in liver cells.

ENZYMES IN VIRAL HEPATITIS

In acute viral hepatitis, ALT and AST are released from damaged liver cells into the blood circulation. High levels of these enzymes are an early sign of liver disease, particularly the condition known as hepatitis. In the early stages of acute hepatitis serum AST levels are usually higher than ALT levels. However, AST stays in the blood circulation for only 18 hours before breaking down, and ALT stays in the circulation for 49 hours. Consequently, after the first one or two days, ALT levels rise higher than AST levels [28].

ENZYMES IN TOXIC HEPATITIS

In acute hepatitis caused by toxins, peak AST and ALT levels usually rise 10–100 or more times the upper reference limit. Typically, the AST:ALT ratio is greater than 1 for the first 1–2 days. The liver enzyme alkaline phosphatase (ALP) is known to also rise dramatically in toxic hepatitis. Patients may also develop a rash, joint or kidney problems and an increased blood eosinophil count. Eosinophils are a type of white blood cell that typically rises in allergic and parasitic reactions. Toxic drug reactions most commonly occur after starting a new drug, but they can occur in someone who has been on a medication for several weeks to several months, and they frequently occur in overdoses of certain drugs, such as acetaminophen.

In acute alcoholic hepatitis the peak ALT rises only 3–5 times the upper reference limit and the ratio of AST:ALT is greater than 2.0. Enzyme levels are useful for determining the cause of acute hepatitis. Enzyme levels and other lab features in acute hepatitis are described further in chapter fourteen.

Causes of chronic hepatitis

Chronic hepatitis was once defined as hepatitis persisting for more than six months. In 2004 the definition was changed. Chronic hepatitis is now defined by the appearance of certain cellular changes that occur in the liver and certain viral components or markers that persist in the blood. A significant disease burden is associated with chronic hepatitis, including vascular diseases and the possible progression to cirrhosis, liver failure, and hepatocellular cancer (HCC).

In the United States, the most common causes of chronic hepatitis are chronic HBV and HCV infection and a metabolic disorder called nonalcoholic steatohepatitis (NASH), which causes a condition of fatty liver. These three causes are responsible for 80–90 percent of cases. Drugs, autoimmune hepatitis, and the iron storage disorder hemochromatosis account for most of the remaining cases [28].

How Is Hepatitis Diagnosed?

Hepatitis is usually suspected when patients seek medical advice for flu-like symptoms or jaundice, a yellowing of the skin and eyes. Blood tests that assess liver damage can determine the source of the jaundice. However, many patients with viral hepatitis never develop symptoms or they develop very mild symptoms. For them, hepatitis is usually detected when they're tested for infectious diseases after volunteering as blood donors or as part of a routine physical or prenatal screen.

If the basic liver test results suggest a diagnosis of hepatitis, other more specific blood tests are used to determine the specific cause. For instance, blood tests for viral markers are used to diagnose or rule out the various types of viral hepatitis. Toxin assays, autoantibody tests and metabolic profiles are used to identify toxic, autoimmune or metabolic causes. Disease severity is assessed by certain other laboratory tests, imaging tests and liver biopsies. These tests are described in chapters fourteen and fifteen.

History of Viral Hepatitis

The first reference to an epidemic of jaundice dates back to 510 B.C. and is found in both the Talmud and in the writings of Hippocrates. Accounts also exist in records from ancient Greece, Rome and China. The first account of hepatitis in Western Europe is described in a letter written in 752 A.D. by Pope Zacharias to St. Boniface, Archbishop of Mainz.

Since, epidemics of infectious hepatitis have occurred regularly, especially during wartime, with major outbreaks occurring about every ten years. Problems related to hepatitis were reported in the Franco-Prussian War, the American Civil War, both World Wars, the Viet Nam War and the Persian Gulf War.

However, the origins of these epidemics remained elusive until the late 19th century when Scandinavian researchers detected the first evidence of the liver cell degeneration that occurs in early hepatitis. These scientists proved that inflammatory jaundice, epidemic hepatitis and a similar condition that had been termed acute yellow atrophy were all the same disease. In the early 20th century, the physician McDonald suggested that a virus was the likely cause [26]. However, it was years before this could be proven. And as late as 1944, hepatitis was described as catarrhal jaundice, implying that the disorder originated in the mucous membranes.

During World War II huge hepatitis epidemics debilitated troops, primarily in the Middle East and Italy. In France, the disorder was called "Jeunisee descamps" and in Germany it was called "Kriegikoruror Soldatengelbsucht." In 1942 the German physician Voegt was the first to demon-

Table 1.1— The Hepatitis Viruses

Virus	Viral Type	Virus Group	Mode of Transmission	Disease
Hepatitis A Virus (HAV)	Small RNA virus lacking an outer envelope	*Picornaviridae*, genus Hepatovirus in the *Heparnavirus* genus	Fecal-oral; enteric transmission of contaminated food and water, uncooked and undercooked shellfish; rarely through sexual intercourse, usually anal and anal-oral sex, and rarely through blood to blood contact	Hepatitis A, Infectious hepatitis, Endemic Hepatitis; HAV usually causes acute infection; acute fulminant infection responsible for about 100 fatalities in the United States annually; very rarely causes chronic infection
Hepatitis B Virus (HBV)	Double-stranded DNA virus with inner core and outer envelope	Hepadnaviridae group of the genus *Orthohepadnaviridae*, similar to woodchuck and squirrel hepatitis viruses	Blood-blood, sexual intercourse; blood products, contaminated medical equipment, needles, childbirth, injecting drug use; chronic infection seen commonly in infants & patients with HIV.	Hepatitis B, serum hepatitis, homologous serum hepatitis
Hepatitis C Virus (HCV)	Single-stranded RNA virus with an outer envelope	*Flaviviridae* group of the genus *Hepacivirus*	Blood-blood; contaminated blood products, medical equipment, intravenous and injecting drug use; rarely through sexual and perinatal contact	Hepatitis C, non-A, non-B (NANB) hepatitis
Hepatitis D Virus (HDV)	Circular, single-stranded RNA virus that requires HBV for its activation	Unassigned group of the Deltavirus family; related to plant satellite viruses and viroids	Blood-blood; primarily injecting drug use, contaminated blood products and equipment; occasionally sexually transmitted	Hepatitis D or Delta Virus

Table 1.1 (cont.)

Virus	Viral Type	Virus Group	Mode of Transmission	Disease
Hepatitis E Virus (HEV)	Single-stranded RNA virus lacking an outer envelope	Calciviridae, genus proposed, closely resembles rubella virus and a plant virus known as beet necrotic yellow vein virus	Fecal-oral; fecal contamination of food and water, primarily in tropical and sub-tropical regions	Hepatitis E, particularly severe, sometimes fatal disease in 3rd trimester of pregnancy
Hepatitis F Virus (HFV)	Virus-like particles	Undetermined	Undetermined	Uncertain
Hepatitis G (HGV); CBV-C	RNA virus related to other positive-stranded flaviviruses	Related to flaviviruses	Blood-blood contact; contaminated blood products, medical equipment	Uncertain; tends to co-exist with hepatitis B and C

strate the infectivity of this disease by injecting volunteers with body fluids taken from patients with hepatitis [25].

Hepatitis viruses

The hepatitis viruses are introduced briefly in this section and more extensively in chapters five through nine. Despite hepatitis's ancient origins, it's only been in recent years that the diversity of infectious agents responsible for hepatitis has come to light. The name hepatitis was implemented in 1912, and in 1953 hepatitis became a reportable disease. However, the era of modern hepatitis virology didn't start until 1966 with the discovery of the hepatitis B virus (HBV).

The hepatitis viruses are a diverse group of viruses that share a remarkable tropism or affinity for the liver. These viruses are profoundly different from one another in their physical structure, epidemiology and mode of transmission.

However, the hepatitis viruses are similar in that they can all cause clinically overt acute hepatitis associated with frank jaundice. Symptoms in viral hepatitis are so similar that one type of viral hepatitis can't be distinguished from another without blood tests for viral markers. Symptoms caused by the hepatitis viruses are generally far more severe than symptoms in hepatitis caused by other viruses such as cytomegalovirus.

While infection with HAV tends to quickly resolve, approximately eleven to 22 percent of patients with HAV infection are hospitalized, and adults who become ill lose an average 27 days of work [17]. HBV usually causes an acute self-limited infection although 51 percent of patients with acute HBV infection never develop symptoms. However, HBV tends to always cause chronic infection in its young and immunocompromised patients, including patients with human immunodeficiency (HIV) infection, which causes AIDS.

Infection with hepatitis C differs in that it tends to cause chronic infection in up to 80 percent of the patients it infects. Hepatitis D differs in that it can only infect persons already infected with hepatitis B. The ability of the hepatitis F and G viruses to cause disease is less certain, and the hepatitis E virus typically only causes a mild acute infection similar to that of HAV. However, HEV is often fatal when it affects pregnant women especially during the third trimester.

Hepatitis A

Early cases of epidemic hepatitis are generally attributed to the hepatitis A virus (HAV). By the middle of the 20th century, researchers recognized that viruses introduced by fecally contaminated food and water were responsible for HAV. The associated condition was called infectious hepatitis, catarrhal jaundice or hepatitis A.

HAV is classified as the type species of the genus *Hepatovirus* of the family *Picornaviridae*. The virus is a small (27 nm) spherical RNA virus that lacks an outer envelope. Chimpanzees, several species of marmosets, and New World owl monkeys can develop HAV following oral or injected inoculation of the virus. In these primates, the disease course is mild compared to that of humans although the infectious course of the disease in both species is similar [38].

HAV is primarily transmitted through fecal-oral contact although it may also be transmitted through saliva, injecting drug use, sexual intercourse and through transfusions of blood products. HAV may also be carried by flies, which serve as vectors. HAV has been found to be concentrated from contaminated coastal waters by filter-feeding shellfish. Consequently, HAV can be transmitted by the ingestion of inadequately cooked or uncooked shellfish.

Hepatitis B

By 1948, another distinct form of hepatitis called serum sickness was linked to blood transfusions and percutaneous (via the skin) injections, but its origins remained elusive until the mid–1960s. Realizing the cause was distinct from HAV, in 1948 the scientist MacCallum classified this disease hepatitis B to distinguish it from what he called infectious hepatitis or HAV. In 1962, in the 10th edition of *The Merck Manual*, researchers describe serum hepatitis as homologous serum jaundice, inoculation hepatitis, transfusion jaundice, viral hepatitis or hepatitis B [44].

Even before its viral cause was discovered, hepatitis B frequently occurred following blood transfusions, intravenous plasma therapy and medical procedures. The term "German shipyard disease" was used to describe hepatitis B in the early 20th century, and it was attributed to the sharing of contaminated needles and syringes by seamen and dock workers.

Unlike hepatitis linked to HAV, the hepatitis B virus is not associated with the presence of viral material in stool samples. When HBV was eventually discovered, the virus particle found in the serum of patients with HBV was labeled the Dane Particle.

HBV belongs to a small group of DNA viruses belonging to the *Hepadnavirus* family. The group includes the hepatitis viruses of woodchuck (WHV), ground squirrel (GSHV), duck (DHBV) and heron (HHV) [38].

In humans HBV is transmitted through body fluids, primarily by transfusions of blood products, contaminated medical equipment, injecting drug use, childbirth, and sexual intercourse. Most cases of HBV infection are mild and anicteric, which means that they do not cause jaundice, and they're unlikely to be detected. However, worldwide, HBV causes the most cases of chronic hepatitis and hepatocellular carcinoma (HCC). About 410 million people or 5 percent of the world's population are carriers of HBV, and more than 51 percent of the world's population has been infected with HBV [38].

THE AUSTRALIA ANTIGEN IN HEPATITIS B

In 1966, Baruch Samuel Blumberg and his colleagues in Philadelphia discovered an unusual antibody in the serum of two haemophiliac patients who had received multiple transfusions and consequently developed hepatitis. Specific proteins known as antibodies develop when the body's immune system, which is described in chapter two, responds and reacts to the protein particles of specific infectious agents.

This particular antibody isolated by Blumberg was found to react with a protein antigen found in a single serum sample from an Australian Aborigine with viral hepatitis, from an area in which hepatitis B infection is endemic. This antigen was named the Australia antigen, and Blumberg won the 1977 Nobel prize for this discovery.

Australia antigen (AusAg) was later determined to be the surface antigen comprising the protein exterior surface of the hepatitis B virion. This antigen is now called the hepatitis B surface antigen (HBsAg). The corresponding surface antibodies, commonly referred to as HBsAb, were once known as Australian antigen antibodies or AusAb. Early tests for hepatitis B antibodies, indicators of current or past infection, were formerly called AusAb tests.

Hepatitis C

Until 1990, patients with clinical symptoms of hepatitis and negative tests for HAV and HBV were said to have non-A, non-B (NANB) hepatitis. By 1987 the causative agent of the non-A, non-B hepatitis virus had been cloned by

Michael Houghton, Qui-Lim Choo, and George Kuo from the Chiron company. This was the first time anyone had cloned a virus before first growing it in tissue culture. These scientists named this virus the hepatitis C virus (HCV).

Studies of patients initially diagnosed with non-A, non-B hepatitis in the late 1961s indicated a 71 percent incidence of hepatitis C [52] in this group. A small number of frozen blood samples from 1949 taken from patients with strepotoccal infection, which were subsequently tested, showed the presence of HCV [52]. No earlier stored blood specimens are available to indicate when HCV first emerged.

HCV is a single-stranded RNA virus of the genus *Flaviviridae* belonging to the *Hepacivirus* family. Today, patients with apparent viral hepatitis with negative screening tests for HAV, HBV and HCV are said to have non-A, non-B, and non-C (NANBNC) hepatitis.

However, when blood tests for HVC were developed it soon became apparent that most hepatitis not related to HAV and HBV was caused by HCV. Subsequent studies show that prior to screening blood units for HCV, approximately 1.5 percent of donors in the United States were infected with HCV [52]. Prior to 1990, transmission of HCV primarily occurred through body fluids, primarily transfusions of blood products and injecting drug use. HCV may also be transmitted sexually but this form of transmission is inefficient. The risk of infection with a regular sex partner is reported to be 1–3 percent annually [56].

The clinical course of HCV is typically mild and often causes no symptoms. Only 25 percent of HCV-infected patients develop jaundice, and fulminant forms of HCV are very rare. However, more than 80 percent of people with HCV develop chronic infection, which can have serious consequences.

Hepatitis D

Hepatitis D virus (HDV), which is often referred to as delta hepatitis or the delta agent, is a defective RNA virus related to plant viral satellites and viroids. HDV requires HBV to reproduce. HDV is coated with the hepatitis B surface antigen (HBsAg) and depends on HBV for its activation. Consequently, blood specimens that test negative for HBV are known to also be negative for HDV. The presence of HDV is an indication of current or recent HBV infection.

HDV can occur as a superinfection when it is superimposed on someone with active HBV infection or as a co-infection, with its own symptoms and following its own disease course. HDV is very infectious and strongly associated with intravenous drug abuse, with 17–90 percent of addicts with HBV testing positive for HDV. However, homosexual men, who typically contract HBV easily, have a very low risk for HDV.

Hepatitis E

Hepatitis E virus (HEV), which primarily occurs in South Asia and Africa, is similar to HAV in that it typically causes an acute illness that permanently resolves. HEV is more severe when it occurs in pregnancy, especially during the third trimester. HEV accounts for sporadic and epidemic hepatitis in tropical areas and in people returning from those areas. Like HAV, it is transmitted through fecal contamination, and younger people are more likely to be infected.

Hepatitis F

Hepatitis F virus (HFV) has been described as the cause of a fulminant giant cell hepatitis. Its ability to cause disease or pathogenicity in humans is controversial and it's thought to rarely cause disease in man. Several cases of hepatitis F have been reported in France.

Hepatitis G and GB

Hepatitis G virus (HGV) is also known as hepatitis GB or hepatitis GB-C. It is an RNA virus that worldwide occurs as a co-infection in more than 20 percent of people with HBV or HCV. It has a very high infectivity rate in recipients of contaminated blood although it has a very low, if any, disease burden. Studies show the presence of HGV in 1.5 percent of the blood supply in the United States [56]. Because of the innocuous nature of the virus, blood products are not routinely screened for HGV. The recently discovered hepatitis GB virus is considered non-pathogenic.

Other causes of infectious hepatitis

Hepatitis may also occur as a result of infection with several other viruses, including cytomegalovirus (CMV), the Epstein-Barr virus (EBV) that causes infectious mononucleosis, the Marsburg virus, herpes viruses, varicella, and the Ebola virus. Hepatitis may also be caused by some types of bacteria, protozoa, fungi, and parasites. These organisms and the hepatic diseases they cause are described in chapter four.

History of Non-Infectious Hepatitis

Long before viruses were discovered to be responsible for most infectious hepatitis, various chemical compounds capable of causing liver disease, such as arsenic, had been identified. Hepatitis due to toxins or metabolic causes, including obesity, is similar to viral hepatitis with the exception that fever is less conspicuous in non-infectious hepatitis.

In toxic hepatitis, jaundice may occur soon after exposure to toxins or considerably later depending on the type of toxin and its dosage. In the case of mushroom poisoning with *Amanita phalloides*, which has a mortality rate greater than 25 percent, symptoms of diarrhea appear quickly, followed by severe liver and kidney failure. In metabolic disorders, liver damage may have an acute onset, occurring in infancy, or it may develop slowly in adulthood.

Autoimmune hepatitis

In 1951, researchers described a form of chronic hepatitis occurring primarily in young women. Because nearly 15 percent of these patients had positive lupus erythematosus cell tests, this disorder was first called lupoid hepatitis. By the 1970s its autoimmune origin was discovered. This form of hepatitis, which primarily affects women between 14 and 25 years, is now referred to as autoimmune hepatitis. Autoimmune hepatitis is described more extensively in chapter ten.

Toxic hepatitis

Chlorinated hydrocarbons, including carbon tetrachloride, were recognized as a cause of liver toxicity shortly after their introduction in the early 20th century. Arsenicals, once used as a treatment for syphilis, have long been known for their ability to damage the liver. Compounds containing yellow phosphorus, typically insecticides and firecrackers, are also known to cause hepatitis. Mushroom poisoning accounts for several hundred cases of hepatitis each year, mostly in Europe.

Many drugs, such as the major tranquilizer chlorpromazine (Thorazine) and the analgesic acetaminophen (Tylenol), are well known for their ability to cause liver disease. In the United States, about 25 percent of all cases of fulminant hepatic failure are reported to be related to medication. The many toxins known to cause hepatitis are described in chapter eleven, and the metabolic causes of hepatitis are described in chapter twelve.

Signs of Hepatitis

Signs are disease characteristics that show up on a physical examination or as a result of diagnostic tests. Hepatitis causes many signs, including jaundice and liver enlargement. Signs, like symptoms, can suggest specific disorders. However, many of the signs and symptoms in hepatitis also occur in a number of different liver disorders. Blood tests are also needed to diagnose hepatitis and determine its cause.

Table 1.2 Signs of Hepatitis

Abnormal blood clotting	Enlarged liver
Abdominal distention, bloating	Enlarged spleen
Ascites	Hypoalbuminemia (low blood albumin)
Bilirubinemia (elevated bilirubin level)	Increased heart rate
Bruises	Pale stools
Dehydration	Jaundice of skin and eyes
Dry mucous membranes	Rash —flat, pustular or hives
Dry skin and hair	Skin changes in the hands
Elevated liver enzymes	Varices (enlarged blood vessels)
Encephalopathy-altered mental status	Vascular spiders

Hepatic encephalopathy and hepatic coma

Encephalopathy is a condition of brain inflammation causing impaired consciousness. Encephalopathy is characterized by swelling and an enlargement of brain cells called astrocytes, similar to the changes seen in Alzheimer's disease. Hepatic encephalopathy has been recognized since ancient times. Hippocrates writes of a patient with hepatitis who barked like a dog and lost the ability to speak.

Patients with hepatic encephalopathy often have memory loss, sleep disturbances, fixed stare, reduction of spontaneous movement, cognitive impairment, personality problems, shortened attention span, loss of balance, apathy, slow reaction times, confusion, tremor, slow or slurred speech, problems controlling temper and mood swings.

Encephalopathy may be mild, causing minor personality changes or it may be severe. In severe encephalopathy, symptoms range from stuporous to violent. In children, encephalopathy often causes mania. Encephalopathy can occur in severe acute hepatitis although it is most likely to occur in patients in liver failure. Acute encephalopathy can be triggered by infection, gastrointestinal or esophageal bleeding, electrolyte imbalances, diuretics, vomiting, excess dietary protein, severe constipation and alcohol withdrawal.

Blood ammonia levels are typically elevated in encephalopathy and also in hepatic coma. However, an elevated ammonia is not considered the cause since an elevated ammonia level does not always cause encephalopathy. The encephalopathy is presumably related to cerebral intoxication by intestinal contents that can no longer be metabolized by the liver. This impaired digestion causes a release of other chemicals such as mercaptans into the blood circulation. Excitotoxins, such as monosodium glutamate, aspartate and aspartame, are also thought to contribute to hepatic encephalopathy [47].

Patients with encephalopathy often progress to hepatic coma. Hepatic coma is often associated with fetor hepaticus, a foul smelling breath associated with impaired digestion. At first, hepatic coma resembles normal sleep but it soon progresses to complete unresponsiveness. In the early stages of coma, patients may be delirious.

Portal hypertension and varices

As liver tissue becomes damaged and scarred in cirrhosis, blood pressure in the liver's portal vein rises, causing a condition of portal hypertension. Normally, almost all of the blood from the digestive organs enters the liver through the portal vein. In cirrhosis, the portal circulation is obstructed. This causes the digestive organs to become chronically congested with stagnant blood that interferes with their function, causing indigestion, constipation or diarrhea.

Portal hypertension can lead to varices. As blood from the intestinal organs fails to properly move through the portal vein, the liver attempts to shunt this intestinal blood into smaller blood vessels, which forces these vessels to expand or bulge. Some of these newly enlarged vessels, called varices, that are located in the stomach and esophagus may become quite large. These smaller vessels were never intended to carry high blood volumes and as varices develop, the pressure within them increases dramatically. Consequently, varices can rupture and bleed, causing severe blood loss.

If the varices are detected early, beta adrenergic blocking agents (beta blockers) can be used to reduce the blood pressure in the portal vein, which helps to prevent rupture. Ruptured varices causing severe blood loss can lead to hepatic encephalopathy or coma. If detected early, ruptured vessels can be treated with a procedure known as an endoscopy, in which the vessels are expended with balloons and tied off. Surgery can also be used and a shunt, directing blood to a different vein in the liver, can be inserted.

Ascites

In patients with end stage liver disease, acute hepatic failure, and conditions causing portal hypertension such as alcoholic hepatitis, serous fluid, a clear fluid that can leak from blood vessels, often accumulates within the peritoneal or chest cavity, causing a condition known as ascites. A condition of severe or gross ascites causes marked abdominal distension, striae or stretch marks, and hernia.

Ascites in patients with cirrhosis is an ominous sign. Up to fifty percent of cirrhotic patients with ascites end up dying within one year. Ascites can be partially controlled with a low sodium diet, diuretics and fluid withdrawal or paracentesis, which involves aspirating fluid from the abdominal cavity.

Jaundice

Jaundice, which is derived from the French *jaunisse,* which means yellow, is a physical sign characterized by a yellow appearance of the eyes, skin and tissues. Jaundice is caused by deposits of a bile pigment known as bilirubin. Jaundice is the most characteristic clinical sign of liver disease, and it becomes clinically apparent when total bilirubin levels, rise to 2–3 mg/dl. Yellowing is most conspicuous in the outer perimeter of the eye and in the mucous membranes of the mouth.

Jaundice is not specific for liver disease. Jaundice occurs whenever blood levels of bilirubin rise. Jaundice may occur in conditions of hemolysis, the breakdown of red blood cells, a condition that accompanies many diseases including autoimmune hemolytic anemia (AIHA) and hemolytic disease of the newborn. The usefulness of bilirubin levels in classifying jaundice is further described in chapter fourteen.

CLASSIFICATIONS OF JAUNDICE

Jaundice can be classified into two major categories, depending on whether the elevation of bilirubin, which is called bilirubinemia, is associated with indirect or direct bilirubin. Total bilirubin and direct bilirubin measurements are used to measure blood bilirubin levels. The difference between total bilirubin and direct bilirubin represents the indirect or unconjugated fraction of bilirubin.

Unconjugated bilirubinemia. Bilirubin primarily results from the normal or abnormal destruction of red blood cells. Unconjugated or indirect bilirubinemia is caused by increases in the type of bilirubin that has not yet been conjugated by the liver. High levels of indirect bilirubin are caused by excess bilirubin production, for instance in hemolytic disease of the newborn and autoimmune hemolytic anemia, and in liver disease that disrupts the liver's ability to conjugate bilirubin. This can be caused by some toxins and drugs and it is also seen in certain conditions such as the physiological defect Gilbert syndrome, Crigler-Najjar syndrome, and neonatal jaundice.

Conjugated bilirubinemia. Conjugated bilirubinemia, an increase in direct or conjugated bilirubin, can be caused by hepatocellular disease, cholestatic disease or post-hepatic disease. Hepatocellular disease refers to conditions in which the liver cell or hepatocyte is injured, such as viral or toxic hepatitis, cirrhosis, and alcoholic hepatitis. Cholestatic disease is caused by defective transport of bilirubin into the liver cell opening or canaliculus. This can be caused by certain drugs, such as chlorpromazine and anabolic steroids, viral hepatitis, and the autoimmune liver disorder primary biliary cirrhosis. Posthepatic causes are those caused by a mechanical obstruction of bile release, including common bile duct disease and pancreatic cancer.

Skin changes

A number of different skin changes, including rash, hives, pruritis (itching), skin discolorations, pigment changes, and nail changes are frequently seen in hepatitis.

HAND CHANGES: PALMAR ERYTHEMA
(LIVER PALMS) AND WHITE NAILS

In liver disease the hands are warm and the palms appear bright red, especially at the bases of the fingers. The soles of the feet may also be affected. The mottling of skin tone recedes or blanches on pressure and the color quickly returns. Patients with palmar erythema may complain of throbbing or tingling palms.

White nails, due to the decreased circulation of the nail bed, are usually seen in cirrhosis although they may also be seen in hepatitis. A pink zone is seen at the tip of the nail.

VASCULAR SPIDERS

Vascular spiders are central lesions with a cluster of radiating spider veins that occur in liver disease, especially cirrhosis, and they may occur transiently in viral hepatitis. Vascular spiders are also known as arterial spiders, spider telangiectasis and spider angiomas, and they may disappear as the liver condition improves or if the blood pressure falls in shock or hemorrhage. Vascular spiders can bleed profusely and typically occur on the neck area, the face, forearms and hands.

Symptoms of Hepatitis

Symptoms are the characteristic changes and physical disturbances noticed by patients. Symptoms associated with specific viruses such as the peculiar skin changes that can occur in hepatitis C are discussed in the specific viral chapter.

Table 1.3 Symptoms Seen in Hepatitis

Abdominal (right upper quadrant) pain	Jaundice
Chills	Insomnia
Constipation	Joint pain
Dark, tea-colored urine	Light or pale feces
Diarrhea	Loss of appetite
Distaste for food and cigarettes	Muscle pain (myalgia)

Table 1.3 (cont.)

Fatigue	Nausea
Fever	Pruritus (itching)
Flu-like symptoms	Vomiting
Headache	Weight loss

Development of Hepatitis

Following viral exposure the virus presumably gains access to the liver via the blood circulation. Viral components have been demonstrated in liver cells, and the liver is considered the primary site of replication for hepatitis viruses.

In toxic and metabolic hepatitis, liver cells are directly damaged or their function is diminished. The source of the liver cell injury influences the disease course with certain toxins, such as phosphorus, causing fatal liver disease in up to 51 percent of affected patients. Many factors, which are discussed in chapter three, also influence the severity and clinical course of hepatitis.

Regardless of the cause, the acute stage of hepatitis usually develops in four distinct phases: an incubation period; a prodromal or symptomatic phase; an icteric phase; and a convalescent or recovery phase. Exceptions are instances of acute fatal poisoning and fulminant hepatitis. Fulminant hepatitis is described later in this chapter. Changes in specific types of viral hepatitis are found in chapters five through nine.

Acute Hepatitis

Acute hepatitis refers to a self-limited condition of liver inflammation that emerges suddenly and typically resolves within several months. Acute hepatitis follows two major pathways: 1) direct damage caused by toxins, primarily the analgesic acetaminophen, and by shock (ischemic hepatitis or shock liver, which can be caused by bleeding, infection, cardiac problems) and 2) direct effects of the infectious agent, including effects caused by the immune response, such as the cellular damage that typically occurs in viral hepatitis and alcoholic hepatitis.

Shock liver is the most common cause of all acute hepatitis in the United States, and hepatitis B is the major cause of acute viral hepatitis [28]. Drug reactions are also an increasingly common cause of acute hepatitis. Toxins are a less common cause of hepatitis, but they are responsible for most fulminant fatal hepatitis.

In chapter fourteen we'll see how the different pathways of damage in acute hepatitis cause different patterns of liver enzyme elevation, and how these tests can be used to determine the cause of acute hepatitis. Viral hepatitis can be divided into four distinct phases:

Phase I: Early or incubation phase

During the early or incubation phase of hepatitis, which averages about four weeks for HAV and up to 6 months for HBV, patients are usually asymptomatic, which means that they have no clinically significant symptoms. However, the hepatitis B and C viruses, which typically cause a more severe infection than HAV, may cause gastrointestinal and influenza-like symptoms. Blood tests taken at this time often show evidence of viral infection or elevated liver enzymes, an indication of liver cell damage.

Liver enzymes are chemicals found in liver cells that help with various metabolic processes including digestion. When liver cells are damaged, these enzymes, which are described further in chapters two and fourteen, spill out into the blood circulation causing elevated liver enzyme levels.

Phase II: Prodromal or symptomatic phase

In the second phase of hepatitis, which typically lasts from 3 days to 3 weeks, patients may experience flu-like symptoms, loss of appetite, nausea, fever, headache, upper abdominal pain and fatigue. Patients may also develop serum sickness-like symptoms, with rash and joint pain.

Phase III: Icteric phase

In the icteric phase, which lasts about 4 weeks, jaundice usually develops. At the onset of jaundice, the urine darkens and stools become pale, followed by yellowing in the skin and eyes. Serum, the liquid portion of blood, darkens, ranging from pale gold to deep brown depending on the severity of the jaundice.

At this time, prodromal symptoms resolve although some patients may develop bradycardia, a condition of slow heart rate. Temporary itching may also develop for a few days. In about 70 percent of patients the liver is enlarged and palpable (easily discerned when the abdomen is touched) with a smooth, tender edge. In about 20 percent of patients the spleen is enlarged and palpable. Spider vessels may appear on the skin and some patients continue to feel discomfort, predominantly gastrointestinal symptoms.

Phase IV: Convalescent or resolution phase

In the convalescent phase, which ranges from a few weeks to a few months, symptoms and jaundice resolve, and liver function tests return to normal. However, some patients will continue to have symptoms of fatigue until there is complete resolution. Evidence of immunity is demonstrated by antibodies to the specific virus. Most patients will experience clinical recovery within six months from the onset of disease. However, patients with HBV and HCV may develop chronic hepatitis.

Fulminant hepatitis

Fulminant hepatitis is a rare form of hepatitis characterized by the severe impairment of liver functions in the absence of preexisting liver disease or the sudden onset of liver failure with altered mental status and abnormal bleeding tendencies in an otherwise healthy person. It usually develops within the first ten days of illness, although the associated bleeding disorder and encephalopathy seen in fulminant hepatitis typically appear within eight weeks from the onset of illness.

CAUSES OF FULMINANT HEPATITIS

Viral infection and drug-induced liver damage are the two most common causes of fulminant infection in adults. In the United States, viral hepatitis causes 50 percent of cases, and acetaminophen toxicity accounts for approximately 20–35 percent of cases. The hepatitis viruses most likely to cause fulminant infection include hepatitis A, hepatitis B, hepatitis D, hepatitis E, and non A-E (NANE) hepatitis. In the United States and Europe about 24 percent of fulminant hepatitis is caused by NANE virus. NANE hepatitis is characterized by a high fatality rate, low rate of spontaneous recovery, and the complication of aplastic anemia, a type of anemia that can be fatal.

In infants, inborn errors of metabolism such as tyrosinemia and hereditary fructose intolerance are the major metabolic causes of fulminant hepatitis. In children, viral infection and Wilson's disease are also common causes.

Fulminant hepatitis may also occur in ischemic shock, surgical shock, infectious hepatitis, after exposure to toxins, after idiosyncratic or hypersensitivity reactions to various drugs, and it may also occur during the advanced stages of chronic hepatitis. It may also be caused by metabolic disorders including fatty liver of pregnancy, and it occurs after heat stroke, severe bacterial infection, infection with the herpes simplex virus, and Reye's syndrome, which is a condition of acute encephalopathy and liver disease that typically develops in children recovering from a viral infection, usually influenza or chicken pox.

In children, fulminant hepatitis is known to occur after infections with Epstein-Barr virus, cytomegalovirus, parymoxovirus, varicella zoster virus, herpes virus, parvovirus, and the adenovirus that causes the common cold. Some children with Wilson's disease show no signs of liver disease and are not diagnosed until they suddenly development fulminant liver disease. In some cases, especially those occurring in children, the cause of fulminant liver disease (or hepatitis) remains unknown.

SYMPTOMS OF FULMINANT HEPATITIS

In early infection, fulminant hepatitis may develop so rapidly and dramatically that jaundice may not have yet developed. Because of its startling presentation, fulminant hepatitis may be confused with an acute psychosis, meningitis or encephalitis. In some instances, marked jaundice develops quickly after a typical acute onset of disease.

Ominous signs in fulminant hepatitis include continuous vomiting, fetor hepaticus, which causes a sweetish, slightly fecal, foul smell of the breath, confusion and drowsiness. Rigidity frequently occurs although a flapping sort of tremor known as asterixis may also develop.

DISEASE COURSE IN FULMINANT HEPATITIS

Patients with fulminant hepatitis move into hepatic coma rapidly, and the clinical picture is that of acute liver failure, with a rise in temperature, an elevated white blood cell count, deepening of jaundice, liver atrophy and occasionally widespread hemorrhages. Liver enzyme and bilirubin levels do not indicate the severity of disease, and in some instances liver enzyme levels fall as the condition worsens. Coagulation disorders frequently occur and the prothrombin level is the best indicator of prognosis.

Patients with viral hepatitis who survive fulminant infection usually have complete recoveries and rarely develop chronic disease. The reason is that in fulminant hepatitis, the immune system launches a complete response. In people who develop chronic illness, the immune reaction is considered incomplete or ineffective.

INCIDENCE AND EPIDEMIOLOGY

In the United States approximately 2000 cases of fulminant hepatitis occur each year, and it affects equal numbers of males and females. The mortality rate may reach 80–90 percent in adults and 50 to 75 percent in children unable to receive liver transplants. The type of viral hepatitis most likely to cause fulminant hepatitis varies in different geographical regions. In the United States, hepatitis C accounts for 44.8 percent of fulminant viral hepatitis cases, hepatitis A accounts for 31.5 percent of cases, and hepatitis B accounts for 24.7 percent of cases. In hepatitis B, fulminant infection develops within 7 days of disease onset, whereas the duration from onset is 10 days for hepatitis A and 21 days for hepatitis C [64].

Subfulminant hepatic failure is the term commonly used to describe the condition in which symptoms of fulminant liver disease occur after a longer period of illness. Subfulminant hepatitis can occur up to 26 weeks after the onset of symptoms.

Hepatitis carriers

Hepatitis carriers harbor the hepatitis virus or, in the case of HBV infection the hepatitis B surface antigen, for more than six months after the onset of infection. Worldwide, about 410 million people are carriers of HBV with prevalence varying in different regions. Almost all infants infected with HBV perinatally become carriers.

In the United States about 1.25 million people are carriers of hepatitis B, and about 3 million people are carriers of hepatitis C. People with a weaker immune response, including men and patients with suppressed immune systems, including patients with HIV, the AIDS virus, are more likely to become carriers. About 10 percent of adults with HBV and 90 percent of infants with HBV go on to become carriers. About 80–85 percent of people with HCV infection become carriers.

Carriers can have a benign disease course with few symptoms or a long-term chronic progressive disease that can result in cirrhosis and liver cancer. Individuals with hepatitis B may eventually clear hepatitis B surface antigen in old age. Hepatitis carriers may also become re-infected after a benign disease course.

Apparently healthy carriers who remain asymptomatic or free of symptoms may show changes on liver biopsy that range from non-specific minimal abnormalities to liver scarring and cirrhosis.

Synctial giant cell hepatitis

Synctial giant cell hepatitis is a type of hepatitis primarily seen in children characterized by cell changes that include a fusion of hepatocytes forming a cell mass with multiple nuclei. Criteria for diagnosis include: 1) clinical features of subacute, chronic or fulminant hepatitis with greater than average symptom severity; 2) biopsy findings of synctial giant cell transformation of the liver cell cords, fusion of liver cells, bridging areas of liver cell destruction, and impaired bile flow; 3) demonstration by electron microscopy of tubular or filamentous particles within the giant cell cytoplasm that resemble the nucleocapsids of Paramyxoviruses. Conditions of giant cell hepatitis may also occur in patients with autoimmune hepatitis, and it has rarely been reported in patients after liver transplants.

Relapses and Complications of Viral Hepatitis

In viral hepatitis relapses can occur and symptoms can persist even when there are no longer signs of viral infection. In some people acute hepatitis progresses directly to chronic hepatitis, with symptoms that persist indefinitely. In others, especially those with HCV, symptoms may be absent until chronic hepatitis develops decades later.

Relapses are reported to occur in 1.8–15 percent of all hepatitis cases

[56]. A course similar to that of the initial disease may occur although symptoms are generally milder. Some patients do not experience any symptoms but have elevated liver enzymes. Relapse may be triggered by large amounts of alcohol or failure to rest and recover. Patients who relapse usually experience a complete recovery although for some relapse may indicate the development of chronic hepatitis.

The following sections describe some of the conditions and complications that can occur after the acute phase of hepatitis has resolved. Complications related to specific types of hepatitis, such as the immune complex vasculitis that develops in HBV, are described in the specific hepatitis virus chapters.

Prolonged cholestasis

Cholestasis is defined as the failure of normal amounts of bile to reach the duodenum. In some cases of hepatitis, jaundice may persist, worsen or recur due to prolonged cholestasis. Cholestasis may co-exist with hepatitis, causing it own symptoms, including sudden onset of jaundice, moderately enlarged liver and, after several weeks, itching. The jaundice of cholestasis typically persists for 8–29 weeks [56].

Post-hepatic syndrome

For several weeks to several months after hepatitis has resolved adult patients may continue to feel below par for variable periods. Associated symptoms include anxiety, fatigue, loss of appetite, alcohol intolerance, and right upper abdominal discomfort. Liver enzymes may rise up to three times the normal range [56].

Aplastic anemia

Aplastic anemia, a type of anemia caused by defective functioning of the organs that produce red blood cells, can occur as a consequence of viral hepatitis. Aplastic anemia associated with viral hepatitis is more common in Japan than in the United States.

Chronic Hepatitis

Chronic hepatitis typically occurs when liver injury persists for more than six months, confirmed by laboratory results for viral markers or by biopsy. In the United States, most chronic hepatitis is caused by HBV and HCV infection and by a metabolic disorder called nonalcoholic steatohepatitis (NASH). NASH is the most severe type of nonalcoholic fatty liver disease (NAFLD) that can occur. These three disorders make up 80–90 percent of all chronic hepatitis. The remaining cases are caused by drugs, autoimmune hepatitis and hemochromatosis.

Chronic hepatitis can take two different pathways: persistent disease and the persistent carrier state. Patients with persistent disease can have symptoms that average from mild to severe with progression to cirrhosis and liver cancer. Persistent disease can spontaneously resolve in some patients although in most patients damage occurs over many years. In the persistent carrier state, patients harbor infectious viral particles and remain infectious although they usually show no apparent signs or symptoms of disease.

Chronic hepatitis includes several different subtypes and stages that are used to classify disease severity and prognosis. These subtypes, which can range from minimal to severe, are briefly described in the following sections and more fully explained in chapter fifteen with liver biopsies. The following subtypes are still used although staging classifications are considered superior.

Chronic active hepatitis (CAH)

Chronic active hepatitis is defined by a piecemeal necrosis (cell destruction or erosion at an interface between connective tissue and liver tissue seen at the edges of portal tracts) on biopsy sections. CAH may range from mild to severe, with severe CAH showing marked inflammation, liver cell swelling, regeneration and collapse. Severe CAH can progress to cirrhosis.

Chronic persistent hepatitis (CPH)

Chronic persistent hepatitis is defined by inflammation of the portal tracts of the liver. Biopsy specimens in CPH show white blood cell infiltration, a typical finding in inflammation. CPH is associated with mild disease.

Chronic lobular hepatitis (CLH)

Chronic lobular hepatitis is defined as substantial necrosis within the lobules of the liver with no portal involvement. CLH is associated with mild disease.

Hepatitis in Neonates and Children

The liver of the newborn can react to different insults, including drugs, chemicals, viruses and bacteria. In the typical response to injury or foreign substances, the giant cells of the liver proliferate, causing a condition once known as giant cell hepatitis. Today, this disorder is called neonatal or idiopathic hepatitis, and it typically causes an increased level of direct bilirubin, a bile pigment produced by the liver.

Perinatal (occurring around the time of childbirth) or neonatal hepatitis usually causes ongoing liver cell destruction, and its causes include: amino acid defects, which are described in chapter twelve, such as alpha 1-antitrypsin deficiency, galactosemia and tyrosinemia; infections such as cytomegalovirus, syphilis, coxsackie virus, rubella, Escherichia coli, hepatitis A, hepatitis B, herpes, and toxoplasmosis; iatrogenic (caused by doctors or treatment) causes, such as total parenteral nutrition and medications; shock; congenital heart disease; and cystic fibrosis.

Symptoms and diagnosis in perinatal hepatitis

Hepatitis B infection in infants, or perinatal HBV infection, does not usually cause symptoms. However, more than 90 percent of infants and 30–50 percent of small children become hepatitis B carriers. Although they usually do not develop symptoms in childhood, they can later develop chronic disease.

Because hepatitis antibodies may be passively transferred and show up temporarily in the newborn's blood circulation, infants of mothers with HBV infection can have false positive test results and because the infant's immune system is still immature, they may not show evidence of early infection. Consequently, infants must be re-tested for hepatitis between 9–15 months of age. The CDC recommends that children of mothers infected with hepatitis B be vaccinated at birth and administered HBIG within their first 24 hours. They must also be re-vaccinated at 9–15 months if their tests for hepatitis B surface antigen and antibody are negative [15].

Babies born to mothers with antibodies to HCV show passively transmitted antibody for their first six months. Transmission of active HCV RNA from HCV positive mothers is rarely seen although it occurs more often in women who have a coexisting HIV infection.

Causes of neonatal hepatitis

NEONATAL CMV INFECTION

Cytomegalovirus (CMV) is a very common infection in neonates and small children. In good hygienic conditions the incidence is 5–10 percent, and in under-privileged regions the incidence is as high as 80 percent. CMV is often acquired in the placenta from a mother who does not have symptoms. CMV can also be transmitted in breast milk and in blood products. CMV may cause mild symptoms or fulminant hepatitis with marked jaundice and neurological defects.

OTHER CAUSES OF NEONATAL HEPATITIS

Both herpes simplex and human herpes virus VI have been found to cause fulminant neonatal hepatitis. Rubella, if contracted in the first trimester of pregnancy, can also cause a fulminant hepatitis. Infections in children are also described in the specific viral hepatitis chapters.

Hepatitis in Pregnancy

Overall, the course of viral hepatitis is not affected by pregnancy, and hepatitis does not cause health concerns to the unborn baby, although some forms of hepatitis can be transmitted during and around the time of childbirth. Viral hepatitis in pregnancy has the same prognosis as in nonpregnant patients. Women with Wilson's disease or autoimmune hepatitis are much less fertile and are likely to have complications during pregnancy. Therefore, it's recommended that women with these conditions receive appropriate treatment to gain control of their disease before becoming pregnant. Despite these complications, babies born to these women are normal.

Special considerations related to specific viruses are described in the viral hepatitis chapters. As a brief summary, hepatitis A in pregnancy causes no effects on the fetus, whereas hepatitis B can be transmitted to the fetus, and hepatitis E is frequently fatal during pregnancy in Africa and Asia. Hepatitis B in infants can be prevented by administering vaccinations.

Although pregnancy does not alter the course of viral hepatitis, several liver diseases, including acute fatty liver and HELLP syndrome, can occur in pregnancy. These conditions can worsen the liver damage associated with hepatitis. For this reason, women with hepatitis should have regular blood tests for ALT. Enzyme elevations should be further evaluated to determine the cause. The conditions that can affect the liver in pregnancy are described in the following sections.

Acute fatty liver

Acute fatty liver (AFL) in pregnancy was first described in 1941. In this condition, the liver cells contain diffuse fat droplets that affect liver function. The onset is typically between the 30th and 38th week of pregnancy. Symptoms include nausea, repeated vomiting and abdominal pain followed a week later by jaundice. The patient with AFL often has high uric acid levels, related to tissue destruction and increased levels of lactic acid. These elevations are not seen in viral hepatitis. In regards to liver enzymes, serum AST levels are typically elevated and gamma GT levels are normal.

In the past, AFL was considered a catastrophic illness with high mortality. With early recognition and prompt treatment, most cases of AFL are mild with fetal and maternal mortality estimated to be 0–20 percent [56]. Death is usually related to causes besides the liver such as disseminated intravascular coagulopathy (DIC), which is a clotting disorder that can cause massive hemorrhage and kidney failure. AFL does not typically occur in subsequent pregnancies.

Toxemias (Eclampsia)

Toxemia in pregnancy typically causes hypertension, fluid retention and increased urine protein levels (proteinuria). Liver damage is only seen in patients with severe conditions. Jaundice is usually hemolytic, which means that it's caused by the breakdown or hemolysis of red blood cells. Rupture of the liver can occur if shock develops.

HELLP syndrome

HELLP syndrome is a rare variant of toxemia that causes hemolysis, elevated liver enzymes and a low platelet count. In about ten percent of women with toxemia, liver disease causes abnormal bleeding and hemorrhage. HELLP syndrome can occur in the absence of hypertension and proteinuria, and it usually resolves after delivery.

Gallstones

About 6 percent of women with hepatitis are at risk for developing gallstones or cholelithiasis during pregnancy. Gallstones can cause pain and jaundice. Gallstones may need to be treated or removed if they do not pass naturally. Otherwise they can contribute to miscarriage or premature birth.

Cholestasis

Cholestasis, a condition of bile obstruction, can cause symptoms of itching especially on the legs and feet of pregnant women. Normally, because of the increased estrogen levels in pregnancy and also with the use of oral contraceptives, some women experience itching and slight jaundice. This is a result of impaired bile flow. Certain women have an inherited susceptibility to this tendency.

Breastfeeding

Women with hepatitis A and B can breastfeed their babies especially if the babies have received the appropriate vaccinations. It is not known whether the hepatitis C virus can be transmitted in breast milk. It is currently considered low risk.

Prevalence of Hepatitis

In the United States the incidence of acute hepatitis has fallen by more than eighty percent since 1994. Today, most cases of acute hepatitis are caused by shock rather than viral infection. Still, an estimated one hundred persons in the United States die annually from acute liver failure due to hepatitis A.

Chronic infection affects up to eighty percent of people with the hepatitis C virus (HCV) and ten to fifteen percent of people with the hepatitis B virus (HBV). An estimated 1.25 million U.S. residents are chronically infected with HBV, and 3.9 million have evidence of HCV infection. Of these patients with HCV, about 2.7 million have chronic HCV infection. More than 410 million people worldwide are chronic carriers of the hepatitis B virus. In some parts of the world, viral hepatitis is considered endemic.

Chronic liver disease is the tenth leading cause of death in the United States and the fourth leading cause of death in males between the ages of thirty and sixty. Chronic hepatitis can also progress to hepatocellular carcinoma (primary liver cancer), which is the fifth leading cause of cancer death worldwide.

2

The Healthy Liver

Since ancient times, the liver has been regarded as having extraordinary powers. In Eastern medicine, the liver is often described as storing the body's *prana* or life force, serving to activate and regulate the vital energy of other organs. In traditional Chinese medicine, the liver organ system is called the "general of the army" because it maintains harmony throughout the body. Indeed, the liver, which is often described as the body's engine or furnace, is essential for life. In both Western and Eastern medical traditions, the liver is considered the central repository and regulator of blood. In liver disease, all of the body's organs and their functions are affected.

Chapter two serves as an introduction to the liver and its many functions. Included are the liver's interactions with other organs and systems, and the liver's role in homeostasis, a system in which the body's organs and systems work together to maintain good health. Chapter two also describes some of the consequences of liver disease.

In addition, chapter two describes the immune system and explains how the immune system keeps the liver healthy by protecting it from microorganisms and toxins and by responding to liver cell injuries. In this chapter readers also learn how the immune system's response contributes to the liver damage that occurs in hepatitis.

Liver Anatomy

Normally, with the exception of the skin, the liver is the largest organ in the body and the most durable, weighing 1200–1510 grams or 3–4 pounds in adults. In adults, the liver represents one-fiftieth or two to three percent of the total adult body weight, and it is usually larger in men than women.

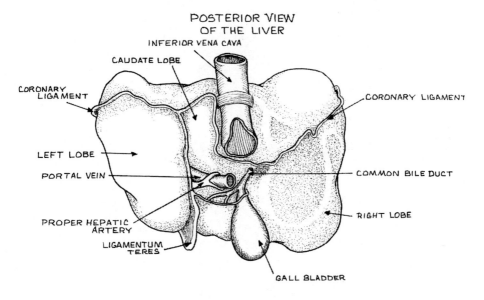

POSTERIOR VIEW
OF THE LIVER

INFERIOR VENA CAVA

CAUDATE LOBE

CORONARY
LIGAMENT

CORONARY LIGAMENT

LEFT LOBE

PORTAL VEIN

COMMON BILE DUCT

PROPER HEPATIC
ARTERY

RIGHT LOBE

LIGAMENTUM
TERES

GALL BLADDER

Posterior view of the liver. (Marvin G. Miller)

In infants the liver is proportionally larger, representing one-eighteenth of the body weight, primarily because of the larger left lobe seen in infancy.

Wedge-shaped, the liver is strategically positioned among the other organs that it communicates with. The liver is located beneath the diaphragm in the right upper quadrant of the abdomen, held in place with ligaments, and situated within the peritoneal (surrounding the peritoneum, the serous lining surrounding the abdomen) cavity. The upper edge of the liver is in line with the nipples. The liver, which is normally dark reddish brown in color, is covered with a sheath of tissue known as Glisson's capsule and it is protected by the ribs.

The liver's lobes

Anatomically, the liver is divided into left and right lobes. The left lobe is about one-sixth the size of the right lobe. The liver's two lobes are separated by the falciform ligament, an anterior or front extension of the peritoneum. The peritoneal folds of tissue that line the chest cavity connect the liver to the diaphragm and anterior abdominal wall. Another ligament, the ligamentum teres, is the vestigial (formed during the early stage of development) remnant of the umbilical vein. The ligamentum teres connects the umbilicus to the inferior border of the liver. In the condition of portal hypertension, which causes increased blood pressure in the portal vein, the umbilicus veins may re-open, causing venous dilation around the umbilicus.

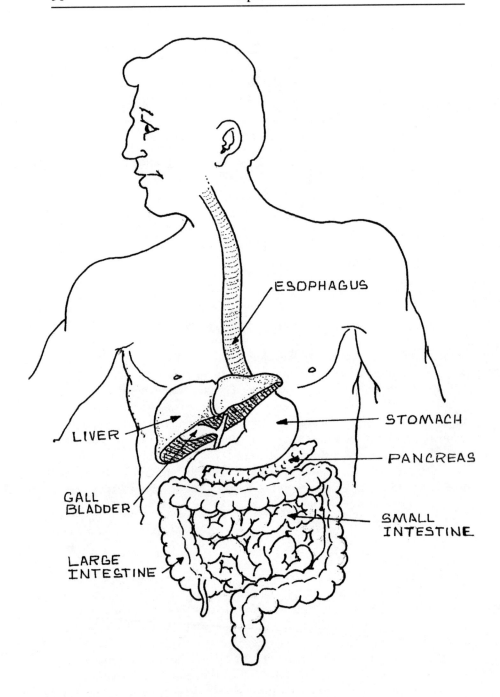

The digestive system (Marvin G. Miller).

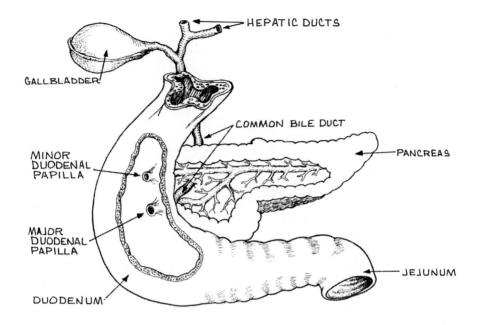

Gallbladder and intestines (Marvin G. Miller).

Two smaller lobes are located on the right lobe. The caudate lobe is found on the posterior surface and the quadrate lobe is found on the inferior surface. The Riedel's lobe, an anomaly, may appear as an anatomical mobile extension of the right lobe of the liver.

The liver's functional units

The liver's lobes are further divided into functional units or lobules bounded by portal triads and central veins. Lobules contain enlarged capillaries or sinusoids interwoven through liver tissue or parenchyma. Each portal triad is the center of a microvascular unit called an acinus. Each acinus is a diamond-shaped mass of liver tissue supplied by branches of the portal vein and hepatic artery and drained by a terminal branch of the bile duct.

The liver's blood supply

The liver has a dual blood supply or two major routes: the portal vein and the hepatic artery. The portal vein carries used blood from the intestines, stomach, pancreas and spleen to the liver, whereas the hepatic artery, a branch of the aorta, brings oxygenated (rich in oxygen) blood from the heart to the liver. After blood transported to the liver has been filtered and processed, it returns to the heart and lungs where it is recycled and reoxygenated.

The body's entire blood supply passes through the liver several times each day. Blood flow through the liver (hepatic blood flow) in normal adults is between 1510–1900 ml/min, which represents about 25 percent of the heart's output. Hepatic blood flow increases after eating and it decreases during sleep and exercise.

Liver tissue

The liver is primarily made up of liver cells known as hepatocytes. Every milligram of tissue contains about 202,000 liver cells. These cells carry out the liver's many metabolic functions. For instance, liver cells absorb nutrients from food transported from the intestines, and they separate the carbohydrate, fat, and protein molecules. Liver cells then transform these compounds into various proteins, hormones and lipids, and they store a number of converted molecules for the body's future energy needs.

The portal system

The portal venous system includes all veins that carry blood from the abdominal part of the alimentary tract, the spleen, pancreas and gallbladder. The portal vein enters the liver at the porta hepatis, a fissure or opening that lies far back on the inferior surface of the right lobe. Here the blood flows into two main branches, one to each lobe.

The portal vein is formed by the union of two veins, the superior mesenteric vein and the splenic vein, which are situated at the head of pancreas. Right and left hepatic veins emerge from the back of the liver and enter the inferior vena cava near its point in the right atrium of the heart. The portal vein supplies about 70% of the liver's blood supply. Blood also exits the liver through the hepatic vein.

The hepatic artery

The hepatic artery is a branch of the celiac axis that runs along the upper border of the pancreas to the first part of the duodenum. The hepatic artery supplies the rest in the form of oxygen-enriched arterial blood. This arterial blood enters through a fissure known as the porta hepatis, which lies far back on the inferior surface of the right lobe.

Sinusoids

Ultimately, both blood supplies connect in the sinusoids. The sinusoids are blood vessels that separate the rows of hepatocyte liver cell plates

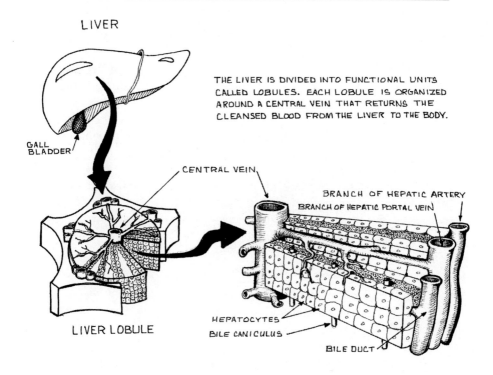

LIVER

THE LIVER IS DIVIDED INTO FUNCTIONAL UNITS CALLED LOBULES. EACH LOBULE IS ORGANIZED AROUND A CENTRAL VEIN THAT RETURNS THE CLEANSED BLOOD FROM THE LIVER TO THE BODY.

GALL BLADDER

CENTRAL VEIN

BRANCH OF HEPATIC ARTERY

BRANCH OF HEPATIC PORTAL VEIN

LIVER LOBULE

HEPATOCYTES

BILE CANICULUS

BILE DUCT

Functional units of the liver (Marvin G. Miller).

comprising most of the liver's tissue. The sinusoids are formed from branches of the portal vein and hepatic artery and they are lined with filtering endothelial cells and phagocytic Kuppfer cells. When the liver is injured and cut off from portal blood, for instance by veno-occlusive liver disease, it becomes dependent on the hepatic circulation. Consequently, in some forms of liver disease, the liver shrinks and atrophies, losing its ability to regenerate.

FENESTRATIONS

The blood vessels in the liver contain holes called fenestrations through which drugs and other substances are transported from blood into the liver cells. Inside the liver cells, the drugs can be processed and metabolized.

The liver's sectors, segments and zones

Anatomically, the liver can be divided into sectors and segments, and functionally, it can be divided into zones. The main portal vein divides into right and left branches, each supplying two subunits or sectors. The sectors on the right side are anterior and posterior and, in the left lobe, medial and lateral, resulting in four separate sectors with their own blood supplies.

The right anterior sector is divided into segments V and VIII and the right posterior sector contains segments VI and VII. The left medial sector contains segments III and IV and the left lateral sector contains segment II.

The functional anatomic unit of the liver is the metabolic lobule or acinus. The acinus lies adjacent to the portal triad, which consists of a branch of the portal vein, hepatic artery and bile duct. The liver's three zones are related to the location of the acini. The zones contain their own blood supplies and cellular components. When the liver sustains injury, cell damage occurs and spreads through these specific zones. Zone 3 is most susceptible to injury and most likely to be affected by hepatitis.

The liver's nervous and lymphatic systems

The nerves supplying the liver come from the stomach's vagus and phrenic nerve systems and from the sympathetic ganglia. The sympathetic nerves or ganglia originate from cell bodies within the spinal cord situated between the seventh and tenth vertebrae.

Lymphatic vessels, which transport lymph fluid to the liver, terminate in the small groups of glands around the porta hepatis and drain into the glands around the celiac axis. A few superficial lymphatic vessels pass through the diaphragm and travel through to the mediastinal glands in the chest cavity.

The liver's regeneration abilities

The liver is able to regenerate or form new cells as needed. This regenerating capacity is one of the most intriguing survival mechanisms the body has. Up to 75 percent of the liver's cells can be surgically removed or destroyed by disease before it ceases to function. When the two largest lobes of the liver are removed and the smaller lobes are left intact, the remaining cells can grow and divide until the liver regains its former size, at which time tissue growth stops.

Normally, liver cells divide slowly. However, when the liver is injured, a vigorous replication of the remaining liver cells occurs. The results range from complete structural and functional tissue integrity to tissue with cellular distortion and functional derangement, including scarring or fibrosis. For instance, after chronic infection with hepatitis viruses, inflammation is followed by early fibrosis. This is not seen in acute hepatitis, even in fulminant cases.

In regeneration, interacting cells, particularly Ito cells and Kuppfer cells, are activated to release various cellular growth modulators. The biology of this regeneration depends on the type of injurious agent, the nature of the liver disease, and the number of hepatocytes that have been damaged.

REGENERATION IN VIRAL HEPATITIS

Depending on the circumstances, there may be a proliferation of normal epithelial cells, or, in the case of viral or toxic hepatitis, an increase in abnormal early cells with a greater propensity to produce the protein alphafetoprotein. Abnormally high levels of this protein are seen in hepatocellular carcinoma. Regeneration of liver tissue damaged by viral hepatitis can also cause an accumulation of mutations in proliferating hepatocytes and early progenitor cells that ultimate lead to hepatomas.

The Gallbladder and Biliary System

The gallbladder

The gallbladder is a pear-shaped organ approximately 9 cm long with a capacity of about 51 ml that functions to store and concentrate bile. Normally, the gallbladder can only be felt (palpable) when it is distended. The

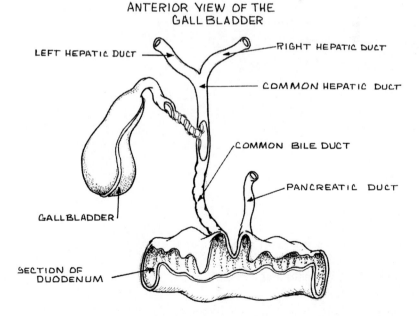

Anterior view of the gallbladder (Marvin G. Miller).

gallbladder, which is tucked beneath the liver and connected to it by bile ducts, lies above the transverse colon in a groove extending from the inferior border of the liver and to the right end of the porta hepatis. The gallbladder releases bile through the bile ducts into the intestines when fatty or rich foods are ingested. Here, the bile breaks down the fat molecules and aids in digestion.

Bile

Bile is a yellow-orange digestive fluid produced and secreted by the liver and stored in the gallbladder. Bile, which has a characteristic bitter taste, is produced primarily during the day with peak production occurring around 9 am. Bile aids in the digestion of fats and helps to neutralize poisons. Bile has the ability to coat some toxins, offering protection until the toxins can be excreted in the feces.

Bile production primarily occurs in the bile canaliculi, which are specialized modifications of the liver cell (hepatocyte) membrane that help form bile ductules allowing for transport. Hepatic bile contains 5 to 15 percent total solids, primarily bile acids, which are sometimes called bile salts, bilirubin, cholesterol, sodium, potassium, calcium and proteins.

Liver cells secrete bile into the duodenum section of the small intestine to help with digestion. The bile ducts of the liver also collect bile and transport it to the gallbladder. The gallbladder then secretes bile through bile ducts into the intestines when it receives a hormonal signal that the digestive system needs help in digesting fatty foods.

Bile acids

Bile acids are chemical compounds synthesized in the liver from cholesterol. Cholesterol is derived from two sources: 1) the metabolized remnants of dietary sources and 2) production within liver cells. Bile acids have three major functions: 1) to regulate cholesterol levels; 2) stimulate bile flow in the biliary system, and 3) emulsify and absorb dietary fats in the intestines.

In the intestines bile acids are conjugated with the amino acids glycine or taurine. Regulating bile acid metabolism is one of the liver's major functions. Bile acids are used for the production of bile and they're also transported to the gallbladder and intestines to aid in digestion. Bile acids are also carried to the bowels and through the portal vein into the blood circulation. Blood bile acid levels rise 51 percent above fasting levels within 90 to 120 minutes after eating.

In acute hepatitis alterations of bile acid synthesis and conjugation are caused by diseased liver cells. This is considered an acquired defect in contrast to the inborn error of bile acid synthesis that occurs in idiopathic neonatal hepatitis.

The bile ducts

The right and left hepatic ducts emerge from the liver and unite in the porta hepatis to form the common hepatic duct. This duct joins up with the gallbladder's cystic duct to form the common bile duct. The biliary ducts are used for the transport of bile. In obstructive liver disease the bile ducts can be blocked.

Microscopic View of the Liver

Liver tissue is shown microscopically to consist of columns or plates of liver cells known as hepatocytes radiating from a central vein. These columns are interlaced in orderly fashion by sinusoid cavities and held together by collagen proteins. The liver tissue has two systems of tunnels, the portal tracts and the hepatic central canals. These tunnels extend in such a way that they never meet.

Hepatocytes

Liver tissue or parenchyma is primarily composed of cells known as hepatocytes. Hepatocytes, which are the main target of the hepatitis viruses, comprise about sixty percent of the liver. In biopsies of patients with hepatitis, the pathologist looks for changes indicating damage to hepatocytes. Hepatocytes have a polygonal shape and are about 30 μm in diameter. The nucleus of the hepatocyte cell is usually single although it may be double and divides by mitosis. The lifespan of liver cells is about 151 days in experimental animals.

Hepatocytes have three surfaces: 1) one facing the sinusoid and the space of Dissë, a tissue space between hepatocytes and sinusoidal lining cells; 2) the second facing the canaliculus, which is a groove on the contact surface of liver cell through which bile is released, and 3) the third surface facing other hepatocytes. The hepatocyte has no basement membrane surface layer although it is surrounded by a supporting cytoskeleton consisting of microtubules and microfilaments.

HEPATOCYTE STRUCTURES

Hepatocytes have several distinct parts, each with specific functions: 1) the nucleus, which contains viral (RNA or DNA) protein, has a double membrane allowing interchange with the surrounding cytoplasm; 2) mito-

HEPATOCYTE
(LIVER CELL)

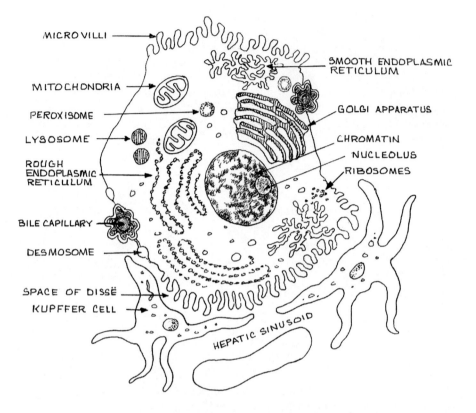

MICROVILLI

SMOOTH ENDOPLASMIC RETICULUM

MITOCHONDRIA

GOLGI APPARATUS

PEROXISOME

CHROMATIN

LYSOSOME

NUCLEOLUS

ROUGH ENDOPLASMIC RETICULUM

RIBOSOMES

BILE CAPILLARY

DESMOSOME

SPACE OF DISSË

KUPFFER CELL

HEPATIC SINUSOID

Hepatocyte (Marvin G. Miller).

chondria, which produce energy and synthesize heme protein used in the production of hemoglobin needed for red blood cells; 3) rough endoplasmic reticulum (RER), which synthesizes proteins, particularly albumin and clotting factors, enzymes, and triglycerides; 4) smooth endoplasmic reticulum (SER), which functions to conjugate bilirubin, detoxify many drugs and other foreign substances, and produce steroids, cholesterol and several amino acids; 5) lysosomes, which act as scavengers and storage areas for copper, ferritin, bile pigment and lipofuscin, the brown pigment seen in liver spots; and 6) the Golgi apparatus which assembles the materials secreted into bile.

Sinusoidal cells

Sinusoidal cells include endothelial cells, Kupffer cells, ito cells and pit cells. Together with hepatocytes, the sinusoidal cells make up liver tissue.

Endothelial cells line the sinusoids, creating a barrier between the sinusoid and the space of Dissë. The Kuppfer cells are attached to the epithelium.

KUPFFER CELLS

Kupffer cells, which make up ten percent of liver tissue, are highly mobile white blood cells of the monocyte/macrophage cell line. They are phagocytes, which means that they are able to engulf and ingest old cells, foreign particles, tumor cells, bacteria, yeasts, viruses and parasites. Kupffer cells become activated when the body is subjected to infection or trauma. However, most viruses are too small to be recognized by Kuppfer cells. The Kuppfer cells must wait until the immune system produces antibodies to the virus. When hepatitis viruses are trapped by these antibodies, the Kuppfer cells are able to destroy the virus-antibody complex.

ITO CELLS

Ito cells, which are also known as perisinusoidal cells, lie in the space of Dissë within the liver and function to store fat. Here, they store up to a two year supply of vitamin A and, when prompted, carry out fibrosis of the hepatic lobule in the process of developing cirrhosis.

Liver Function

The liver has many functions that it carries out simultaneously. The liver receives all digested food, drugs, chemicals, toxins and non-viable blood cells, and it must sort, process, detoxify, recycle or eliminate these substances. The liver also produces or synthesizes a number of different proteins, hormones, and clotting factors, and it stores many carbohydrates, vitamins and minerals. In addition, the liver helps regulate blood sugar, energy, and hormone levels and it helps build muscles.

Table 2.1 The Liver's Functions

Alcohol metabolism
Albumin Production
Bile production and transport
Bilirubin conjugation and metabolism
Blood cell recycling and elimination
Building muscle
Carbohydrate metabolism
Cleansing the blood of toxins and excreting them as wastes
Clotting factor production
Converts fat into cholesterol and triglycerides
Converts food into energy
Converts glucose into glycogen
Detoxification of drugs and toxins

Disposal of bile pigments
Drug metabolism and regulation of blood drug levels
Fatty acid production and metabolism
Fighting infections within the gastrointestinal tract
Filters and detoxifies chemicals
Hormone production and regulation
Immune system chemical production
Iron and mineral storage
Lipid (cholesterol, lipoprotein) production and metabolism
Processes and stores proteins, fats, and carbohydrates
Production of bile and bile acids
Stores vitamins, minerals and sugar (glycogen)
Regulating bile acid metabolism
Regulating blood drug levels
Regulates fat stores and their transport

The Liver's Key Players

Liver cells

The liver's functions are carried out by the various cells that make up the liver tissue or parenchyma, with most of the functions carried out by cells known as hepatocytes and to a lesser extent the Kupffer cells, Ito cells and sinusoidal cells. When the liver's cells are damaged or destroyed, they're unable to carry out their functions.

Enzymes

Enzymes are proteins that act as catalysts for certain chemical reactions. Liver cells contain many different enzymes that aid in various metabolic functions, such as protein production. Depending on the type of liver disease present, one or more enzymes are released from damaged cells, and the blood levels of these enzymes rise. Some diseases also inherently cause increased production of certain enzymes. Enzyme levels, which are described in chapter fourteen, can be used to help diagnose the type of liver disease that's present.

TRANSAMINASE (AMINOTRANSFERASE) ENZYMES

The two transaminases, along with another enzyme alkaline phosphatase, are the most common liver enzymes used to diagnose liver disease. The transaminases include: 1) aspartate transaminase or aspartate aminotransferase (AST), formerly known as serum glutamic oxalacetic transaminase (SGOT); and 2) alanine transaminase or alanine aminotransferase (ALT), formerly known as serum glutamic pyruvate transaminase (SGPT). AST is found in other tissues besides the liver, including bones, the intestines, and the placenta, and elevations may occur in disorders affecting any of these organs. ALT is present in liver, heart and skeletal tissue, but primarily in liver tissue. Therefore, an increased ALT is more specific for liver damage than an increased AST.

OTHER LIVER ENZYMES

Alkaline phosphatase (ALP) enzymes are present in liver and bone, and elevations are seen in disorders affecting both organs. A fractionation test can be performed to determine if elevated alkaline phosphatase levels are a result of liver or bone damage. Gamma-glutamyl transpeptidase (gamma GT or GGT) is another liver enzyme that's usually elevated in alcohol abuse and biliary cholestasis. Glutathione-s-transferase (GST) is an abundant enzyme in liver tissue. GST is rarely measured in the clinical laboratory although it may be used in research studies. Levels of GST rise rapidly in hepatitis and return to normal quickly.

The Liver's Metabolic Functions

Metabolism refers to the processes of change or biotransformation, the building up and breaking down of new chemical compounds. The liver synthesizes many compounds and changes many others into byproducts or metabolites and removes them through excretion into bile or urine.

Drug metabolism

Most drugs are only soluble (able to be dissolved) in lipids or fats. When they're ingested, they're taken up by fat or protein molecules in the intestines and transported to the bloodstream. Once drugs cause their intended effects, they're transported to the liver to be prepared for excretion. Drugs move through openings known as fenestrations found within the blood vessels of the liver.

THE CYTOCHROME P 450 ENZYME SYSTEM

Drug metabolism primarily occurs in the smooth endoplasmic reticulum of the hepatocytes with the help of several enzyme systems, including mono-oxygenases, cytochrome c-reductase and cytochrome P450 enzymes. The cytochrome P450 system, the phases of drug metabolism, and the development of drug toxicity are described in chapter eleven.

Bilirubin conjugation

After an average lifespan of approximately 120 days, circulating red blood cells (RBCs) are engulfed and destroyed by other cells in the spleen, liver, and bone marrow. During this process, the protein known as hemoglobin or haem found in RBCs is released into the blood circulation. Haem is also produced by the metabolism and breakdown of a few other proteins, including several respiratory and liver enzymes and myoglobin, a protein found in muscle.

Haem, which is released into the blood circulation, is quickly broken down into several other compounds, primarily a chemical substance known as unconjugated bilirubin. About 80 percent of the bilirubin produced each day is caused by the normal destruction of RBCs.

Unconjugated or indirect bilirubin, which is only soluble in lipids, is transported through the bloodstream by other proteins and carried to the liver cells. Here, bilirubin is rapidly conjugated or linked with glucuronic acid to produce water soluble, conjugated bilirubin compounds. The conjugated or direct bilirubin compounds are then excreted into bile.

UROBILINOGEN

Some of the bilirubin conjugates are re-absorbed by the intestines and converted into urobilinogen compounds. Most of this urobilinogen is taken up by the liver and re-excreted in the bile. A small amount, roughly 2–5 percent, is taken up by the general circulation and appears in the urine along with small amounts of conjugated bilirubin. An increase in urine urobilinogen occurs whenever liver function is decreased or there is an excess of urobilinogen in the gastrointestinal tract that exceeds the liver's capacity to re-excrete it.

HYPERBILIRUBINEMIA

Hyperbilirubinemia and bilirubinemia are terms used to describe elevated blood levels of bilirubin. Hyperbilirubinemia can result from defects or disturbances in the production, metabolism, transport or excretion of bilirubin. Excess unconjugated or indirect bilirubin blood levels can occur when too much bilirubin is produced, for instance from an increased breakdown of red blood cells or muscle cells. Hyperbilirubinemia caused by an increase in conjugated or direct bilirubin occurs when liver function is impaired or there is a bile duct obstruction. The use of bilirubin blood tests to help diagnose liver disease is described in chapter fourteen.

Protein synthesis

The liver is the body's primary site of plasma protein synthesis. Proteins synthesized by the liver include: albumin; prealbumin; immunoglobulin (Ig) proteins used for antibody production; beta2-microglobin; transferrin; haptoglobin; alpha 1-antitrypsin; C-reactive protein; C3 complement; lipoproteins; and various protein factors essential for blood clotting, such as fibrinogen.

Most drugs, hormones, nutrients, and minerals are transported through the body circulation via these proteins. The molecules of hormones and drugs are linked to albumin, prealbumin and other carrier proteins. When liver disease limits protein synthesis, drug levels may be altered and nutritional deficiencies can occur. In some cases, for instance in the case of gamma globulins, these proteins are released from damaged liver cells and blood levels rise. Blood levels of these proteins, which are described in chapter fourteen, help diagnose liver disease.

Lipid metabolism

Most of the body's cholesterol is produced in the liver. This cholesterol, along with smaller amounts of dietary cholesterol enter the hepatic pool. Here they are converted to bile acids or used to produce hormones and membranes for new liver cells. Approximately 33 percent of the fatty acids originating from adipose tissue enter the liver. Here they are transformed into triglycerides or oxidized. Excess triglyceride production results in a condition of fatty liver, which can lead to hepatitis.

Ammonia metabolism

Ammonia is a breakdown product of protein, and most of the body's ammonia is produced in the gastrointestinal tract, including the portal vein. Normally, most of the ammonia produced in the portal vein is metabolized, with the help of urea enzymes, to the compound urea. Urea is then excreted in urine. In liver disease this process may be impaired, and ammonia levels rise as a result. Excess ammonia injures the central nervous system, causing conditions of memory impairment and cognitive disturbances.

High ammonia levels are usually only seen in advanced liver disease, the condition of Reye's syndrome, fulminant hepatitis, hepatitic encephalopathy, and inherited disorders of urea metabolism and cirrhosis.

Excretory function

The liver's cells are efficient when it comes to clearing foreign substances known as xenobiotics, such as synthetic dyes or chemicals. Some of these substances remain intact as they're shuttled off into the bile pool, while others are broken down before they're cleared. This rapid clearance is considered an active transport system. The ability of liver cells to clear these substances is impaired in hepatitis.

Older invasive tests for liver function called dye excretion tests, such as the bromsulfophtalein (BSP) clearance test, were once used to measure liver function but because these procedures can cause fatality, they're no longer used. Today more sensitive laboratory tests that don't require the injection of dyes are used.

The Immune System

The immune system is the body's gatekeeper. Immune system cells act like soldiers defending the body against toxins and microorganisms and launching a response to destroy these foreign agents. Physically, the immune system is a network of organs and blood cells with specific functions that work together to keep us healthy. The immune system's key players are white blood cells known as lymphocytes and proteins known as cytokines, which include interferon, interleukin and various growth factors.

The most important immune system organ is the bone marrow, the pulpy tissue stored within bone. The bone marrow is the manufacturing plant or site of production for the body's red and white blood cells. Other immune system organs, such as the lymph nodes, spleen, tonsils, thymus, and adenoids serve as storage sites, maturation sites and transport points for the white blood cells necessary for guarding against infection.

The thymus gland

The thymus gland is a small gland situated in the upper chest cavity behind the sternum and between the lungs. The thymus gland reaches its maximum size during puberty. After puberty, in a process of involution, the thymus gland tends to shrink with age. By age 30, the thymus gland has typically decreased its size by two-thirds and its T lymphocyte stores by 90 percent. An endocrine gland, the thymus gland produces and secretes thymic hormones and thymic peptides.

Peptides are attached amino acids that act as transmitters, communicating with organs and cells. Thymic peptides have important immune system functions. They directly influence antibody production and T lymphocyte maturation. In addition, they coordinate the interaction of the immune, endocrine and central nervous systems.

White blood cells known as T lymphocytes are transported to the thymus for maturation. Here, T lymphocytes are programmed by thymic peptides to recognize specific foreign antigens. Some T lymphocytes are programmed to defend against specific bacteria and other T lymphocytes are programmed to protect us from specific viruses. In infection, the thymus gland increases its production of thymic peptides in an effort to assist the immune response.

The immune response

Thousands of white blood cells known as T lymphocytes travel through the blood circulation scouting for foreign substances, such as bacteria and viruses. T lymphocytes can be further divided into two major subtypes known as CD4 and CD8 cells. The CD4 cells are helper cells, the soldiers in the army that scout for microorganisms. The CD8 cells are suppressor cells, the warriors that destroy infected or damaged cells. When the CD4 T lymphocyte cells encounter foreign substances, they initiate a series of events known as the immune response. In the immune response, other white blood cells, including B lymphocytes and natural killer (NK) lymphocytes rush to the site of attack.

IMMUNE SYSTEM CHEMICALS

During the immune response, certain white blood cells release chemical compounds known as cytokines and complement. Cytokines include various growth factors, interleukins and interferons that help the body fight infection and help modulate the immune response.

ANTIGENS AND ANTIBODIES

The immune system initiates an immune response when its cells encounter protein particles from viruses, pollen and other substances that they recognize as foreign. These protein particles are collectively known as antigens. The body's own proteins that make up our cells and tissues are recognized by the immune system as self antigens. Normally, the immune system tolerates self antigens and doesn't respond to them.

When the immune system cells encounter foreign antigens, they initiate a chain reaction that results in the production of specific antibodies. These antibodies are usually able to destroy or neutralize the specific type of antigen that caused their production.

The immune response in hepatitis

The immune system responds to injury or foreign antigens, proteins not normally found in the body, by launching a response. Injured and infected cells are destroyed. But what about the foreign antigens? Viruses contain either DNA or RNA that identify them as specific viruses. Viruses also have a number of protein components or antigens. The immune system responds to these proteins and produces antibodies capable of neutralizing or destroying the viral particles. In the laboratory, these antigens and their corresponding antibodies are recognized as signs of infection. Tests used to measure these antigens and antibodies are called viral marker tests.

Viral RNA and DNA

Levels of viral RNA in HCV infection and DNA in HBV infection can be detected with screening tests. These test results help diagnose infection. The amount of virus present can also be quantitatively measured in tests for viral load. These tests help determine the severity of infection and the response to treatment. The genotype or specific DNA or RNA pattern can also be determined with molecular genetic techniques. Blood donors are typically screened for viral DNA and RNA because these tests are the most sensitive for detecting hepatitis. RNA and DNA proteins show up early in infection, days or weeks before the viral antigens and antibodies can be detected.

Immune system markers

Early in viral infection, specific viral protein particles or antigens appear. Tests for viral antigens are particularly important in hepatitis B. The antigen protein found on the outer surface of HBV is called the hepatitis B surface antigen, which is commonly shortened to HBsAg. The HB represents the hepatitis B virus, and the sAg represents the protein antigen found on the surface of the virus.

Hepatitis B also has a core antigen, HBcAg, and a pre-core or e antigen designated HBeAg. Although core antigen is not found in the blood, HBsAg and HBeAg are found in active infection. In active infection HBcAg can be found in liver cells and in some white blood cells.

Antibody production in hepatitis

The immune system cells responds to these protein antigens by producing specific antibodies. These antibodies are capable of destroying or neutralizing the viral antigens. The antibody to the hepatitis B surface antigen is called the hepatitis B surface antibody or HBsAb. Here, HB represents hepatitis B and sAb represents the antibody directed against the surface antigen protein. In most cases, hepatitis antibodies form and appear in the blood circulation around the same time as the virus clears. In this sense, antibodies are indicators of immunity.

IgM and IgG antibodies

Antibodies are formed by B lymphocytes from the body's stores of immunoglobulin (Ig) proteins. The first antibodies to show up belong to the immunoglobulin M class and are called IgM antibodies. Weeks or months later the IgG antibodies appear. IgM antibodies appear during the active stage of infection and disappear during recovery. IgG antibodies persist for many years and usually for one's lifetime. In hepatitis B, HBcAb, the antibodies to core antigen, appear before surface antibodies develop.

IgM antibodies to core, HBcIgM Ab occur during active infection, but because of their short half-life, they clear after infection has resolved.

Tests for IgM antibodies are positive during active infection whereas tests for IgG antibodies are positive both in active infection and after infection has resolved. HBcIgM antibodies are seen in active hepatitis B infection, and HAV IgM antibodies are seen during active HAV infection. In hepatitis B, tests for HBc IgM indicate active infection whereas tests for HBcIgG can be positive in both active and prior infection. Hepatitis B core antibodies are not detected after vaccinations.

Immunity

Immunity refers to protection from disease. For instance, if we're exposed to the hepatitis B virus (HBV) or given a vaccine containing treated HBV, our immune system cells produce HBsAb antibodies capable of neutralizing or destroying HBV. If we're exposed to HBV at a later time, our HBV antibodies destroy HBV antigens, thereby protecting us from HBV infection. Our HBV surface antibodies are a sign of immunity. If we have HBsAb in our blood circulation, we have immunity from HBV either from past infection or as a result of vaccination.

The hepatitis B core and e antibodies, which were briefly described in this section and more extensively in chapters six and fourteen, help to show if we have a current hepatitis B infection or if we were infected with hepatitis B in the past. HBsAg normally clears from the circulation within 3 months. The continued presence of surface antigen, HBsAg, for more than six months is an indicator of chronic HBV disease.

How Hepatitis Affects the Liver

Liver injury in hepatitis is primarily due to the effects caused by the immune response. In hepatitis, lymphocytes rush to the liver tissue causing a condition of inflammation or swelling. Immune system chemicals released by these lymphocytes during the immune response destroy infected and damaged hepatocytes. There is evidence that free radicals generated by inflammatory cells in the liver also contribute to liver cell damage [30].

In hepatitis, liver cells are destroyed or necrotized. In biopsy specimens from patients with viral hepatitis, hepatocytes appear swollen, a condition sometimes referred to as balloon degeneration. As the number of functioning hepatocytes is diminished, liver function declines.

Consequently, patients with hepatitis may have difficulty digesting fatty foods and they may develop nausea. However, symptoms in hepatitis are often vague and non-specific and aren't a reflection of the severity of the liver disease. Blood tests are better indicators. In hepatitis liver enzymes stored within hepatocytes are released from dying cells, causing elevated blood enzyme levels. In addition, conjugated bilirubin is unable to move through the cell canaliculus into bile. This causes bilirubin levels to rise.

Other Organs and Systems Affected By Hepatitis

The spleen

In hepatitis, the spleen is generally enlarged with increased activity or hypersplenism. This results in an increased destruction of red blood cells in the spleen. Red cells that survive may have membrane defects (changes in the red blood cell surface) that hastens their destruction. The diminished number of red blood cells causes a condition of anemia.

The coagulation system

The liver synthesizes or produces ten different proteins, such as fibrinogen and prothrombin. These proteins interact together to form the fibrin clot, which is necessary for blood clotting. Without this ability to clot, wounds would not stop bleeding. Blood tests that measure the length of time needed for blood to clot, such as the prothrombin time (PT), can be used to help determine the severity of liver disease and to evaluate the patient's risk for bleeding during a liver biopsy.

Other Complications of Hepatitis

Aplastic anemia

Aplastic anemia, a potentially fatal condition of low red blood cells, is a rare complication of acute viral hepatitis, usually type non-A, non-B, non-C. Typically, this condition, which primarily affects males younger than 20, occurs a few months after disease onset when the hepatitis is resolving.

In hepatitis, aplastic anemia is an ominous sign. Aplastic anemia, which is caused by a deficiency in cellular growth factors and precursor cells, is associated with a severe reduction in the amount of bone marrow tissue that can produce blood cells. This results in a deficient production of blood cells and other blood components including platelets. The clinical course of aplastic anemia may be acute and fulminating or chronic.

Platelet disorders

Platelets are small blood components essential for the clotting process. Low platelet counts and diminished platelet function often occur in viral hepatitis, folic acid deficiency and alcohol excess.

Gallbladder system

The gallbladder is mutually dependent on the liver. The liver produces bile and transports it to the gallbladder where it is stored and secreted as needed to aid in digestion.

Hormone production

The liver is responsible for breaking down cholesterol molecules and producing many of the body's hormones including thyroid hormone and steroid hormones. Normally, the liver regulates the production and breakdown of these substances. In liver disease, hormonal disturbances are common. For instance, many men with hepatitis have increased estrogen levels, causing a condition of breast enlargement known as gynecomastia.

Vascular system

The pro-inflammatory chemicals fibrinogen, homocysteine, C-reactive protein, and lipoprotein a, which is shortened to Lp(a), are all produced by the liver. When liver cells become inflamed and imbalanced, high levels of these substances are found in the blood. Lp(a) prevents the normal breakdown of fibrinogen, a condition that leads to clot formation and inflammation within blood vessels. Lp(a) also resembles low density lipoprotein (LDL) cholesterol, in that it promotes plaque formation within blood vessels.

In hepatitis, high blood levels of these chemicals contribute to both cardiovascular and vascular diseases, including heart attack and stroke.

Cholestasis

Cholestasis refers to the interruption or blockage of normal bile flow. Viral and toxic hepatitis often result in cholestasis, which causes elevated blood levels of bile acids and bilirubin and accompanying jaundice. This condition resolves when the offending drug or toxin is removed or when liver inflammation resolves.

3

Risk Factors

Chapter three focuses on the risk factors for hepatitis. Risk factors include a number of different substances and circumstances, such as injection drug use, incarceration, and dialysis that increase the risk of developing hepatitis. Guidelines and recommendations prepared by the Centers for Disease Control and Prevention (CDC) to help reduce the risk of hepatitis in these circumstances are also described in this chapter. In addition, this chapter includes an overview of blood products and the steps that are taken to reduce the risk of hepatitis from transfusions and organ transplants.

Toxins

Toxins are substances capable of injuring the body. Hepatotoxins are toxins that injure the liver. Toxins can cause hepatitis, although some of the hepatotoxins are seemingly innocuous or only affect a small number of people. In this section some of the less obvious causes of hepatitis are described. Toxins are described in greater detail in chapter eleven.

Molds

Aflatoxin, a toxin produced by the mold *Aspergillus flavus*, is found in moldy plants, especially peanuts, soybeans, corn and rice stored in hot, humid conditions for extended periods. Aflatoxins are a well known cause of toxic hepatitis and hepatocellular cancer (HCC). In patients with viral hepatitis, aflatoxins are presumed to contribute to the development of HCC. Aflatoxin is thought to also cause a trademark cytochrome P54 mutation when ingested in large amounts. This mutation is frequently seen in HCC epidemics in Africa and in sporadic cases of this cancer in other regions.

Aflatoxin toxicity is a well known causes of hepatitis in dogs. In dogs, hepatitis is also caused by infection with the canine virus CAV-1, toxins and poisons, and metabolic disorders such as copper accumulation. It is likely that other viruses besides CAV-1 are responsible for canine hepatitis, but none have yet been identified.

Mushrooms

The mushroom *Amanita phalloides*, a toadstool commonly known as the death angel or death cap, can cause a fulminant fatal type of hepatitis.

Prescription and over-the-counter medications

More than 1,000 different medications have the potential to cause hepatotoxicity (liver damage). Some individuals have a genetic inability to metabolize certain potentially hepatotoxic drugs, such as phenytoin (Dilantin), a drug used to treat seizure disorders. Individuals with impaired kidney function often are unable to properly metabolize drugs into their less toxic byproducts or metabolites.

Alcohol has a synergistic effect with many medications, including the analgesic acetaminophen. Taken together with alcohol or another hepatotoxic medication, many medications are more likely to cause liver damage than if they were taken alone. Mild liver disease can affect drug metabolism. Certain conditions such as hepatitis C may increase the toxicity of certain analgesics including ibuprofen and acetaminophen. Fasting and malabsorption disorders can also increase susceptibility to acetaminophen-induced liver disease.

Expired medications and antibiotics

Certain expired medications, primarily tetracycline derivatives, cannot be properly metabolized by the liver. With impaired metabolism, these compounds interfere with protein synthesis and interfere with the normal transport of fats. Consequently, expired and also high doses of tetracyclines can act as toxins causing accumulations of phospholipid fats. This causes a condition known as microvesicular fat disease or steatosis. Infiltrated with fatty deposits, liver function becomes impaired. Vomiting and apathy are prominent symptoms in microvesicular fat disease.

Analgesics

Both acetaminophen, which is found in Tylenol(r) and other over-the-counter analgesic preparations, and acetylsalicylic acid found in aspirin can cause a potentially fatal form of fulminant hepatitis. Salicylates are often used in high therapeutic doses for acute rheumatic fever, juvenile and adult rheumatoid arthritis, and systemic lupus erythematosus. Even with serum salicylate levels that are therapeutic, some patients can develop acute hepatic injury and chronic active hepatitis [46].

Recreational drugs

Recreational drugs such as cocaine and Ecstasy are well known causes of toxic hepatitis. Cocaine overdoses cause a syndrome of liver damage, rhabdomyolysis, a condition causing a rapid breakdown of muscle tissue, disseminated intravascular coagulation (DIC), which is a breakdown of the normal clotting process, hypotension, which is a condition of low blood pressure, and hyperexia, which is a condition of increased body temperature. The liver damage in cocaine toxicity causes liver tissue necrosis and fat deposits in the central part of the lobes.

The CDC reports that intranasal cocaine use has been independently associated with the development of hepatitis C, presumably due to the use of contaminated straws or related paraphernalia [19].

The amphetamine-like compound 3, 4-methylenedioxymetamphetamine (MDMA, Ecstasy) is well known for causing drug-induced hepatitis. MDMA toxicity causes symptoms similar to those of cocaine toxicity, including fulminant hyperthermia, disseminated intravascular coagulation, rhabdomyolysis, and acute renal failure. Occasionally, severe dehydration occurs, causing excessive fluid intake and water intoxication. Persons with a genetic deficiency of the cytochrome P450 enzyme system (five percent of the white population) are suspected of being predisposed to MDMA-related hyperthermia and liver disease.

Either sporadic or regular ingestion of MDMA can cause isolated, severe acute liver toxicity over a period of days or weeks. Hepatitis can occur as part of the syndrome seen in cocaine toxicity or as a delayed systemic fulminant hepatitis with no other accompanying symptoms. The liver damage caused by MDMA can result in a fulminant fatal form of hepatitis. Liver biopsies of MDMA associated hepatitis show necrosis in the central and mid-zonal regions of the liver. In delayed hepatitis, massive or focal necrosis with inflammation may be seen.

Herbal medicines

Many herbs can injure liver cells, especially combinations of Kampo preparations used in traditional Chinese medicine, sarsaprilla, sassafrass, and herbs containing pyrrolidizine alkaloids, such as heliotropium, senecio, crotalaria, and symphytum. A complete list of herbs known to cause liver toxicity is found in chapter eleven.

Toxins found in Asian medicines that can cause hepatitis include aconite, acorus, borax, borneol, bufonis, cinnabar, calomel, litharge, minium, myiabris, orpiment, realgar, Socrpion, strychnos nux vomica, semen strychni, and toad secretion [23].

Environmental chemicals

A number of environmental chemicals including pesticides, glue, and cleaning solvents can cause toxic hepatitis. Two of the most widely recognized environmental causes of hepatitis include carbon tetrachloride and vinyl chloride.

Carbon tetrachloride, a solvent used in chemical research, fire extinguishers and dry cleaning can be inhaled or mixed in drinks. People who work with this solvent should be routinely tested for liver enlargement and tenderness and with liver enzyme tests [56]. The metabolism of carbon tetrachloride produces a toxic chemical that induces liver cell necrosis. This toxicity is reduced in protein malnutrition, which explains the resistance seen in natives of underdeveloped countries who are treated with carbon tetrachloride for helminth (worm) infestation.

Vinyl chloride, a chemical used in the plastics industry, causes liver damage after chronic exposure. The earliest changes caused by vinyl chloride include fibrosis in zone 1 of the liver, portal hypertension, and enlarged spleen. Advanced changes include liver tumors and peliosis or nodular hepatitis. Toxins are described further in chapter eleven.

Age, Gender and Ethnicity

People of advanced age and the female sex are at increased risk for hepatic drug reactions. The effects of estrogens on liver function are considered partly responsible for the increased risk of toxic hepatitis in women. Certain ethnic groups, particularly Asians, are more susceptible to liver disease and hepatitis, and certain forms of hepatitis are more prevalent in different countries. For instance, in Greece and Hong Kong, there is a significantly higher incidence of hepatitis B and a higher rate of hepatitis B carriers among blood donors than in the United States or the United Kingdom [56].

Age

Drug reactions causing liver disease are rare in children with the exception of accidental acetaminophen overdoses. Children appear to have a natural resistance to drug-induced hepatic injury. Children are less likely to experience liver damage from the same blood level of acetaminophen as adults with similar blood levels. Children infected with hepatitis C through blood transfusions are more likely to clear the virus than adults.

Risk for chronic infection with HBV is associated with age at infection. About 90 percent of infected infants and 61 percent of infected children less than 5 years old become chronically infected compared with 2–6 percent of adults.

The elderly are likely to experience decreased rates of phase 1 but not phase 2 drug transformation. This is related to diminished hepatic volume and blood flow through the liver. Adults are more likely to develop liver injury from certain drugs known to cause liver toxicity such as isoniazide (INH), a drug commonly used to treat tuberculosis.

Gender

Hepatitis due to drug toxicity is more likely to occur in females than males. Females are reported to have lower levels of cytochrome P461 enzymes, which may be why they're more likely to develop liver disease when using drugs that can cause chronic hepatitis such as methyldopa, a drug used to treat hypertension. Females are also ten times more likely than men to develop autoimmune hepatitis.

Men infected with hepatitis B are more likely to become carriers because of the weaker immune response seen in men. People who become carriers typically have a poorer immune response and are not as competent at producing the immune system chemical interferon.

Ethnicity

In the United States and other developed countries, the incidence of HAV has declined in recent years with highest rates seen in low socioeconomic areas. However, in many developing nations, the incidence of HAV still remains high, especially in children.

In different parts of the world, there are dramatic differences in the prevalence rates for hepatitis B. In parts of Southeast Asia and sub-Saharan Africa, more than 90 percent of the population show evidence of current or past HBV infection. Within the United States, approximately 5 percent of the population show evidence of current or past HBV infection, and rates increase with age and in low socioeconomic areas. In the United States, the rate of HBV infection is higher in African Americans, Hispanics and Asian Americans than in whites.

Hepatitis D is significantly more prevalent among hepatitis B carriers from Middle Eastern and Mediterranean countries. Outbreaks of HDV with high mortality have been reported among the indigenous populations of Venezuela and other South American countries. In the United States, HDV is strongly associated with illicit drug use and the use of multiple blood products.

Different strains of hepatitis C are seen in different parts of the world. Nevertheless, the incidence of hepatitis C is particularly high in Taipei, Taiwan, and Africa. In the United States, persons of color have a higher prevalence rate of HCV infection than whites.

Hyperthermia

Hyperthermia or heat stroke, a condition of dangerously increased body temperature stroke, can cause liver cell damage. In approximately 10 percent of victims of heat stroke, hepatitis is severe and potentially fatal. The damage is caused by a loss of oxygen and direct thermal injury. Obesity is a risk factor in hyperthermia.

Exertional heat stroke (related to exercising in high temperatures) causes collapse, convulsions, hypotension or low blood pressure and high fever. In addition patients may experience complications such as rhabdomyolysis, which contributes to a breakdown of muscle, including heart, tissue and brain damage [56].

Injection Drug Use

Studies consistently show that illegal drug use accounts for about 61 percent of all new cases of hepatitis C viral (HCV) infection. While most of these cases are related to injection drug use, studies show that snorting cocaine is also an independent risk factor for HCV, which may be related to sharing straws.

Injection drug use is responsible for a significant number of new cases of hepatitis B viral (HBV) infection although the rates of HBV infection in the U.S. have declined since peaking in the 1980s. In 2000, 17 percent of all new HBV infections were attributed to injection drug use [14].

Injection drug users often jointly purchase drugs and prepare solutions together. These solutions, the water used to dissolve the drugs, mixing containers, cotton filters, syringes and needles may all serve as sources of viral transmission. Injection drug users often drink alcohol, which adds to their risk of severe disease.

Hemodialysis

Patients with renal disease are routinely treated with a procedure known as dialysis or hemodialysis to remove toxins that would normally be cleared by the kidneys and excreted with urine. The number of patients treated by maintenance hemodialysis has increased dramatically since 1970. Chronic hemodialysis patients are at high risk for hepatitis because the procedure involves extended periods of vascular intravenous access. Furthermore, equipment may be contaminated, personnel may transmit infectious agents, and toxins may be introduced through the water supply used in the process.

Hepatitis B transmission

The CDC began conducting national surveillance for hemodialysis-associated hepatitis in 1972. Rates of hepatitis B transmitted by dialysis ranged from 6.2 to 30 percent [18]. Subsequent recommendations for the control of hepatitis B, such as the requirement for HBV vaccinations for hemodialysis staff, resulted in a sharp decline of hemodialysis associated hepatitis, but still the risk of hepatitis remains high.

The hepatitis B virus is relatively stable in the environment and remains viable for at least 7 days on environmental surfaces at room temperature even in the absence of visible blood. The hepatitis B antigen has been detected in dialysis centers on clamps, scissors, dialysis machine control knobs and doorknobs [18]. In 1977, the CDC recommended that hemodialysis patients with hepatitis B be segregated, using different equipment, than patients without hepatitis B. This resulted in a 70–80 percent reduction of HBV infection among hemodialysis patients. Still, outbreaks of HBV continue to emerge at hemodialysis centers.

Hepatitis C transmission

Since 1990, limited data indicate the rate of hepatitis C infection occurring among hemodialysis patients is 0.7 to 3 percent annually [18]. None of these patients had blood transfusions or reported injecting drug use during this period. However, not all hemodialysis patients are tested for HCV, a disease that often does not initially cause symptoms. Recent studies of hemodialysis patients in the United States show that the prevalence of antibodies to HCV among these patients ranges from 10–36 percent in adults and approximately 18.5 percent among children [18].

Risk factors for HCV in hemodialysis patients include a history of blood transfusion, the volume of blood transfused, and the years of dialysis. The time patients spend on dialysis increases their risk for HCV infection, ranging from 12 percent for patients on dialysis less than 5 years to 37 percent for patients treated with dialysis for more than 5 years [18].

Incarceration

Approximately 0.7 percent of the U.S. population is incarcerated in correctional systems. This group has a disproportionately greater burden of infectious diseases, including hepatitis [16]. Recent estimates indicate that 12 percent to 40 percent of all Americans with chronic HBV or chronic HCV infections were released from prison during the previous year [16].

In recent years, public health and correctional professionals have come to realize the significance of including incarcerated populations in community-based disease prevention and control strategies. These strategies are also directed toward correctional staff, a group that has an increased risk for occupational exposure to bloodborne pathogens.

Reported risk factors for viral hepatitis transmission among the incarcerated population include illicit drug use, sexual activity, and other percutaneous exposures such as tattoos and body piercings with contaminated needles.

Tattoos and Acupuncture

Hepatitis C is efficiently transmitted through contaminated acupuncture and tattoo needles, and contaminated tattoo dyes. It's important to use only certified acupuncturists and tattoo artists whose businesses are inspected and licensed. Although several case-controlled studies indicate that tattooing is not a risk factor for HBV or HCV results from these studies may not apply to all populations. One study of a limited number of injecting drug users suggested an increased risk of HBV and HCV infection in individuals receiving tattoos in prison [16].

The hepatitis B virus is also transmitted through tattoos and it's thought that ritual tattooing ceremonies may be responsible for the high rate of HBV infection in endemic areas [6]. Before the discovery of HBV and its transmission, the needles used in this process were regularly used on successive clients in the United States.

Hepatitis can be spread through other rituals including ritual circumcision, cicatrix formation on the skin, acupuncture, and the rituals used to denote "blood brothers" or "blood sisters."

Blood Products

From the time of the earliest transfusions of blood from one person to another, there was evidence that transfusion carried risk. Advances in blood typing, immunology and sterile collection of units eliminated some of the risk, but disease transmission remained a problem through the 1941s.

At this time blood units began being tested for syphilis. Until the 1970s this was the only test performed on blood donors.

In 1972, tests for hepatitis B surface antigen were implemented, and most Blood Banks performed tests for hepatitis A, although its risk for blood transfusion remains low. Despite this implementation, there was still a risk for "non-A, non-B" hepatitis, with the risk of this disease reported to be as high as 12 percent and higher when paid donors were used. This led to the requirement by the Code of Federal Regulations to label the source of blood as being from volunteer or non-volunteer donors (42).

When HIV emerged in the 1980s, blood safety concerns escalated. Blood donors became scrutinized more closely and physicians began restricting the use of blood products, using them only when there was a critical need. However, people with blood factor deficiencies, such as hemophiliacs, receive concentrated clotting factors made from multiple donors. This puts them at high risk for hepatitis B and hepatitis C.

The role of the FDA

Since 1979 the Food and Drug Administration (FDA) has been a part of the U.S. Department of Health and Human Services. The FDA is authorized to regulate and assure the safety of consumer products. The Center for Biologics Evaluation and Research (CBER) is the branch of the FDA that regulates biological products, including blood products. In 1973, the FDA required all Blood Banks to register as drug manufacturers for their transfusion services.

The relationship between the FDA and Blood Banks remained collegial until the 1980s because of criticism and concerns regarding blood safety. In response, the FDA began inspecting Blood Banks, and in 1992, it classified blood products as pharmaceuticals requiring current good manufacturing practices (CGMPs).

Lookback procedures for HCV

Early efforts to identify patients exposed to the HIV virus that causes AIDS through transfusions consisted of identifying infected donors and "looking back" at records to identify patients who received blood products from these donors. This was a voluntary program endorsed by the blood bank community in 1984.

Once HIV and the hepatitis C virus (HCV) were identified and tests became available, the FDA recommended lookback to identify patients possibly exposed to units from infected donors. In high risk areas, lookback was recommended by the CDC.

However, the first generation of tests for HCV were not specific or sensitive. This caused inaccurate information to be released to recipients of blood products. Improved tests for HCV, the second generation tests, became available in 1992. Furthermore, a mobile population made it difficult to follow up with blood donors and some recipients had died by the time contaminated units had been identified. HCV had also been present for decades before it was identified, and many of the donors with HCV may have had chronic infection but no evidence of disease, giving false reassurance to blood recipients.

With increased knowledge regarding HCV and improved tests, in 1998 the FDA decided it was important to identify patients who had contracted HCV through blood transfusion. Lookback for HCV required contacting blood recipients who might have been received blood products more than a decade ago. The results, however, have been disappointing. In 2000, the CDC reported that only 1.5 percent of recipients notified by targeted lookback discovered their positive HCV status through lookback.

The American Association of Blood Banks (AABB)

The AABB is an organization comprised of physicians, scientists, medical technologists, nurses, and public relations specialists established in 1948 as an international association dedicated to promoting excellence in transfusion medicine. Most Blood Banks are inspected and certified by the AABB and follow their standards, which comply with those of the FDA, but usually are even more stringent. Hospital Blood Banks are also accredited and inspected by the Joint Commission on Accreditation of Healthcare Organizations (JCAHO) and the College of American Pathologists (CAP).

Blood product safety

With the implementation of nucleic acid testing (NAT) for hepatitis in 1999, the risk of contracting HCV through transfusion of blood products is 1 in 2 million, compared to 1 in 103,000 when antibody tests alone were used [52]. With NAT testing, viral material is detected, eliminating the "window period" that limited antibody tests. The window period refers to the time in which persons have been infected with hepatitis until they begin producing hepatitis antibodies.

The incidence of HBV has also declined considerably, but with HBV it's more difficult to determine the exact decrease because antibody testing for hepatitis B had been available for a longer time. Furthermore, HBV is more common in certain areas such as Taiwan and Greece, and the incidence of transfusion related HBV is higher in these areas.

Before 1990, blood transfusion was one of the most common causes of HCV infection. However, between 1985 and 1990, the number of cases of non-A, non-B hepatitis related to transfusion had declined by more than 51 percent due to improved screening of blood donors [52]. For instance, donors who had received tattoos, acupuncture or ear piercing were prohibited from donating for one year, and donors admitting to injecting drug use were permanently rejected. Since 1994, the risk of transfusion related hepatitis has been low.

Organ transplant donor safety

Organ transplant safety is regulated by the Organ Procurement and Transplantation Network and the United Network for Organ Sharing. Prior to transplant organ donors undergo screening tests for hepatitis.

Contaminated RhoGam

RhoGam is a product containing Rh immune globulin that's given to Rh negative mothers to prevent them from developing antibodies to the Rh factor. Rh antibodies have the potential to cause fatal blood incompatability reactions in future offspring who are Rh positive. In the 1970's a large batch of RhoGam was contaminated with the hepatitis C virus (confirmed years later when tests for hepatitis C became available). Among several hundred Irish women infected with the contaminated lot, half still had demonstrable virus in 1998, many had evidence of liver fibrosis and two had developed cirrhosis.

The primarily benign course of hepatitis C in the women in this study may not be an accurate portrayal of the effects of hepatitis C in the general population. Studies of morbidity and mortality in blood donors of various ages infected with hepatitis C from transfusions show that 15–20 percent of HCV-infected patients were affected by morbidity associated with death [55].

Contaminated Equipment

Surgical, acupuncture and dental instruments

Improper or inadequate sterilization techniques can transmit hepatitis in surgical, acupuncture and dental patients. Patients have also been infected with contaminated solutions due to re-use of needles and the use of radioactive tracer and saline solutions by multiple patients. Vaccine guns can also transmit hepatitis and are thought to be the cause of the high incidence of hepatitis C in veterans.

Beauty shop and tattoo parlor equipment

Hepatitis can be transmitted from scissors and razors contaminated with traces of blood from nicks. Pedicure and manicure equipment can be similarly contaminated. Contaminated tattoo needles and contaminated dye solutions can also transmit hepatitis. Needles used to pierce ears and body parts may also be contaminated. Cleaning solutions for needles, scissors and combs may be contaminated if the solution is too dilute or old.

Occupational Hazards

Certain occupations cause an increased risk for hepatitis. These include employees, students, contractors, public-safety workers and volunteers whose occupation involves contact with patients or with blood or other body fluids from patients in a healthcare, laboratory or public safety setting.

An exposure that might place individuals at risk for hepatitis is defined as a percutaneous injury (needlestick or cut with a sharp object) or contact of mucous membrane or non-intact skin (skin that is chapped, abraded or inflicted with dermatitis) with blood, tissue, semen, vaginal secretions or other body fluids.

In studies of individuals who sustained injuries from needles contaminated with blood containing HBV, the risk of developing clinical hepatitis if the blood was positive for both hepatitis B surface antigen and HBe antigen was 22–31 percent. HBV has been shown to survive in dried blood at room temperature on environmental surfaces for at least one week.

Bloodborne infection risk is reduced by universal precautions, which include the use of protective equipment such as latex gloves and masks, when working with patients, blood and body fluids. Hepatitis B and hepatitis A can be prevented by vaccinations. Under provisions of the Ryan White Act, postexposure treatment and follow-up testing for infectious diseases such as hepatitis and AIDS is provided to individuals who incur occupational exposures.

Sex Workers

Sex workers have an increased risk for hepatitis A and B, both of which can be prevented with vaccines and consistent use of prophylactics. Sex workers also have a slight risk of HCV infection. HAV is primarily transmitted through oral-fecal contamination during sex. HBV is easily transmitted during sexual intercourse whereas HCV is rarely transmitted through sexual intercourse.

4

Infectious Hepatitis

Infectious diseases are caused when our body's cells become infected by infectious agents. Under certain conditions, these agents can be transmitted from the infected individual (or his blood and other body fluids) to other persons. These newly infected individuals develop the same infectious disease or become disease carriers.

In the years before microbiologists developed methods of classifying the infectious causes of disease into specific groups of bacteria, fungi, protozoa and viruses, all infectious agents were referred to as viruses. The word virus stems from the Latin word for poison, and early scientists had observed that the diseases resulting from infection appeared to cause effects similar to those caused by poisons.

More than 90 percent of the cases of infectious hepatitis are caused by the hepatitis viruses A–E, which are described in chapters 5–9. These hepatitis viruses primarily damage liver cells although other organs may be affected in the process. Hepatitis is also caused by other infectious agents such as cytomegalovirus (CMV) that primarily affect other organs and occasionally affect the liver. Infectious hepatitis can also be caused by an assorted variety of bacteria, fungi and parasites. Chapter four describes these other (non A–E virus) infectious causes of hepatitis and the disease course seen when the liver is affected.

Causes of Infectious Hepatitis

Liver Abscesses

An abscess is an isolated accumulation of pus associated with a localized infection. Abscesses may cause tissue destruction, pain, swelling and inflammation. If large or multiple areas of liver tissue are affected, abscesses can cause a condition of hepatitis. A number of microorganisms can cause abscesses. Bacteria normally present in the biliary tree can reach the liver via the portal vein, the system circulation or directly, for instance, during trauma, perforated peptic ulcers, or appendicitis. Abscesses are most often seen in elderly patients with gastrointestinal diseases.

Liver abscesses often have a bacterial origin, with *Enterobacter* infections predominating. In immunosuppressed patients, mycobacterial infections and fungal infections can also cause abscesses. The ameba *Entamoeba histolytica* is a frequent cause of abscess in tropical regions.

Liver abscesses are diagnosed with abdominal ultrasound, magnetic resonance imaging (MRI), or computerized axial tomography (CT) scans. Blood tests for liver function typically show an elevated alkaline phosphatase level. Aspiration of the abscess can allow the wound drainage to be further examined and the responsible organism identified. Drainage is also used as a therapy. In bacterial infection, broad spectrum intravenous antibiotics are generally recommended.

Protozoa

Protozoa are single-celled organisms known to cause parasitic infections in humans. While parasites are more common in underdeveloped countries, the incidence of parasitic infections has increased in the United States in recent years due to a relaxation of control efforts, introduction of parasites from immigrants and visitors from foreign countries, and the use of immunosuppressant and chemotherapeutic medications. Protozoa that can cause intestinal infection or hepatitis include: *Giardia lamblia*; *Entamoeba histolytica*; *Dientamoeba fragilis*; *Balantidium coli*; *Toxoplasma gondii*; *Plasmodium* species (cause of malaria), and *Isospora* species.

ENTAMOEBA HISTOLYTICA AND AMOEBIC LIVER ABSCESS

The amoeba *Entamoeba histolytica* can cause various clinical diseases, most commonly amebic dysentery, amebic colitis (inflammation of the colon), and liver abscesses. Liver abscesses occur in up to 10 percent of patients with amebic colitis. *Entamoeba* reaches the liver via the portal vein. In the liver, *Entamoeba* destroys or necrotizes liver tissue. The cell destruction causes the tissue to become spongy and the abscess produces a thick reddish pus. Secondary bacterial infection can occur, confusing the clinical picture. The primary treatment for amoeba is metronidazole.

Amebic abscesses can develop many years after travel to tropical areas, and they are more often seen in males. The reason for this period of latency preceding abscess formation is unclear. Symptoms include right upper quadrant pain, fever, chills, biliary obstruction, liver enlargement and mild jaundice. Lesions near the diaphragm can cause right shoulder discomfort. Rarely, amebic abscesses can rupture within the lung or pericardium. *Entamoeba* can be diagnosed by ultrasound, examinations of stool samples for parasites and for serology tests that detect the presence of antibodies to *Entamoeba histolytica*. Most infections with *E. histolytica* are acquired by ingestion of contaminated food or water although an outbreak in 1982 in the United States was caused by a contaminated colonic irrigation machine.

Amoebic hepatitis. Amoebic hepatitis may occur in some cases of *Entamoeba histolytica* infection or amebiasis. Amoebic hepatitis is characterized by an enlarged tender liver in someone with intestinal amebiasis. It is uncertain whether hepatitis is a result of bacterial, toxic, or direct amoebic involvement of the liver. Rarely, amoebic abscesses may also appear in other organs, such as the lung and brain, either by direct spread from the intestinal disease or by a secondary spread from a liver abscess.

TOXOPLASMA GONDII

Toxoplasma gondii is an intracellular protozoan with felines as the definitive host. Infection in humans occurs after ingesting raw or undercooked or meat or by ingesting cysts excreted by felines. Usually, toxoplasmosis causes asymptomatic or benign disease in hosts with suppressed immune systems. In progressive disease, the predominant symptom is encephalitis, causing cerebral (brain) mass lesions that are seen with computed tomography (CT) or magnetic resonance imaging (MRI) procedures. In some cases, the liver, heart, eye, lung, and liver may also be affected. Liver involvement results in hepatitis. Diagnosis is made with blood tests for-Toxoplasma antibodies.

Helminthic liver parasites

Helminths are parasitic worms known to infest humans. Helminths are classified into nematodes, which are roundworms; and platyhelminths, which are flat worms. Platyhelminths are also known as trematodes or flukes. Adult worms vary in size from barely visible to the naked eye up to 10 meters in length.

The life cycles of helminths may be direct or indirect. Direct development requires only one host, which harbors the adult worms, and eggs or larvae are passed in the stools. In some instance, the larvae are infective when passed. Others may require a soil maturation period before the larvae become infective. Indirect cycles involve intermediate hosts, in which the larval stages develop, and definitive hosts, which harbor the adults.

Most living organisms, including humans, serve as definitive and/or intermediate hosts for many parasitic helminthes. Adult and larval stages can occur in the intestinal lumen or tissues of the host. Helminths can reach the liver through the portal system and mesenteric veins. Signs and symptoms of infestation are caused by adults, larvae, eggs, or host reactions to them or their products. Helminths that cause intestinal infection and hepatitis include: *Trichuris trichiura*; *Ascaris lumbricoides* (which can cause biliary colic and obstruction, cholangitis, and intrahepatic abscesses); *Strongyloides stercoralis*; *Fascioloa hepatica*; and *Schistosoma* species.

TRANSMISSION OF HELMINTHS

Infections caused by liver helminths are transmitted through food. It's estimated that worldwide more than 40 million people have acquired food-borne helminth infections. Common infectious agents include *Fasciola* species, which causes severe liver disease, *Paragonimus westermani*, which is sometimes confused with tuberculosis, and *Schistosoma* species. Individuals who have resided in endemic areas who develop hepatitis often have a history of eating raw fish or uncooked water plants. Symptoms of infection include upper abdominal pain, indigestion, diarrhea, and hepatomegaly (enlarged liver). Diagnosis can be made by detecting helminth eggs in stool samples submitted for ova and parasite testing.

SCHISTOSOMA

Schistosomes belong to the group Platyhelminthes, *family Schistosomatidae*, a group of flattened trematodes. Schistosoma flukes require definitive and intermediate hosts to complete their life cycles. Schistosomes are a significant cause of liver disease in endemic areas. Worldwide, they have infected more than 200 million people. Studies of Egyptian mummies indicate that schistosome infection dates back to the predynastic period of 3100 B.C.

Liver involvement is particularly seen with *Schistosoma japonicum* and *Schistosoma mansoni*, but it can also occur with *Schistosoma haematobrium*. In the early stages of disease, a hypersensitivity reaction with increased blood eosinophils is seen, but over time, if untreated, *Schistosoma* can cause extensive collagen deposits that lead to portal fibrosis, portal hypertension and enlarged spleen. Other symptoms include rash, diarrhea and urinary obstruction. Diagnosis can be made by serology tests for *Schistosoma* antibodies or by the presence of *Schistosoma* eggs (ova) in fecal or urine specimens. In one of the largest outbreaks of viral hepatitis in the world, thousands of individuals at a vaccine clinic for Schistosoma were infected with hepatitis C.

Transmission of schistosomes. Schistosomes penetrate the skin directly and transform into intermediate forms that migrate through tis-

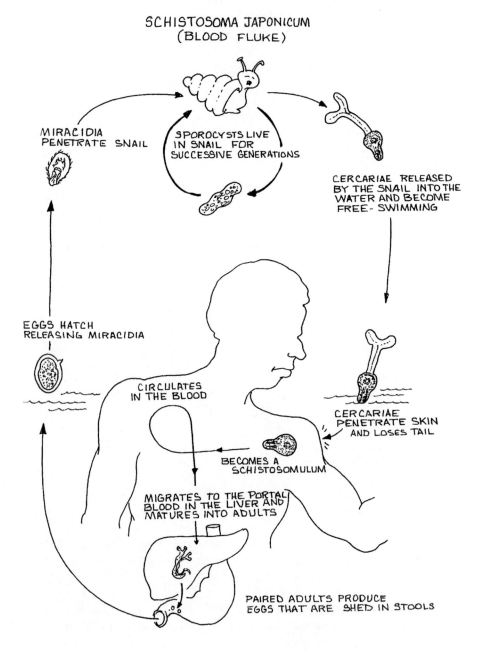

SCHISTOSOMA JAPONICUM (BLOOD FLUKE)

MIRACIDIA PENETRATE SNAIL

SPOROCYSTS LIVE IN SNAIL FOR SUCCESSIVE GENERATIONS

CERCARIAE RELEASED BY THE SNAIL INTO THE WATER AND BECOME FREE-SWIMMING

EGGS HATCH RELEASING MIRACIDIA

CIRCULATES IN THE BLOOD

CERCARIAE PENETRATE SKIN AND LOSES TAIL

BECOMES A SCHISTOSOMULUM

MIGRATES TO THE PORTAL BLOOD IN THE LIVER AND MATURES INTO ADULTS

PAIRED ADULTS PRODUCE EGGS THAT ARE SHED IN STOOLS

Schistosoma infection (Marvin G. Miller).

sue and invade blood vessels through which they travel to the lungs and liver. Once within the liver sinusoids, the worms begin to mature into adults capable of laying eggs and reproducing. The eggs release a number of proteins that produce abscesses in the infected tissues. Schistosome eggs can pass through the wall of the intestine. They are then filtered by the liver.

Hepatosplenic schistosomiasis. Schistosome infection in the liver and spleen is called hepatosplenic scistosomiasis. Liver invasion causes severe liver disease with symptoms of fever, abdominal pain, diarrhea rash, liver tenderness and general malaise. Eggs deposited in the portal triads of the liver stimulate an immune response that can cause fibrosis of the tissue surrounding the portal tracts. The fibrotic tissue is white and hard and has been referred to as Symmers' pipestem fibrosis [2].

FASCIOLA HEPATICA

Fasciola hepatica is commonly referred to as a liver fluke. *Fasciola* is a parasite of domestic and wild animals, including cattle and sheep, and accidentally, of man. After ingestion, the adult parasite travels to the biliary tree where it lays eggs that are passed in feces. These parasitic cysts also release larvae that penetrate through the intestinal wall into the peritoneal cavity. They then migrate to the liver and bile ducts, where they mature or live.

Young larvae cause few symptoms during migration. In the liver they elicit an inflammatory response in the bile ducts. Bile flow may be impaired, resulting in the formation of bile stones and the development of jaundice.

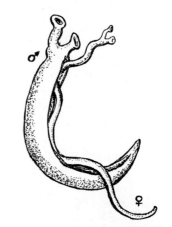

SCHISTOSOMA JAPONICUM
(BLOOD FLUKE)

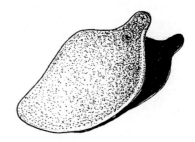

FASCIOLA HEPATICA
(LIVER FLUKE)

Schistosoma and fasciola (Marvin G. Miller).

ASCARIS LUMBRICOIDES

Ascaris lumbricoides is the largest nematode that can be found in the human intestinal tract. Infection (ascariasis) is endemic in many parts of the world, with more than half a billion people infected. Ascaris is transmitted through soil and occurs in areas where sanitation is poor. Ascariasis varies from asymptomatic infection to severe hepatitis. Migration of ascaris to the common bile duct can cause biliary colic and obstruction, leading to intrahepatic abscesses. Diagnosis is made by finding ascaris eggs in feces. Female ascaris typically lay up to 200,000 eggs every 24 hours.

Causes of Bacterial Hepatitis

Hepatitis can be caused by bacterial infection of the biliary tract, portal system or through systemic blood infection. Many different bacteria can infect the liver causing hepatitis or complicating disease when hepatitis is already present.

For instance Campylobacter colitis, an inflammatory bowel disease associated with the microbe *Campylobacter jejuni*, can be related to a non-specific acute form of bacterial hepatitis [56]. In "septic shock syndrome," systemic infection with *Staphylococcus aureus* can infect the liver as it filters the contaminated blood. Bacterial hepatitis should be suspected in cases of hepatitis accompanied by high fever (>101°F). Other symptoms of bacterial hepatitis, which can persist for months, include recurrent fever, elevated white blood cell count, chest pain and right upper quadrant pain.

Before the discovery of antibiotics, most bacterial infection was caused by infection of the portal circulation caused by appendicitis. Today, bacterial infection can still occur after pelvic, urinary tract and infections of the large intestine. Bacteria known to cause acute hepatitis include: *Borrelia* species; *Brucella* species; *Campylobacter jejuni*; *Escherichia coli*, *Listeria monocytogenes*; *Meningococcus* species; *Mycobacterium tuberculosis* (the organism responsible for tuberculosis); *Salmonella* species, *Staphylococcus aureus*; *Streptococcus* species; and *Treponema pallidum*, the organism responsible for syphilis. Blood infection or sepsis with almost any infectious agent may also cause conditions of hepatic ischemia, an inability of the liver to circulate oxygenated blood. Some of the more common causes of bacterial hepatitis are described in the following sections.

Treponema Pallidum: Syphilitic hepatitis

Syphilis is caused by the spirochete bacterium *Treponema pallidum*. Nearly all cases of syphilis are acquired by direct contact with the lesions that occur in individuals with primary or secondary syphilis. Syphilis causes a systemic disease that can affect all of the body's organs and symptoms. While hepatitis can occur in secondary syphilis, it is most often seen in children with congenital syphilis.

Mothers can transmit syphilis to newborns during delivery and during pregnancy through uterine infection. The risk of congenital syphilis is directly related to the stage of maternal syphilis. It is extremely high during the first four years after initial infection and then decreases during late syphilis. Congenital syphilis can occur following maternal infection at any time in gestation, with the risk of fetal infection increasing as the stage of pregnancy advances. In congenital syphilis, the liver, kidneys, bones, pancreas, spleen, lungs, heart, and brain are the organs most likely to be affected.

Liver involvement in affected infants occurs as inflammation confined to the portal triads with rings of collagen deposited about the portal ducts and blood vessels. In some cases, focal inflammation and scarring are scattered throughout the liver tissue. In the most severe cases, the inflammatory infiltrates produce a diffuse hepatitis with separation of liver plates and eventual scarring. Silver stains of liver tissue often show heavy infiltration with *Treponema* spirochetes. In two-thirds of untreated infants, the clinical signs of early congenital syphilis, including hepatitis, begin to appear in the third to the eight week of life. In nearly all cases, the clinical signs appear within three months.

Diagnosis can be made with blood tests for *Treponema* antibodies.

Tuberculosis of the liver

The liver may be affected by *Mycobacterium tuberculosis* infection, especially in miliary tuberculosis, an acute systemic (affecting the blood and organs) condition in which small tubercules or pustules are formed in one or more organs of the body. Although tuberculosis primarily causes a respiratory disease, it can affect the liver and other organs, especially when the body's immune system is suppressed due to HIV infection, aging, malnutrition, drugs or other factors.

Tuberculosis of the liver may present as an abscess, nonspecific hepatitis, or as a granulomatous (with small lesions composed of tissue and white blood cells) liver disease. Rarely, enlarged abdominal lymph nodes may compress the biliary tree, causing symptoms of biliary tract obstruction. Patients with liver tuberculosis often have symptoms of fever and weight loss due to the point of wasting. The liver is generally enlarged but not extensively. In severe conditions, patients may present with liver failure.

Liver tuberculosis typically causes an elevated alkaline phosphatase level and a low albumin. Granulomas present in the liver can resemble those of sarcoidosis or *Listeria* infection, although in TB the granulomas may contain giant cells. Anemia is common, and both the erythrocyte sedimentation rate and C-reactive protein level are elevated. Diagnosis is made by abdominal ultrasound and cultures of wound drainage.

Leptospirosis

Leptospira icterohaemorrhagiae is responsible for Weil's disease or leptospirosis, a type of infectious hepatitis. This organism is typically found in rat, dog or pig urine, making it a hazard for farm and sewage workers and those who use contaminated waters for recreational purposes.

In leptospirosis (*Leptospira* infection) resulting in hepatitis, the liver shows cholestasis and swelling of hepatocytes with very little necrosis. Classic Weil's disease causes a cluster of signs and symptoms (Weil's syndrome) that includes hemorrhages, jaundice, circulatory collapse, increased urine protein, acute liver failure, and high mortality. In Weil's disease, kidney disease may be more pronounced than liver disease.

Protective clothing is used to help prevent occupational exposure, and it has been recommended that sewage workers carry cards to remind their physicians of the possibility of leptospirosis if they become ill. The patient's occupation or leisure activities may suggest this diagnosis in patients with symptoms.

The septic stage of disease has an abrupt onset and may include high fever, muscle pain, nausea, vomiting, headache, conjunctivitis (inflammation of the eyelids), enlarged liver and jaundice. The white blood cell count is elevated, usually in the range of 30,000, and the platelet count may be decreased. Blood levels of bilirubin and alkaline phosphatase are elevated. In contrast to viral hepatitis, the ALT and AST levels may be normal or only moderately elevated.

During the second or immune disease stage, fever resolves although there may be signs of myocardial (heart) involvement and impaired renal (kidney) function. In the third or convalescent stage, a steady clinical and biochemical improvement occurs. Both liver and kidney function usually return to normal and cardiac function improves. Minor relapses of symptoms, particular muscle pain and fever, can occur.

Leptospirosis may be diagnosed by identifying *Leptospira* in urine or blood samples or by the presence of antileptospiral antibodies, with increasing titers occurring during the convalescent phase.

Tropical pyomyositis and Staphylococcus aureus

Staphylococcus aureus is a common bacteria known to occasionally cause a condition of tropical pyomyositis, a primary infection of skeletal muscle accompanied by fever and intramuscular abscesses. *S. aureus* is the cause of tropical pyomyositis in up to 90 percent of all cases. Although this condition can occur in temperate areas, it is most common in tropical regions. Rarely, this condition progresses to hepatitis and causes hepatic encephalopathy, especially in patients that abuse alcohol.

Lyme disease and relapsing fever

Lyme disease is caused by the spirochete *Borrelia burgdorferi*, which is transmitted by Ixodid ticks. Injected in the skin, the organism produces a red rash (*Erythema chronicum Migrans*) that persists for 1–2 months and characterizes the first stage of disease. The rash is accompanied by symptoms of hepatitis, nervous system fatigue, and musculoskeletal pain. In the second stage of disease, the brain and heart may be affected, causing neurological and cardiac (heart related, such as elevated heart rate) symptoms. The third stage is characterized by arthritis, and the hepatitis persists, causing elevated ALT and AST liver enzyme levels.

Relapsing fever is caused by the spirochete *Borrelia recurrentis*, and it is transmitted by the louse, pediculus humans. Symptoms include recurrent high fever, joint pain and inflammation, muscle pain, nausea, vomiting, petechia (small, purple bruises on the skin and eyelids), enlarged liver and jaundice.

About 10 days into the disease, these symptoms begin to resolve and symptoms of circulatory collapse, with hemorrhage and uncontrolled bleeding, develop. In another 10 days, circulatory collapse recurs in the absence of fever. Fatalities are related to bleeding complications, liver failure, cardiac failure or ruptured spleen. Liver enzyme levels are elevated and bilirubin may be as high as 15 mg/dl. Both Borrelia disorders are effectively treated with penicillin, tetracycline or erythromycin antibiotics.

Rickettsial hepatitis — Rocky Mountain Spotted Fever

Rocky mountain spotted fever is caused by organisms known as rickettsia that are transmitted by ticks that penetrate the skin through bites. This disease was first reported in Montana in 1873. Before the introduction of antibiotics, mortality was reported to be as high as 23 percent. In infection, symptoms develop after an incubation period of 2–14 days. Early symptoms include fever, malaise, and vomiting, and in one-third of patients jaundice develops. Early treatment with tetracycline, doxycycline or chloramphenicol antibiotics have reduced mortality to 3 percent.

Viruses

In 1898, the scientists Friedrich Loeffler and Paul Frosch discovered that foot-and-mouth disease in livestock was caused by an infectious particle smaller than any bacteria. Their studies confirmed earlier reports that tobacco mosaic disease, later determined to be plant virus, could be transmitted through a filtered preparation of the infectious agent. Some other infectious agent, smaller than bacteria, was evidently causing disease. These were the first clues that viruses existed.

A few years later in 1901, while working with yellow fever patients, the scientist Walter Reed succeeded in filtering viruses from blood samples. Reed described viruses as ultra-microscopic organisms capable of causing disease. Since, researchers have found that viruses range from simple lifeless forms to complex viable microorganisms. To date there are more than 151 different viruses that can cause disease in man.

The origins of virology

Virology, the study of viruses and the diseases they cause, emerged in 1950 when John Enders and his collaborators reported successfully growing viruses in tissue cultures. Viruses are bundles of genetic material occurring in a wide variety of sizes and shapes that require living hosts for their replication and ultimate survival. Smaller than bacteria, viruses contain a nucleic acid genome of either single or double-stranded RNA or DNA usually surrounded by a polyhedron-shaped (multi-sided) protein coat or capsid. Each viral species has its own unique capsid. Some viruses are also surrounded by an outer protein envelope. Unlike bacteria, viruses lack cell walls and nuclei.

Viruses are classified by similarities in size or shape, physiochemical and physical properties, genome, proteins, antigenic properties, presence or absence of a capsid base of RNA or DNA, number of strands, and type of replication. Viruses thrive in human, animal, bacterial, fungal, or plant cells, where they reproduce. When not infecting a host, viruses can remain dormant, persisting for many years on cell or other surfaces or moving within air currents or water. While dormant, they wait to come into contact with a life form containing the host cells they need to thrive.

In doing so, viruses are able to transfer some of their genetic material into that of the host cell. For this reason, viruses are extensively used in genetic engineering.

Survival mechanisms

To persist within an infected individual or a host population, viruses, particularly RNA viruses such as HCV, must replicate continuously. Each infection cycle within a host cell typically takes 1–3 days and during this time several different copies or mutations of the virus genome can occur. Mutated viruses are sometimes able to escape detection by laboratory tests and they may develop resistance to treatment. Viral survival depends on coping skills not found in plants or animals.

Virions

Virions are complete infectious viral particles consisting of the RNA or DNA viral core surrounded by a protein coat and occasionally external envelope proteins. Virions are the extracellular (outside of the cell) infective form of viruses capable of infecting host cells. In viral hepatitis, virions are highly infectious and remarkably stable in the environment.

Viral replication

When virions enter living hosts, they use the host cell's chemical energy, protein, and nucleic acid synthesizing ability to reproduce. After the infected host cell makes viral components the host cell is often destroyed or transformed into a cancerous state. In viral hepatitis, the infectious virion replicates within the liver cells that it infects.

DNA AND RNA VIRAL MODES OF REPLICATION

Deoxyribonucleic acid (DNA) is the principal component of chromosomes. DNA contains the genetic material or life code for the organism. DNA viruses, which contain single or double strands of DNA, reproduce within host cells, efficiently making copies of themselves from a single replicative strand acting as a template. These copies, made during viral replication, can occasionally deviate from the original DNA structure, forming mutant strains.

Ribonucleic acid (RNA) is a type of messenger protein used in the intermediate steps leading to DNA production. RNA viruses, which contain single or double strands of RNA, reproduce with the help of specific viral enzymes. Copies of the RNA strand with a negative strand serve as templates for the production of positive strand RNA. Because these copies are made from a template, variations of the genome are not unusual. Strains with modified genomes can occasionally result during viral replication, producing mutant strains. This is one of the reasons vaccines for RNA viruses are difficult to produce.

Tropism

Tropism is a property of affinity or attraction. Viruses show tropism in that specific viruses have a specific affinity for specific types of host cells. For instance, the hepatitis viruses have a tropism for liver cells. This property allows these viruses to seek out liver cells once they inhabit the body.

Causes of Viral Hepatitis

Other viruses besides the hepatitis viruses can have tropism for the liver although the liver is not their primary target. For instance, cytomegalovirus (CMV), which primarily causes rash, retinitis, and deafness, can target a variety of host cells, including stomach and liver cells. Depending on the general health of the patient, viruses with a predilection for multiple cell types tend to seek out the most susceptible organs. In patients with livers already damaged by toxins or infection, these viruses are most likely to target the liver cells.

Other viruses known to infect the liver and cause hepatitis include: adenovirus; coxsackievirus; echovirus; enterovirus; Epstein Barr virus (EBV); hantavirus; herpes simplex virus; herpes zoster virus; human immunodeficiency virus (HIV); human papillomavirus (HPV); human herpes virus-6 (HHV-6); Marburg virus; Lassa virus; paramyxovirus; parvovirus B19; reovirus 3; rubella virus; and varicella.

Cytomegalovirus (CMV)

Cytomegalovirus (CMV), a member of the herpesvirus family, is a double-stranded DNA virus. CMV can cause mononucleosis, hepatitis, retinitis, pneumonitis, colitis, and congenital cytomegalic inclusion disease. Infection with CMV is usually caused by contact of virus with cells of the oropharynxy (relating to the mouth and throat) or the genital tract or by transfusion of contaminated blood. When leukocyte reduced blood products are used, which is customary in most hospital Blood Banks in the United States, CMV cannot be transmitted in blood products.

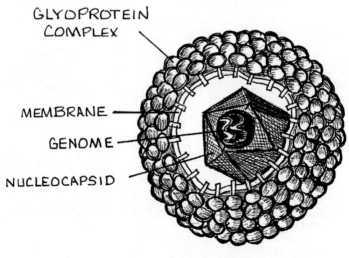

CYTOMEGALOVIRUS

Cytomegalovirus (Marvin G. Miller).

Clinical disease usually results from the host's inflammatory response to the virus. CMV is found in about 51 percent of the adult population and in about 0.5 to 5 percent of infants. CMV can establish a period of latency within white blood cells known as monocytes and reactivate at a later time when the conditions for replication are more favorable, such as during treatment with immunosuppressant drugs.

CMV can target many different cells although most cells do not permit CMV to replicate. CMV can replicate in the brain, eye, blood vessels, lungs, heart, lymphocyte cells, liver, adrenal glands and pancreas. Infants infected during pregnancy or at birth often develop enlarged spleens and livers and they may develop bilateral hearing loss and mental retardation.

CMV can be detected through culture techniques and with tests that detect viral DNA. IgG antibodies to CMV can be detected in blood tests but they cannot differentiate past from recent infection. Patients with CMV hepatitis are usually treated with the antiviral drugs gancicolvir or phosphonoformate (Fosarnet).

Marburg virus

The Marburg virus, the agent of Marburg hemorrhagic fever, is an RNA virus of the filovirus family, a species which includes the Ebola virus. The Marburg virus, which is indigenous to Africa, was first recognized in 1968 when it caused outbreaks of hemorrhagic fever in several European laboratory workers who had been exposed to African green monkeys or their tissues. Since, several cases have been reported in travelers to South Africa, and an outbreak occurred in gold mine workers in Durba, Democratic Republic of the Congo.

Despite numerous studies, the actual animal host of the Marburg virus is unknown. However, it's known that infected persons can spread the virus to other people through droplets of body fluids.

After an incubation period of 5–10 days, the disease onset is sudden and is marked by fever, chills, headache, and myalgia. Around the fifth day after the onset of symptoms, a flattened rash appears, which is most prominent on the trunk. Nausea, vomiting, chest pain, sore throat, abdominal pain and diarrhea follow. Symptoms may become increasingly severe and may include jaundice, hepatitis, inflammation of the pancreas, delirium, shock, liver failure and multi-organ dysfunction.

Recovery from Marburg hemorrhagic fever may be prolonged and accompanied by recurrent hepatitis. Other possible complications include inflammation of the testis, spinal cord, eye, and parotid gland, or by prolonged hepatitis. The case-fatality rate for Marburg hemorrhagic fever is between 23–25 percent. Infection with the Marburg virus is detected by an

ELISA test for detecting IgM-capture antibodies, PCR tests for viral DNA and virus isolation. Tests for IgG-capture antibodies can be used to diagnose past but not current infection.

Treatment includes supportive therapy, replacing lost blood and clotting factors with appropriate blood and blood product transfusions, and treatment for complicating infections. Laboratory workers who have contact with non-human primates associated with this disease are at risk. The World Health Organization (WHO) recommends that barrier nursing techniques and universal precautions should be used in these laboratories.

Epstein-Barr virus (EBV)

The Epstein-Barr virus (EBV) was first discovered in 1964 and found to be the cause of infectious mononucleosis and Burkitt's lymphoma. EBV is present worldwide and childhood infection is common especially in less affluent socioeconomic groups. In lower socioeconomic areas, 80 percent of five-year olds show past evidence of infection compared to 40–50 percent of five-year olds in high socioeconomic areas.

Primary EBV infection is always followed by a permanent carrier state. Hepatitis from EBV can develop as a complication of acute infection or from a later relapse. Diagnosis is made by the presence of IgG antibodies to early antigen. Antibodies to early antigen show evidence of active viral replication.

Lassa virus

Lassa virus, the cause of Lassa fever, a hemorrhagic fever with a high mortality rate, belongs to the family *Arenaviridae*. Lassa virus is endemic in West Africa and has been reported in Sierra Leone, Guinea, Liberia, Nigeria. It is rarely seen in the United States and Europe and all cases have occurred in people who have traveled to Africa.

Lassa fever was first discovered in 1969 when two missionary nurses died in the town of Lassa in Nigeria, West Africa. In West Africa, the Lassa virus causes about 100,000 to 300,000 infections annually and approximately 5,000 deaths. The viral host is a small rodent of the genus Mastomys with a hairless tail. The virus is shed in rodent urine and droppings and can be transmitted through inhalation of air contaminated with viral particles (airborne transmission), direct contact of the virus with open wounds, introduction through contaminated medical equipment, or eating food contaminated with rodent urine or droppings. The virus is not transmitted through casual contact.

The incubation period for Lassa fever is 6–21 days. About 80 percent of infected persons are asymptomatic. The remaining cases have severe multi-system disease, in which the virus attacks multiple organs, including the liver and spleen. Symptoms include fever, chest pain, sore throat, back pain, cough, abdominal pain, vomiting, diarrhea, conjunctivitis, facial swelling, elevated urine protein, hepatitis and neurological symptoms including hearing loss.

Death occurs in 15–20 percent of hospitalized patients. Mortality is particularly high in the third trimester of pregnancy and for 95 percent of the fetuses carried by infected pregnant mothers. Lassa fever is usually treated successfully with ribavirin, especially when it is prescribed early in the course of infection.

NANE (non-A/non-E) hepatitis virus

Worldwide, at least 300,000 cases of community-acquired and transfusion-related viral hepatitis occur each year that are not caused by hepatitis viruses A, B, C, D or E or by other viruses commonly known to cause hepatitis. The viral cause, which is referred to as the NANE virus in studies, has not yet been determined although there have been several promising candidates. This novel virus, which is still being researched, has been found to cause both acute and chronic hepatitis, and it is transmitted through blood and blood products. The NANE virus is described further in chapter nine.

Causes of Fungal Infections

Fungi known to cause hepatitis include Histoplasma, Cryptococcus, Aspergillus, Blastomyces, and Candida albicans. Fungal hepatitis is most likely to occur in individuals with suppressed immune systems, including patients with AIDS and patients on immunosuppressant medications. In hepatitis caused by fungal infections, liver abscesses are often seen and the mortality rate is high.

Candida albicans

Candida albicans is a fungus known to cause an infection known as candidiasis primarily affecting mucosal surfaces such as the mouth and vagina. Candidiasis is likely to occur during or following antibiotic therapy, during pregnancy, in immunosuppressed individuals and in patients with indwelling venous catheters. Candidiasis can also cause a systemic infection, persisting in the blood and infecting internal organs, including the liver. This can result in a condition of hepatitis. Candidiasis can be confirmed by the presence of *Candidia albicans* in blood cultures and in tests for Candida IgM antibodies.

Histoplasmosis

The fungus *Histoplasma capsulatum* causes histoplasmosis, a disease usually characterized by a mild respiratory illness. However, some patients, especially immunosuppressed individuals, may develop a recurrent systemic disease affecting several different organs, including the liver. The hepatitis caused by histoplasmosis may be severe and associated with a septic-shock like syndrome. Diagnosis is made with imaging studies of the chest, or with blood or urine tests for *H. capsulatum* antibodies. The hepatitis caused by histoplasmosis is usually treated with amphotericin B.

5

Hepatitis A

The hepatitis A virus (HAV) is distinguished as the first of the hepatitis viruses to be discovered although it was not formally identified until 1973. Unquestionably an ancient disease, hepatitis A is also distinguished as being the most common preventable infectious disease in the world, with HAV vaccines available since 1995.

In the United States, HAV is responsible for 50 percent of all cases of acute hepatitis [38] and it is the seventh most commonly reported infectious disease. Approximately 141,000 new HAV infections are reported to the CDC each year. In the developed world Hepatitis A accounts for 20–25 percent of all clinical hepatitis. Worldwide, an estimated 1.4 million cases of hepatitis A are reported annually.

Hepatitis A typically causes an acute self-limited infection that resolves within several months. However, in extreme cases, hepatitis A can cause a fulminant fatal disease, and on rare occasions it can cause chronic disease due to persistent liver damage rather than persistent infection.

In this chapter readers will learn about the hepatitis A virus (HAV), its discovery, its infectivity, and its geographic distribution. Readers will also learn about the disease caused by HAV, including the incubation period, epidemiology, disease course, symptoms, diagnosis, serological markers, treatment, risk factors, and complications.

The Hepatitis A Virus (HAV)

The hepatitis A virus is an ancient virus found in all parts of the world. Risk of infection is highest in developing countries, especially in areas of low socioeconomic status. Hepatitis typically runs a mild acute course with symptoms ranging from mild fatigue, nausea, vomiting and fever. It can also cause jaundice, especially in infected adults, and in rare instances it can lead to fulminant hepatitis and acute liver failure.

Hepatitis A is classified as the type species of the genus *Hepatovirus* of the family *Picornaviridae*, which includes the polio virus. HAV was initially classified as an enterovirus because of its symptoms until the entire nucleotide sequence of its viral genome determined it to be a hepatovirus, a type of virus that requires liver cells as its host. HAV enters the body through ingestion and spreads through the bloodstream to the liver, its target organ. From there, HAV is excreted into the bile and passed into the feces.

Electron microscopy examination of fecal extracts from patients in the early stages of HAV infection reveals a small (27 nm), spherical particle lacking an outer envelope. The HAV is approximately 7.5 kb long, symmetrical and single stranded and it contains 7510 nucleotides of positive sense RNA, making it a single-stranded RNA virus.

HAV surveillance

In the United States, hepatitis A is a reportable disease, which means that all states are required to report all cases of HAV infection to local or state health departments. From there, cases meeting specific requirements are reported to the CDC. This allows for: 1) tracing contacts of infected patients who might require prophylactic treatment; 2) detecting and responding to outbreaks; 3) determining the effectiveness of HAV vaccinations; 4) monitoring disease incidence among different age groups; 5) determining the epidemiological characteristics of infected persons, including the source of infection; and 6) determining missed opportunities for vaccination.

HAV viability

The hepatitis A virus is resistant to environmental factors, including temperatures as high as 57°C and as low as 0°C, acids with pHs as low as 3.0, and certain chemicals including ether. Depending on conditions, HAV can remain stable in the environment for months. At room temperature, HAV persists for about 30 days. Boiling water destroys HAV and heating foods at temperatures higher than 185°F for more than one minute is also effective. Disinfecting surfaces with a 1:100 dilution of sodium hypochlorite (household bleach) is needed to inactivate HAV [32].

HAV cell cultures

Another unique property of HAV is its ability to be propagated in experimental cell cultures efficiently. Furthermore, in cell cultures, unlike its cousin, the poliovirus, HAV doesn't destroy the culture cells that allow for its growth. These properties have made it possible to study viral replication and develop conventional vaccines for HAV.

HAV strains

Although HAV is widespread and found in all parts of the world, strains collected in different regions show no significant changes. While various genotypes of HAV exist, there is only one serotype or specific antibody produced in response to HAV infection. Antibodies to HAV effectively neutralize every strain of HAV. Virion proteins 1 and 3 are the primary sites of antibody recognition by the virus.

Chimpanzees, several species of marmosets and New World owl monkeys are susceptible to HAV and may be infected through either oral or percutaneous (through skin puncture) inoculation. Although disease symptoms are milder in these animal models than in humans, the disease course is similar. Studies of infected animals have been useful in determining viral replication and liver cell injury in HAV infection.

Replication and shedding

HAV replicates within the liver, in cells known as hepatocytes, and is shed in high concentrations in the feces from two weeks before to one week after the onset of clinical illness. Although viral shedding slows down immensely after jaundice develops, active virus is still shed in feces in smaller amounts. Recent data suggest that HAV also replicates within cells of the small intestine [38].

Within the infected host liver cell, the HAV virion acts as a messenger ordering the production of a large polyprotein molecule. This molecule is processed via RNA translation with the help of a specific HAV enzyme into both structural and nonstructural proteins that are assembled into RNA copies.

The RNA copies produced through translation serve as templates, allowing for the synthesis of many more HAV RNA particles. Large numbers of virus particles are found in the feces during the incubation period of HAV infection, beginning as early as 10–14 days after exposure. Viral shedding within feces reaches its maximum near the end of the incubation period just prior to the onset of symptoms. At this time the individual is most infectious. As virus clears from the feces, IgM and later IgG antibodies to HAV show up within the blood. Antibodies to HAV, which are produced by the immune system, neutralize and destroy HAV, causing the disease to be self-limiting.

Discovery of HAV

Although the first reports of hepatitis A date back to 510 BC, epidemic jaundice was first formally described by the physician Rokitansky in 1842 who called it acute yellow atrophy. A viral cause for hepatitis was first suspected by the physician McDonald. In his writings, he described the likelihood of there being a special virus capable of injuring liver tissue that was already damaged by other causes.

A specific virus capable of causing hepatitis in healthy persons was formally referred to in a 1931 paper by H.C. Brown and colleagues. By exposing himself to blood taken from infected patients, Brown contracted hepatitis within less than five weeks, a timeframe that corresponds to the incubation period of hepatitis A.

Similar experiments in which the German physician Voegt transmitted hepatitis A to volunteers by feeding them duodenal juice taken from infected patients confirmed that HAV could be transmitted orally. In the United States, Havens and colleagues at Yale University transmitted jaundice by feeding either serum or a filtrate of stool extract from infected patients to four conscientious objectors who volunteered for the study. They developed hepatitis after a 20–30 day incubation period. Although stool samples from the volunteers collected during their recovery periods were not infectious, stools collected 5 days after the onset of symptoms were infectious [25].

Hepatitis A and Hepatitis B

In parallel studies at Yale, patients also developed hepatitis after receiving inoculations of serum from patients hospitalized with hepatitis. Hepatitis in these volunteers developed after 51 days. The longer incubation period indicated that there was a second form of hepatitis transmitted through blood. In the 1941s, the British physician F.O. MacCallum proposed using the terms hepatitis A for epidemic hepatitis and hepatitis B for the type of hepatitis found to be transmitted through blood.

In a series of experiments conducted in the 1960s by the Willowbrook State School, an institution for the mentally disabled on Staten Island prone to hepatitis outbreaks, researchers inadvertently confirmed that there were two distinct hepatitis viruses. The experiments also demonstrated the usefulness of measuring AST levels in patients without symptoms to diagnose hepatitis.

The hepatitis A virus was first visualized by electron microscopy in 1973 by Stephen M. Feinstone and his colleagues at the National Institutes of Health (NIH). They accomplished this by aggregating fecal material taken

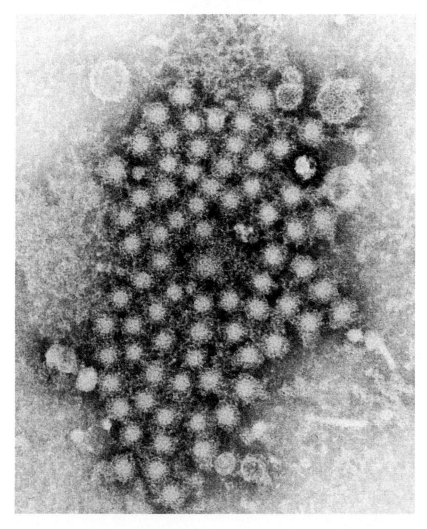

Hepatitis A virus (Centers for Disease Control Public Health Imaging Library).

from prisoners in Joliet, Illinois, with serum samples containing specific HAV antibodies taken from persons infected with HAV. This technique was then used in further tests for anti–HAV antibodies in patients recovering from hepatitis. These researchers also successfully grew the virus in cultures of Marmoset monkey cells.

Around the same time, using these cell cultures researchers at Merck defined and characterized the genome of the hepatitis A virus. In 1996, Merck's Dr. Hilleman developed the first hepatitis A vaccine by modifying the cultured virus in such a way that prevented it from causing active disease.

Endemic and Epidemic HAV Infection

Hepatitis A is endemic or common to certain regions. Epidemics of hepatitis A occur when outbreaks of infection occur in specific populations.

Endemic hepatitis A

The endemic form of hepatitis A is hard to recognize because it usually affects children at an early age, and children usually do not develop symptoms. Furthermore, young children still in diapers easily transmit HAV. In the developing world, where sanitation is limited, infection is almost universal. In one study, 100 percent of Egyptian children 1 to 3 years old showed serological evidence (HAV IgG antibodies) of past infection. Similar results were seen in studies in Pune, India and Nicaragua [25].

Epidemics of hepatitis A

Long before the discovery of HAV, epidemics of jaundice were carefully studied by researchers. Early on it was noted that epidemics of hepatitis A usually began in the fall, peaked in winter, and then waned until the following year. This seasonal pattern still holds true although the reasons for it are unclear.

EPIDEMICS OF HEPATITIS A IN WARTIME

Reports of hepatitis epidemics are common throughout military history. One of the first reported epidemics in the United States debilitated troops during the War of 1812. In World War I, British, French, and other Allied forces reported epidemics of jaundice starting in 1915 and continuing with intermittent outbreaks. Either hepatitis A or hepatitis E are thought to be responsible for these cases depending on the location of the battle. Because of its late entry into the war, United States troops escaped most of these epidemics. According to some historians, this led American troops to be unprepared for hepatitis during World War II.

During World War II, epidemics occurred in British troops serving in Palestine during 1941 and 1942 and in Allied Forces in North Africa in 1942 and 1944. At the peak of the epidemic in November 1942, nearly 2,000 men were hospitalized with jaundice compared to 3,000 men hospitalized with battle casualties. Overall, there were approximately 200,000 recognized cases of hepatitis among army soldiers alone [25]. In 1942 Germany, an estimated 10 million cases of hepatitis occurred among military personnel and civilians.

In more recent years, outbreaks of hepatitis A have also occurred among troops serving in the Viet Nam War and the Persian Gulf War. In the civilian population, outbreaks have occurred in healthcare facilities, day care centers and among football teams and restaurant customers.

Transmission of HAV

Hepatitis A can occur sporadically in random isolated cases or in an epidemic form. In either case, HAV is primarily spread by the fecal-oral route, most commonly by person-to-person contact, usually in conditions of poor sanitation and overcrowding. HAV is most often transmitted by the ingestion of fecally contaminated food transmitted by infected food handlers. Failure to wash hands and poor hygiene contribute to the problem, which also frequently affects daycare centers.

During the first two weeks of infection, the time of peak infectivity, individuals with HAV do not yet have symptoms and do not realize they're infective. In addition, flies are known to act as vectors, carrying HAV from fecal material to food and water sources. In rare instances, viremic (evidence of viral particles in their blood circulation) blood donors can transmit HAV through blood and blood products although Blood Banks today screen all donors for HAV.

In industrialized communities, water-borne transmission is rare but outbreaks of HAV caused by contaminated food occur sporadically. HAV can also be transmitted through sexual contact, especially in men who have sex with men. Recent studies show that saliva may also contain small amounts of HAV and serve as a possible source of HAV transmission [38].

Because children infected with HAV often do not have symptoms, they play an important role in HAV transmission and serve as a source of infection for others. Parents and child-care workers handling soiled diapers can contract or transmit the disease without recognizing that they've been exposed. In one study of adults without an identified source of infection, 53 percent of households included a child less than 6 years and further studies showed that in many cases the child was associated with HAV transmission within the household. In this study up to 41 percent of the children showed serological evidence of current HAV infection. [32].

Transmission via contaminated foods

Certain foods such as raw oysters, mussels, and clams are common sources of HAV. The hepatitis a virus is known to survive for extended periods of time in seawater. In one study, viral nucleic acid was present for 232 days in seawater. Steaming clams may not kill the virus because the temperature reached inside the clams is not sufficiently high. An outbreak of hepatitis A in Shanghai in 1998 caused by the ingestion of raw clams affected almost 300, 000 people [71].

In an October 2003 outbreak of hepatitis A at a Chi-Chi's Mexican restaurant in Pennsylvania [46], a 38-year-old man died, and nearly 200 other people were affected. In 1997, frozen strawberries caused 263 cases of hepatitis A among people in 5 states. In October 2003 a hepatitis A outbreak in several restaurants in Georgia, North Carolina, and Tennessee was linked to scallions, a type of green onion. Transmission of HAV has also been reported as occurring through ingestion of sandwiches, orange juice, raw or undercooked fruits and vegetables, potato salad and meat.

In both the United States and Europe hepatitis A outbreaks have been caused by consumption of contaminated lettuce, ice slush beverages, frozen strawberries, and salad. The practice of using global food items that cannot be heated to inactivate the virus may be a major cause of future outbreaks.

High risk groups and high risk factors

Other groups at high risk for HAV infection include men who have sex with men, staff and residents of institutions for the mentally handicapped, day care centers for children, injecting and non-injecting drug abusers, sewage workers, laboratory workers in contact with HAV, certain health care workers, and low socioeconomic groups. Transmission of HAV through blood products is extremely rare, but it can occur following transfusion of blood products from a donor who is in the incubation stage of the disease. Use of human sewage for soil fertilization can result in frozen-fruit-related epidemics of HAV [56].

Spread of HAV is related to overcrowding, poor hygiene and poor sanitation. With improved standards of living, the incidence of HAV has decreased in recent years. In urban areas of Bosnia, up to 96.9 percent of adults show antibodies to HAV, indicating prior infection. In underdeveloped countries up to 90 percent of children have antibodies to HAV by age 10 [56].

In highly endemic areas, most children are infected early in life although they usually have few if any symptoms. Fewer than 10 percent of the incidences of HAV infection in children younger than 6 years cause jaundice [71]. The age 5–14 year age group is most affected by HAV, and adults are often infected by spread from children.

The risk for HAV is highest in developing countries, areas of low socioeconomic status and areas without adequate sanitation. High infection rates also occur in settings where fecal-oral spread is likely, such as day-care centers and nursing homes.

Other groups with a high risk for HAV include international travelers, injecting and non-injecting drug users, hemodialysis patients, military personnel stationed abroad, missionaries, homosexual men, sewage workers, and certain daycare and healthcare workers. Residents of American Indian reservation or native Alaskan villages also have higher rates of HAV infection. Travelers to Mexico account for 84 percent of the cases of hepatitis A in the United States associated with international travel.

Close contacts including sexual contacts of infected individuals are also at risk. The secondary infection rate for HAV in household contacts of patients with HAV is approximately 20 percent. Approximately 10 percent of the cases of HAV in the United States occur in men who report having sex with men. Approximately 51 percent of persons with HAV infection do not have an identified source for their infection.

TRANSMISSION IN HEALTHCARE SETTINGS

Transmission of hepatitis A from hospitalized patients with unsuspected disease to staff and other patients is well recognized. Nocosomial infections are infections that occur in healthcare settings. Documented nocosomial hepatitis A infection has occurred in an adult patient with diarrhea following an elective cholecystectomy surgery, premature infants with prolonged viral excretion, burn patients incubating HAV in hospital settings, and an immunosuppressed patient with negative tests for HAV antibodies due to a weakened immune response [25].

TRANSMISSION VIA BLOOD TRANSFUSIONS

Once considered rare, parenteral (intravenous) transmission of hepatitis A from blood and blood products has been documented many times. Blood from a single donor who became ill one week after donating blood transmitted disease to 11 recipient neonates and an additional 45 persons who had contact with the infants. Recently, in Italy clotting factor concentrates were found to be contaminated with HAV. The solvent-detergent method of viral inactivation typically used for blood products was considered inadequate for nonenveloped viruses such as HAV. Experimentally, vapor heating of clotting factors can successfully eradicate HAV.

TRANSMISSION VIA SEXUAL PRACTICES

Certain sexual practices are associated with high risk for HAV transmission. According to the CDC, inapparent fecal contamination is commonly present during sexual intercourse. Like other enteric infections, hepatitis A can be transmitted during sexual activity, especially that involving oral-anal contact and insertive anal contact. Measures used to prevent other STDs such as condoms and good personal hygiene have not been successful in preventing outbreaks of hepatitis A.

Hepatitis A outbreaks among men who have sex with men have been reported frequently. Cyclic outbreaks have been reported in urban areas of the United States, Canada, Europe, and Australia. Studies show that persons with evidence of HAV infection report more frequent oral-anal contact, longer duration of homosexual activity, and a larger number of sexual partners than persons without serologic evidence of HAV infection (positive tests for anti-HAV IgG) [32].

However, hepatitis A differs from most sexually transmitted diseases (STDs) in that prior infection confers permanent immunity, vaccines are available to prevent disease transmission, and the period of infectivity is relatively short compared to that associated with other STDs.

Transmission via drug abuse

In both the United States and in Europe, outbreaks of HAV have been reported among injecting and noninjecting drug users. In the late 1980s, 10–19 percent of reported cases of HAV occurred among persons with a history of injecting drug use. Since then, outbreaks have been reported in the midwestern and western United States among users of methamphetamine. Transmission among injecting drug users likely occurs through contaminated needles and related equipment and through fecal-oral routes [32]. Hepatitis A can be spread through contaminated syringes and from rectally carried drugs as well as by unsanitary living conditions, crowding and poor personal hygiene.

Studies show that approximately 41 to 51 percent of drug users in northern Europe have evidence of HAV infection. At Johns Hopkins Hospital in Baltimore, Maryland, injection drug users had rates of HAV infection twice as high (67 percent) as in homosexual men (27 percent) and correlated with poverty.

Racial and ethnic groups

The CDC reports that in the United States, the highest rates of HAV infection are seen in American Indians/Alaskan Natives, and the lowest rates are seen among Asians. The rates of HAV in Hispanics are higher than among non–Hispanics [32].

Geographic distribution

In the United States, over the past several decades, the highest rates of hepatitis A have occurred in a limited number of states and counties. Rates have been substantially higher in the western states than in other U.S. regions. Consistently elevated rates of hepatitis A from 1967–1997 occurred in Arizona, California, New Mexico, Oregon and Washington [32]. Native American Indian reservations also have high transmission rates.

Hepatitis A is common in countries with under-developed sanitation systems. Outside of the United States, hepatitis A is common with increased transmission rates seen in Canada, Japan, Australia, New Zealand and the Western European countries.

HAV Infection

HAV infection typically causes a mild, self-limiting acute form of hepatitis. Most cases of hepatitis A result from person-to-person transmission during community-wide outbreaks. The most frequently reported source of infection, representing 12–26 percent of all cases in the United States, is either household or sexual contact with a person infected with HAV [32].

Epidemiology

HAV infection occurs endemically in all parts of the world, with frequent reports of minor and major outbreaks occurring about every decade, often in the fall. The exact incidence is difficult to determine because many infections are not recognized, especially because some patients never develop jaundice. The United States is an area of low HAV prevalence although its nearest southern neighbor, Mexico, is an area of high prevalence.

Tests for HAV antibodies, which are used to diagnose HAV infection, have made it possible to study disease incidence in different countries. These studies show that, unlike infection with hepatitis B or hepatitis C, chronic infection with HAV does not typically occur and there are no carriers of HAV.

The number of people with antibodies to HAV has declined since World War II in many countries although large epidemics still occur. In the United States, approximately 33 percent of the population has serologic evidence of prior HAV infection. This rate increases directly with age and reaches 75 percent among persons older than 70 years. Cyclic increases of hepatitis A have occurred every decade in the United States, with the last nationwide increase occurring in 1995. In 1997, 30,021 new hepatitis A cases were reported to the National Notifiable Diseases Surveillance System (NNDSS) [32].

Disease Course in HAV

Hepatitis A is usually mild, especially in children where it may not be recognized or merely deemed to be influenza. Typically, viral particles emerge in the stool during the incubation period. These persist until about the time the immune system begins producing IgM antibodies to HAV. The clinical course of acute HAV infection is typically that of a mild flu-like illness that lasts for a few days to a few weeks.

Only about 10 percent of children infected with HAV develop jaundice. Among older children, 41–51 percent develop jaundice, whereas 70–80 percent of adults with HAV develop jaundice. Viremia, which is the presence of viral material within blood, occurs early in infection and can persist for several weeks after the onset of symptoms.

Three phases of acute HAV infection

Hepatitis A causes acute hepatitis, which typically includes an incubation period, a prodromal state, an icteric or symptomatic stage, and a recovery or convalescent stage.

INCUBATION PERIOD

The incubation period of HAV ranges from 15 to 51 days with a mean of 28 days. Large numbers of virus particles can be found in feces during the incubation period with peak levels occurring about 10 days before the onset of symptoms. HAV gradually declines in feces and viral particles are rarely seen after the first few weeks when antibodies to HAV appear in the blood. During the incubation period patients with HAV are highly infectious because of the high levels of HAV in their stool samples.

Serological markers. An IgM antibody to HAV (anti–HAV IgM) appears early in the course of illness and persists for two to twelve months. Immunoglobulin M antibodies (IgM) directed at the invading microorganism are the first antibodies to appear in infection. The presence of HAV IgM antibodies indicates current or active HAV infection. An IgG antibody (anti–HAV IgG) appears toward the end of the acute illness, persists for one's lifetime, and conveys lifelong immunity. The test for HAV IgM is used to diagnose current infection, and the test for HAV IgG is used to determine immunity to HAV.

HAV IgM antibodies— positive results are an indicator of current infection
HAV IgG antibodies— positive results are an indicator of recovering or past infection
Equivocal HAV IgM results occur when results fall slightly below the testing cutoff. Equivocal results occur in early infection, while antibody production is rising and in recovering infection when IgM antibody titers are falling. Results are reported as equivocal with a footnote recommending that the test be repeated in 1–2 weeks.

PREICTERIC (PRIOR TO JAUNDICE) OR PRODROMAL PERIOD

The incubation period is followed by a preicteric or prodromal period lasting an average 5 to 7 days, although the timeframe varies from one day to more than two weeks. During the prodromal period patients can develop nonspecific flu-like symptoms including low grade fever, malaise, headaches and muscle pain. Loss of appetite, nausea, and vomiting may also occur. Diarrhea can also occur but it is more likely to be seen in children. In one study in approximately 15 percent of cases, a prodromal period was absent. In these cases, patients developed jaundice right after the incubation period.

ICTERIC OR SYMPTOMATIC STAGE

Less than 10 percent of children younger than 3 years develop symptoms of HAV infection. Most infected adults develop symptoms, with the most severe symptoms reported in older patients. During the icteric phase jaundice (icterus) may develop along with one or more other symptoms. The most common signs and symptoms in HAV infection include fatigue, nausea, vomiting, fever, hepatomegaly (enlarged liver), liver tenderness, jaundice, dark urine, pale stools, joint pain, lack of appetite, aversion to tobacco and greasy foods, and rash. Less frequently, patients may develop chills, muscle pain (myalgia), joint pain (arthralgia), cough, upper respiratory symptoms, constipation, diarrhea, itching (pruritis) and hives (urticaria). The symptomatic phase of HAV infection averages about 30 days and ranges from 7 to 90 days.

In patients who develop jaundice, the urine darkens before jaundice becomes clinically apparent. Other symptoms often resolve when jaundice develops. Jaundice lasts an average of 7 days and ranges from 4 to 25 days. Average total bilirubin levels peak at about 6.5 mg/dl. Serum aminotransferase (ALT and AST) levels rise and are similar to those seen in HBV infection although they do not persist for as long. Most people with HAV will have normal ALT and AST enzyme levels by six weeks after the onset of symptoms. Occasionally, minor enzyme elevations can persist for up to 3 months or longer.

In up to 70 percent of children younger than 6 years, infection with HAV causes no clinical symptoms [32]. The disease is more prolonged and causes graver illness in patients older than 51 years and in patients debilitated by other medical disorders, including other types of hepatitis. In some adults, cholestasis can occur, causing severe jaundice and pruritis (itching) of several weeks duration. A relapsing form of HAV infection has been reported in up to 11.9 percent of patients [25].

Pancreatic involvement. The association between hepatitis and pancreatitis is well known. The severity of pancreatitis may range from an abnormal appearance on ultrasound to clinical symptoms of frank pancreatitis and is more likely to occur in the elderly. In fulminant hepatic failure, up to 35 percent of patients show signs of pancreatitis.

HAV in the elderly

The later in life HAV infection occurs, the greater severity of symptoms. HAV outbreaks in nursing homes are particularly devastating. Evidence shows that while past infection usually causes lifelong immunity, re-infection may occur in elderly patients who no longer have detectable IgG antibodies to HAV. Data from the Shanghai outbreak showed that most of those affected requiring hospital admission were older than 41 years.

Mortality Rate of HAV

The overall case-fatality rate for HAV ranges from 0.03 percent in younger patients to 2.7 percent for patients older than 51 years. In the United States, approximately 100 persons die each year from acute liver failure caused by hepatitis A.

Children younger than 5 years, especially those with other medical disorders, and adults older than 51 years have the highest mortality rates. People with other significant diseases including other liver diseases are more likely to die from HAV infection than other people. This was apparent in the Shanghai outbreak in which a high incidence of hepatitis B surface antigen and hepatitis C antibody were seen in those who died.

Fulminant HAV infection

Fulminant hepatitis is a potentially fatal manifestation of hepatitis. Fulminant infection follows a different clinical course in hepatitis A, B, and C. Pyrexia, an elevation of normal body temperature commonly known as fever, is most frequently seen in fulminant HAV infection. Fulminant infection is most often seen in adults although it can be seen in children. Fulminant hepatitis A may be related to the dose of virus, a particularly virulent HAV strain, or to impaired immune system function.

Fulminant hepatitis is a life-threatening condition caused by massive necrosis (destruction) of liver cells or sudden and severe impairment of liver function. Most patients do not have a past history of liver disease although fulminant liver failure may be the first presenting sign of Wilson's disease, autoimmune chronic active hepatitis or delta superinfection in patients with chronic hepatitis B.

In hepatitis A, fulminant liver disease is characterized as developing within 2–8 weeks from the onset of jaundice and typically includes hepatic encephalopathy. Hepatic encephalopathy may initially manifest itself as personality changes, including anti-social behavior, nightmares, delirium, mania, violent behavior and tremor.

Chronic hepatitis A

The classic medical view is that hepatitis A does not cause chronic disease or a chronic carrier state. With the advent of HAV RNA tests, it's clear that HAV can persist for longer than previously suspected. There are reports of HAV causing elevated liver enzyme titers for as long as two months after the onset of symptoms. In addition, HAV IgM antibodies have occasionally been found to persist for many months, but this may be due to a slowly declining titer rather than persistent infection.

Chronic hepatitis A describes persistent liver damage due to HAV infection in someone who has recovered from hepatitis A rather than a persistent state of HAV infection. A prolonged course of HAV infection may be confused with other chronic liver conditions such as autoimmune hepatitis.

Cholestatic hepatitis A

Cholestatic hepatitis, a condition of impaired bile flow, can occur in adults with hepatitis A. In this case, jaundice persists for as long as 42–110 days and itching is severe. Both IgM and IgG HAV antibodies remain positive for the duration of cholestatic hepatitis. Prednisolone has been reported to speed recovery of cholestatic hepatitis [56].

Relapsing hepatitis A

Approximately 3–20 percent of patients with HAV may relapse from 21–180 days after their original symptoms resolve. However, studies show that even though the original disease symptoms resolve, transaminase enzyme levels (ALT and AST) do not return to normal in patients who eventually relapse.

The relapse follows a course similar to the original disease although there may be flares with heightened symptoms. The length of time between flares typically increases as the disease resolves. Relapse typically lasts for three to nine months before resolving, and the presence of HAV can be found in stool specimens until the condition resolves. Anti–HAV IgM persists in the blood for the duration of relapse.

On rare occasions, relapse can cause symptoms of arthritis, nephritis (kidney inflammation), vasculitis (blood vessel inflammation), and elevated cryoglobulin levels (further described in chapters 6 and 7), causing a condition of cryoglobulinemia, which is often seen in hepatitis B carriers [56]. Liver transplants have been performed in relapsing patients when liver failure threatens. Corticosteroid treatment has been used to improve symptoms, although in most cases treatment isn't needed.

Extraheptic symptoms in HAV infection

Extrahepatic refers to organs other than the liver. Besides pancreatic involvement, the extrahepatic manifestations of HAV infection include hemolysis, a premature breakdown of red blood cells, gallbladder inflammation (cholecystitis), renal failure, reactive hepatitis, and neurologic symptoms. In addition, autoimmune thrombocytopenic purpura, an autoimmune disorder causing low platelet levels, can occur.

Immune complex disorders such as vasculitis, kidney disease, postviral encephalitis and arthritis can also occur. These symptoms improve as hepatitis A resolves. HAV is also associated with the later development of autoimmune hepatitis.

Diagnosis of HAV

Diagnosis of HAV infection cannot be made on the basis of clinical or epidemiologic features alone. A diagnosis of HAV is based on blood test results showing HAV IgM, which are the first HAV antibodies to develop after infection with HAV. Test results for anti–HAV IgM are positive at about the time symptoms first appear and usually stay elevated until the first rise in alanine aminotransferase (ALT) levels.

Anti–HAV IgG antibodies appear early in the course of infection and remain elevated for years, generally persisting for life. Their presence, in the absence of anti–HAV IgM, indicates past infection or immunization but not active HAV infection. Individuals with anti–HAV IgG who are re-exposed to the hepatitis A virus can respond by producing more anti–HAV IgG, demonstrated by higher antibody titers, but re-exposure in persons with HAV immunity does not result in clinical disease symptoms.

The length of time that the IgM anti–HAV test remains positive varies. In most studies, IgM HAV becomes negative an average of seven months after the onset of symptoms although negative tests can occur after four months. Equivocal IgM results are reported when the testing value is within a specific range from the positive cutoff. Equivocal results may occur in early infection, recovering infection or as a false positive. Tests should be repeated in 1–2 weeks. In repeat testing positive results occur in patients who were initially tested during the early stage of infection.

Laboratory tests

Hepatitis A cannot be distinguished from other causes of hepatitis without serological tests for hepatitis antibodies. Blood tests are used to diagnose HAV and determine the severity of disease and response to treatment. Laboratory tests are described briefly in this section and more extensively in chapter 14.

HAV ANTIBODY TESTS

The anti–HAV IgM test remains positive for at least 3–6 months in most patients, although in up to 25 percent of patients, anti–HAV IgM persists for as long as 12 months. Levels of anti–HAV IgM persist longer in patients with relapsing HAV infection, usually until the duration of the disease. IgG HAV antibodies indicate past infection or vaccination. HAV IgM antibodies must be present to diagnose acute HAV infection.

LIVER ENZYME TESTS

Elevations of alanine aminotransferase (ALT) and aspartate aminotransferase (AST) are seen in acute hepatitis A infection. Levels may exceed values of 10,000 mIU/ml. ALT levels are generally higher than AST levels. Both levels decline, returning to the normal reference ranges over a course of 5–10 weeks although in about 10–20 percent of cases, enzyme elevations persist for up to 3 months and occasionally longer. Levels of the enzyme alkaline phosphatase (ALP) rise in HAV infection and continue to rise during the cholestatic phase of the disease, returning to normal within 6–10 weeks or longer if cholestasis persists.

LIVER FUNCTION TESTS

Bilirubin levels, both direct and indirect levels, begin to rise in the blood soon after the appearance of bile in urine. Levels remain elevated for several months. Levels that remain elevated for longer than 3 months indicate cholestatic HAV infection.

Prothrombin levels typically remain normal during HAV infection although in severe disease, the prothrombin level may rise. This is considered an ominous sign in patients who show signs of encephalopathy (neurological changes). Albumin levels typically fall modestly in HAV infection. The complete blood count (CBC) may show a mild elevation of lymphocytes, a decrease in red blood cells and a low platelet count.

Imaging tests

Imaging tests are not usually needed for a diagnosis of HAV infection.

Biopsy specimens

In acute HAV infection the liver shows widespread liver cell injury. This alters the normal radial appearance of the liver plates and squeezes the sinusoids closed, which is called lobular disarray. Hepatocytes appear lysed and they may contain eosinophilic (filled with granules that stain red with eosin) deposits known as Councilman bodies. These cells may be ingested by macrophage cells.

Increased numbers of enlarged Kupffer cells may be seen along with an increased number of lymphocytes. During the recovery phase, regenerated hepatocytes may be seen. Liver biopsies are described more extensively in chapter fifteen.

Complications of HAV

Complications in HAV infection include dehydration, relapsing disease, renal failure, coagulation defects, cerebral edema, and fulminant liver disease. Approximately 3–8 percent of fulminant liver disease is caused by HAV infection; however, only 1–2 percent of all cases of HAV infection in adults progress to fulminant hepatic failure.

Other conditions reported to rarely occur in association with HAV infection include interstitial nephritis (inflammation of kidney cells), pancreatitis, red blood cell aplasia (type of anemia), agranulocytosis (low level of segmented white blood cells), bone marrow aplasia (low production of blood cells), transient heart block, Guillain-Barré syndrome, acute arthritis, Still disease, autoimmune hepatitis, and Sjögren syndrome. In adults with HAV, up to 20 percent of patients may require hospitalization.

Prevention of HAV

HAV prevention is rooted in control at the source, with an avoidance of sources of contact. Travelers to endemic areas should avoid uncontrolled water sources, raw shellfish and uncooked food. Fruits should be washed and peeled before eating. Boiling water or adding iodine inactivates the virus.

Because avoidance does not always work, HAV infection can also be effectively prevented immunologically in two ways. It can be prevented with 1) passive immunization using nonspecific injections of immune serum globulin containing hepatitis A antibodies after exposure to HAV and 2) by active immunization with the hepatitis A vaccine. Active immunization causes the immune system to react as if it has been exposed to HAV by producing HAV antibodies that provide immunity to HAV.

Immune serum globulin (gamma globulin)

Purified preparations of gamma globulin containing at least 100 IU/ml of hepatitis A antibody derived from large pools of human plasma are used in intramuscular injections to provide passive immunity in patients exposed to HAV. These preparations are also used in patients for whom there may be inadequate time for vaccines to work prior to exposure.

Immune serum globulin is a form of passive immunization and is considered effective when used within 14 days of exposure. Because circulating antibodies, like all proteins, eventually break down within several months gamma globulin injections only offer limited protection. They are used in an effort to provide immunity until patients begin producing their own HAV antibodies as a result of vaccination. After a period of 6 months, travelers to endemic areas require a second dose of gamma globulin unless antibody tests show that they have developed HAV antibodies as a result of vaccination.

The dosage of gamma globulin should be at least 1 IU of hepatitis A antibody per pound of body weight or 2 IU/kg of body weight. In pregnancy and in patients who already have liver disease the dosage may be doubled [71]. Gamma globulin is available in preparations that contain thimerosal (mercury-based) preservatives and in preparations that are free of thimerosal. When administration of gamma globulin is indicated for infants or pregnant women, preparations free of thimerosal should be used [32].

Doses of passive immunoglobulin for travelers to endemic areas are also determined by the length of stay, with periods of stay longer than 3 months requiring 2–2.5 times the dose required for stays less than 3 months. Individuals less than 56 lbs or 25 kg are given 51 IU (0.5 ml) anti–HAV for periods of stay less than 3 months and 100 IU (1.0 ml) anti–HAV for longer visits. Individuals from 56–67 lbs or 25–30 kg are given 100 IU (1.0 mg) anti–HAV for stays less than 3 months and 251 IU (2.5 ml) for longer stays. Individuals weighing more than 110 lbs or 51 kg are given doses of 200 IU (2.0 ml) anti–HAV for stays less than 3 months and 510 IU (5.0 ml) anti–HAV for longer stays [70]. Preparations include BayGam (15–18 percent), which neutralizes circulating myelin antibodies through anti-idiotypic antibodies, and Gammagard S/D, an IgA depleted product.

Patients who receive passive immunization can become infected with HAV but typically only develop subclinical or mild disease. Mild infection allows the immune system to produce antibodies to HAV, which confer active immunity. Passive immunization with serum globulin offers protection for approximately 6 months. Reports of immunoglobulin capable of transmitting hepatitis C have caused some concern in recent years [38].

The HAV vaccine

The foundations for HAV vaccines came to light in 1975 with the demonstration that an injection of formalin-inactivated HAV prepared from extracts taken from the liver of infected marmosets caused the production of protective antibodies in susceptible marmosets. These protected marmosets showed resistance to disease when they were challenged with live virus. Subsequent studies showed that vaccines could be prepared from fetal monkey kidney and human fibroblasts.

HAV vaccines, which are currently only available through injection, are reported to have an efficacy from 80–100 percent after two doses. While healthcare workers and others at risk are not routinely vaccinated, people with chronic liver disease and people traveling to endemic areas should consider HAV vaccination. Currently two HAV vaccines are available and one combination vaccine for hepatitis A and hepatitis B has recently been introduced.

INACTIVATED VACCINES

Inactivated vaccines include Havrix(r) (manufactured by SmithKline and Beecham Biologicals) and Vaqta(r) (manufactured by Merck & Co., Inc.). Both vaccines come in two different formulations, one intended for children and another for adults. The HAV vaccines may be given along with passive immunoglobulin injections without affecting efficacy. Adults are given initial doses and boosters at 6 months for Vaqta and at 6–12 months for Havrix. Pediatric patients are given in smaller doses at similar timeframes.

The safety of HAV vaccines during pregnancy has not been established. Vaccines should be used with caution in acute infection or febrile illness. Hepatitis vaccines should be administered intramuscularly into the deltoid muscle, using a needle size appropriate for the person's age and size.

RECOMBINANT VACCINES

Recombinant vaccines are made by growing the infectious strain into a new organism such as yeast. A recombinant HAV vaccine has been prepared using the viral protein (VP1) of the HAV virus grown in yeast cultures.

SIDE EFFECTS

In clinical trials, the most frequently reported side effects of the HAV vaccine in adults included soreness at the injection site, headache, and malaise occurring up to three days after vaccination. In children, side effects included soreness at the injection site, feeding problems, headache, and injection-site swelling.

Serious side effects reported in persons receiving the vaccine in Europe and Asia prior to its introduction in the United States in 1995 include anaphylaxis, Guillain-Barré syndrome, brachial plexus neuropathy, transverse myelitis, multiple sclerosis, encephalopathy and erythema multiforme [32]. However, for conditions in which surveillance rates were available such as Guillain-Barré syndrome and brachial plexus neuropathy, rates weren't higher than those seen in the non-vaccinated population.

From the time of its introduction in 1995 until 1999 in the United States, the HAV vaccine was responsible for 248 reports of unexplained adverse events occurring within 6 weeks of vaccine administration. These events included neurologic, hematologic and autoimmune syndromes In one-third of these reports, other vaccines were administered simultaneously. None of these events could be conclusively linked to the vaccines. Adverse effects related to vaccines can be reported to the Vaccine Adverse Events Reporting System, VAERS at (800) 822–7968 or through their web page at http://www.fda.gov/cber/vaers/vaers.htm.

PRECAUTIONS

The Hepatitis A vaccine should not be administered to persons with a history of a severe reaction to a prior dose of hepatitis A vaccine or to a vaccine component such as alum. The safety of hepatitis A vaccine during pregnancy has not been determined although the risk to the developing fetus is expected to be low [32]. The CDC recommends that the risk associated with vaccination be weighed against the risk for hepatitis A in women who may be at high risk for exposure to HAV [32]. Because the vaccine is inactivated, no special precautions are needed when vaccinating patients with immune deficiency.

RECOMMENDATIONS

The CDC recommends routinely vaccinating children age 2 years and older who live in areas where rates of hepatitis A are at least twice the national rate. This includes states, counties or communities where the average annual hepatitis A rate from 1987–1997 was 20 cases/100,000 population or higher. The CDC recommends considering vaccination for children in areas where the average annual hepatitis A rate for 1987–1997 was 10 cases/1000,000 population or higher.

The CDC also recommends vaccination for persons at high risk such as persons traveling to or working in areas that have high or intermediate endemicity of infection; men who have sex with men; illegal-drug users; persons with occupational risk such as workers in laboratory settings with exposure to HAV; persons with chronic liver disease; and persons who have clotting-factor disorders who are administered solvent-detergent-treated clotting factor concentrates. Vaccination is also recommended for people living in communities with hepatitis A outbreaks.

Treatment of HAV

Patients with hepatitis A generally require only supportive care and are not usually given special restrictions for diet or activity. However, alternative medical treatments and lifestyle and dietary recommendations described in chapters seventeen and eighteen offer benefits for patients infected with HAV.

Patients who become dehydrated due to nausea and vomiting or who develop symptoms of liver failure may require hospitalization. Treatment consists of low doses of acetaminophen to reduce fever and pain not to exceed 4 grams daily, and antiemetics for nausea such as metoclopromide (Reglan).

Patients who develop fulminant hepatic failure should be considered for referral for liver transplantation to help speed up the process if transplant is needed. However, up to 61 percent of patients with fulminant disease recover without transplantation. Recurrence of HAV infection after liver transplant has not been reported.

Economic impact

The annual costs of treating HAV infection and controlling outbreaks in the United States is estimated to be about three million dollars [32]. Adults with HAV infection miss an average 27 days of work, and between 11 percent and 22 percent of persons with HAV infection are hospitalized. Restaurants and other places of business associated with HAV outbreaks also suffer financial losses.

6

Hepatitis B

The hepatitis B virus (HBV) was the second hepatitis virus to be discovered, and it accounts for approximately 34 percent of all cases of viral hepatitis in the United States. HBV can cause acute infection, chronic liver and kidney disease, and a persistent carrier state. Of the 200 million HBV carriers worldwide, 80 percent live in Asia and were infected during childhood. In this chapter readers will learn about the characteristics, discovery, transmission, and geographic distribution of this virus. Readers will also learn about the disease caused by HBV, including the incubation period, epidemiology, disease course, symptoms, diagnosis, treatment, risk factors, and complications.

The Hepatitis B Virus (HBV)

Smaller than most viruses, hepatitis B is one of the most destructive viruses known to man although in most cases it causes few if any symptoms. Worldwide, HBV is the most common cause of chronic hepatitis, a condition that can lead to cirrhosis and primary liver (hepatocellular) cancer (HCC). More than 2 billion people (51 percent of the world population) have been infected with HBV. About 5 percent of the world population, including more than one million people in the United States, are carriers of HBV. Carriers may have no clinical symptoms of hepatitis although they are able to infect other individuals. In endemic areas, such as east Asia and sub–Saharan Africa, 61–85 percent of individuals show evidence of HBV infection, and 8–25 percent of the population are HBV carriers.

The hepatitis B virus, which affects humans as well as chimpanzees and gibbons, belongs to the class of hepadna viruses. This viral class also

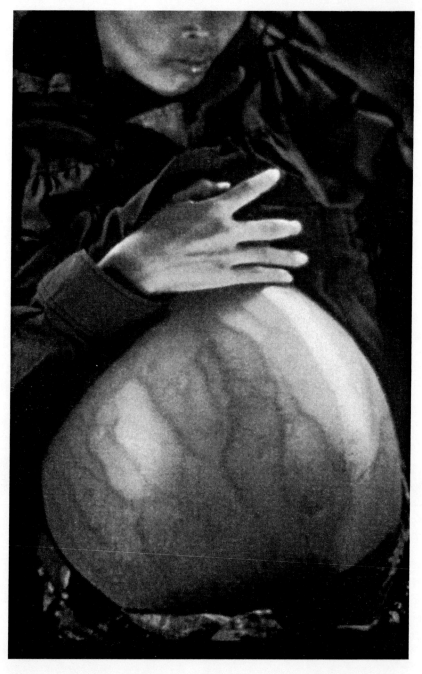

Cambodian woman with hepatoma and distended abdomen from hepatitis B infection (Centers for Disease Control Public Health Imaging Library).

includes the hepatitis viruses of woodchuck (WHV), ground squirrel (GSHV), duck (DHBV) and heron (HHV).

The HBV virion

The hepatitis B virion or infectious particle (Dane particle) is a complex double-stranded 42 nm DNA particle with an electron-dense core structure or nucleocapsid, 27 nm in diameter. HBV also contains a DNA polymerase enzyme, two core proteins, core and e, and an outer envelope containing surface protein. This surface protein, which is highly infectious, is known as the hepatitis B surface antigen (HBsAg). In HBV infection, large amounts of HBsAg can be found in the blood circulation.

In HBV infection, HBsAg becomes firmly embedded in a lipid membrane derived from the host liver cell. During its process of viral replication in the host, HBsAg is produced in excess by infected liver cells and then secreted from the cells in the form of 22 nm particles. In HBV infection, viral DNA and DNA polymerase enzyme are also found in the blood circulation.

The HBsAg particles include infectious Dane particles and many more non-infectious, spherical or elongated particles lacking in DNA. These

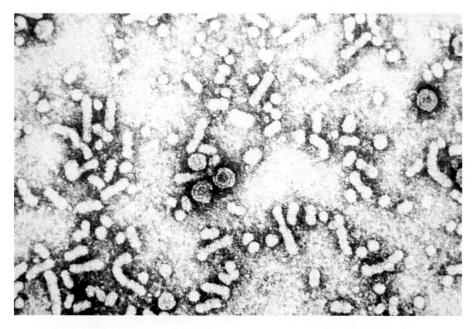

Hepatitis B virions (Dane particles) electron micrograph (Centers for Disease Control Public Health Imaging Library).

secreted viral particles are composed of the major surface protein along with some middle proteins. The presence of HBsAg in the blood correlates with viremia, a condition of systemic viral infection. People who do not clear HBsAg from the blood after infection resolves are known as hepatitis B carriers.

Components of the HBV viron

Hepatitis B surface antigen (HBsAg). Hepatitis B surface antigen, HBsAg, is a specific outer protein cover or envelope that covers the entire hepatitis B virus. Protein particles of HBsAg can be detected in blood, and their presence is a good indicator of HBV infection.

The hepatitis B surface antigen was initially known as the Australia antigen after its discovery by Baruch Blumberg in 1966. HBsAg consists of three separate proteins, pre-S1, pre-S2 and S. HBsAg also consists of small non-infectious particles that do not replicate or contain DNA, and they cannot cause infection.

The hepatitis B virus contains about 1,000 as many non-infectious particles as infectious particles. These non-infectious particles can be isolated and separated from the infectious particles and then used to manufacture HBV vaccines.

The purpose of these non-infectious particles is not well understood. It's been proposed that they protect the virus from the immune system allowing the virus to persist in the host for extended periods. The immune system presumably first attacks these small particles allowing the infectious particles to escape detection for long periods, causing chronic infection. HBsAg that persists for longer than six months indicates chronic infection, either persistent disease or the carrier state.

The Hepatitis B nucleocapsid. The nucleocapsid or central core of the hepatitis B virion consists of the viral genome (DNA) surrounded by the core antigen, HBcAg. The HBV genome is composed of two linear strands of DNA held in a circular configuration. More than 12 HBV genomes have been cloned. Each genome shows surface antigen and a core and pre-core region, which is responsible for the secretion of the hepatitis Be antigen (HBeAg). A fourth region, known as x, which codes for HBx protein, functions to activate viral transcription.

Hepatitis B genes

The hepatitis B viral genome consists of a partially double-stranded circular DNA of 3.2 kilobase pairs that encodes 4 overlapping open reading frames. The four major genes of these frames include *S*, *C*, *X*, and *Pol*.

relapsing course, with progression to cirrhosis and poor responsiveness to interferon therapy. In this mutant form of infection, superinfection with the hepatitis D virus is better tolerated than in infection with the wild-type HBV virus.

SURFACE ANTIGEN MUTATION

A mutation in the surface region affects infants born to carrier mothers causing them to become HBsAg positive despite vaccination. Mutated virus can also cause infection in vaccinated adults. Depending on the assay used, the mutated HBsAg may not be detected. This escape mutant affects the *a* determinant of HBsAg, the antigen primarily targeted by HBV vaccinations. By 2004, several of these mutations had been seen in the United States.

HBx MUTANTS

HBx mutants have been identified in renal dialysis patients where they have been shown to cause low level replication eventually evolving into HBsAg positive wild-type infections [4].

THE YMDD MUTATION

In the YMDD mutation HBV shows resistance to the drug lamivudine. Patients with this mutation show a reduced viral load when they begin taking the drug and then show high titers of viral HBV DNA later in the course of therapy.

HBV Surveillance

Hepatitis B is a reportable disease in the United States. Studies of disease data for hepatitis B allow investigators to assess risk factors, assess the effectiveness of vaccines, offer prophylactic services to patient contacts, and to determine groups in which offering the vaccine would offer protection. Surveillance initiatives have helped in investigating HBV outbreaks, finding sources of infection such as reusable finger-stick devices and initiating preventive changes. In addition, surveillance measures aid in monitoring the effectiveness of prenatal programs, the effectiveness of vaccines for the prevention of perinatal infection, and the effectiveness of educational programs.

HBV PREVENTION INITIATIVES

The goals of the Healthy Project 2010, a federal initiative aimed at reducing specific diseases and providing health services to underserved populations, include reducing the incidence of hepatitis among persons younger than 19 years by more than 99 percent and reducing hepatitis B in high risk groups by more than 75 percent [29].

A 1992 Occupational Safety and Health Administration (OSHA) rule requires providers of health care services to offer hepatitis B vaccines to employees. This has significantly reduced the number of HBV infections in healthcare workers since 1993.

HBV viability

The hepatitis B virus is extremely resistant and is able to withstand extreme temperatures and conditions of humidity. It can survive for at least 15 years in blood samples stored at -20°C or for 2 years at -80°C. At room temperature, the virus is stable for six months, and at 45°C it is stable for 7 days.

HBV is susceptible to many disinfectants. It may be destroyed by 1 percent solutions of sodium hypochlorite (bleach), 70 percent ethanol, and formaldehyde.

HBV cell cultures

Hepatitis B virus does not grow in tissue medium. However, studies of its genome have allowed scientists to clone the organism in yeast and in *Escherichia coli* cultures. These cloned forms are used to manufacture hepatitis B virus.

HBV replication

Once HBV enters the body it passes quickly to the liver where it infects a liver cell. It accomplishes this by attaching to the cell membrane and allowing the viral core particle to enter the cell. The core particle then releases its DNA and DNA polymerase into the liver cell nucleus.

Inside the host cell, the viral DNA replicates through a process of reverse transcription in which an intermediate RNA molecule is produced under the direction of DNA polymerase enzymes. Through this messenger RNA, the host liver cell can make copies of HBV DNA. Mistakes made while producing viral copies result in mutations.

Studies suggest that HBV also replicates within the tubules of the kidney. During the infectious phase of HBV, viral antigens are shed into the blood circulation, inducing an immune response and HBV antibody production. The virus along with its viral antigen and antibody forms a large immune complex. This complex, which has a lattice-like formation becomes trapped by the glomeruli as they work to filter waste materials from the blood. The trapping of immune complexes leads to thickening of the kidney's basement layer, inflammation, and progressive kidney disease.

SIMILARITY TO HIV

The ability of HBV to form mutations is similar to that of the human immunodeficiency virus (HIV) responsible for acquired immune deficiency syndrome (AIDS). Replication in HBV is also similar to that of HIV except that the DNA form is exported from cells in HBV infection. In HIV infection, the RNA form is exported from infected cells. Because both viruses require reverse transcriptase enzymes for replication, anti-retroviral compounds such as lamivudine are effective treatments in these infections.

Discovery of HBV

In his early years as a physician, Baruch Blumberg developed a keen interest in the genetic polymorphisms and environmental factors that influence disease development. In particular, he was interested in the lipoprotein subtypes that predispose certain individuals to heart disease. As a scientific researcher, Blumberg, while studying these protein fractions, encountered an unusual protein in the serum of Australian aborigine patients with serum hepatitis.

In 1966, Blumberg and colleagues named this protein the Australia antigen and in subsequent studies determined it to be the Hepatitis B surface antigen. In 1976, for his work leading to this discovery, 1976 Blumberg won the Nobel Prize in Physiology or Medicine [6].

In 1970, the British scientist Dr. D. S. Dane along with his colleagues reported visualizing the entire hepatitis B virus particle, including its nucleic acid. This infectious virion is known as the Dane particle.

Transmission of HBV

One ml (about ½ a teaspoon) of blood from an individual infected with HBV can contain up to 1.5 million viral particles. HBV is also found in lesser amounts in other body fluids, including saliva, semen, wound drainage exudates, vaginal fluids and breast milk. Most HBV infections, however, are related to transmission of blood and other body fluids that are contaminated with blood.

HBV is efficiently transmitted by percutaneous (entry through skin) or mucous membrane exposure to infectious body fluids. HBV can be transmitted through four general modes: percutaneous, sexual, perinatal, and horizontal.

The approximately 510 million HBV carriers worldwide, including the 1.25 million HBV carriers in the United States, serve as the major source of HBV infection. The HBV carriers with HBeAg in their blood have the highest HBV titers and have traditionally been considered the most infective. However with the increased prevalence of HBV mutations, viral load titers are a better indicator of infectivity.

The hepatitis B virus is transmitted when the virus gains entry into the bloodstream parentally through childbirth; through sexual intercourse; through transfusion of contaminated blood products; through direct contact with contaminated medical instruments and equipment; and through skin puncture causing percutaneous exposure to infectious bodily fluids.

Perinatal transmission

Perinatal transmission refers to the transmission of HBV occurring perinatally, that is, around the time of childbirth. Infants born to mothers who are HBeAg positive have the highest risk (70–90 percent) of infection. Among the children who become infected with HBV, about 90 percent will go on to develop chronic HBV infection. Infants of HBeAg negative mothers have a 10–41 percent risk of developing HBV infection. Among these children, the risk of chronic infection is 41–70 percent.

Children born to HBV positive mothers who are not infected perinatally have a higher risk of developing infection during early childhood. Perinatal transmission has been found to be more common in Asia than in Africa, and infection typically develops within 3 months, whereas in Africa infection typically develops within the first 6 months. While reasons for the higher infection rate in Asian women are not yet certain, HBsAg-positive women in Asia are more likely to be HBeAg-positive than HBsAg-positive women in Africa.

Although infection may occur in the uterus, studies show that most infections are acquired at the time of birth. Transmission may be caused by direct contamination of the infant's circulation with maternal blood at the time of delivery.

High risk groups and high risk factors

Other groups with a high risk for HBV infection include health care workers and emergency response personnel with exposure to blood and blood products, recipients of multiple blood transfusions, patients with clotting factor deficiencies who receive regular transfusions of clotting factors, sexually active homosexuals, persons born in endemic areas, heterosexual persons who have multiple partners or a history of sexually transmitted disease, institutionalized persons, prisoners, hemodialysis patients and household contacts or sexual partners of HBV carriers.

TRANSMISSION VIA SEXUAL PRACTICES

In low prevalence areas such as the United States, most HBV infection is caused by exposure through sexual or blood contact with a chronically infected person. In the CDC's study of acute HBV infections in sentinel countries, heterosexual contact with multiple partners accounted for 41 percent of all cases and homosexual contact accounted for 15 percent of all cases [15].

The most common risk factors for heterosexual transmission include multiple sex partners (more than one partner in a six-month period) or a recent history of a sexually transmitted disease. Risk factors for infection among men who have sex with men include multiple sex partners, engaging in unprotected receptive anal intercourse and having a history of other sexually transmitted diseases.

TRANSMISSION VIA BLOOD TRANSFUSIONS
AND BLOOD PRODUCTS

Prior to 1982, the risk of developing hepatitis B after blood transfusions was high especially in patients multiply transfused with clotting factors made by multiple donors. With improved screening procedures and the use of HBV DNA tests for screening donors, transmission of HBV through blood products is extremely rare.

However, many people in the United States have chronic HBV infection as a result of blood products transfused before 1982.

HORIZONTAL TRANSMISSION

Many studies show that "horizontal" transmission to young children is probably the most common means of HBV transmission worldwide. Horizontal transmission refers to the development of infection in individuals living in households of infected persons who do not have sexual, perinatal, or percutaneous contact with the infected person. Some studies show that the virus, which can be found in saliva, may be transmitted through bites, and it is suspected that repeated inapparent percutaneous exposures through saliva and blood, including sharing of toothbrushes, may be responsible.

TRANSMISSION VIA INJECTION DRUG USE

Injection drug use is one of the primary risk factors for HBV transmission. The CDC estimates that 17 percent of the new cases of HBV that occurred in 2000 in the United States occurred among injection drug users [14]. Within 5 years of beginning injection drug use, approximately 51–70 percent of injection drug users become infected with HBV [65].

Alcohol and HBV. The prevalence of HBV infection is two to four times higher in alcoholics than in corresponding control groups. The prevalence of HBV markers in cancerous tissue is also significantly higher in alcoholics with cirrhosis and liver cancer than in sections of liver tissue not affected by cancer [7]. The mild immune system suppression seen in alcohol abuse may also influence a move into the carrier state after acute HBV infection. Alcohol also induces free radical production, another contributing factor for liver cancer.

The liver cell injury caused by alcohol involves several different factors, including diet, nutrients, the immune response and cellular changes. Liver cell damage caused by alcohol is thought to contribute to HBV-related liver damage in infected individuals. Chronic alcohol consumption is also known to contribute to the development of cirrhosis in patients with hepatitis B. A study of HBsAg positive blood donors who were moderate or heavy drinkers indicated a 5–8 fold greater risk of developing HCC than donors who were non-drinkers [40].

Alcohol abuse may also increase the tendency of chemical carcinogens to induce liver cancer by several mechanisms. These include the conversion of procarcinogens to carcinogens by inducing certain cytochrome P-461 enzymes. This is pronounced in people following low carbohydrate diets [31]. Changes in the metabolism of fatty acids caused by alcohol are suspected of also playing a role. Alcohol also affects the normal process of liver regeneration that occurs in liver disease. This results in fibrosis and increased production of ductules and mutated cells rather than hepatocytes.

TRANSMISSION IN CORRECTIONAL SETTINGS

The prevalence of current or past HBV infection among prison inmates ranges from 13 to 48 percent and varies by region. Prevalence is higher among women than men. Chronic HBV infection is seen in 1.0–3.7 percent of inmates, which is 2–6 times higher than the national prevalence estimate of 0.5 percent in the United States.

The majority of HBV infections among incarcerated persons are acquired outside of the prison community although some infections occur in the correctional setting primarily through injecting drug use and sexual intercourse. Among patients with acute hepatitis B reported to CDC's Sentinel Counties Study of Viral Hepatitis, 5.6 percent had a history of incarceration during the incubation period [16].

TRANSMISSION IN HEMODIALYSIS PATIENTS

The CDC recommends that all patients scheduled for dialysis be tested for both hepatitis B and hepatitis C. Patients with HBsAg should be isolated and confined to dedicated rooms and equipment. Staff members caring for these patients should not care for susceptible patients at the same time including the period when dialysis is terminated on one patient and initiated on another [18].

Patients who clear HBsAg can be moved into the general patient population. Vaccinations for HBV are recommended for hemodialysis patients who are negative for HBV.

TRANSMISSION VIA AFLATOXIN B

Aflatoxin B is a plant mold common in areas with high mortality from HCC. Studies have shown a strong interaction of chronic HBV infection with aflatoxin B exposure and HCC. While aflatoxin alone increases the risk of HCC fourfold and HBV increases the risk about seven times, persons with both HBV infection and aflatoxin metabolites in their urine were sixty times more likely to develop HCC than persons negative for HBV and without aflatoxin B exposure [40].

Geographic distribution

In the United States, the incidence of HBV is considered low. Approximately 200,000–300,000 new cases occur annually and 1.25 million people are carriers [40]. Many of the carriers are immigrants from high or moderate prevalence areas. New infections in the United States result in 10,000 or more hospital admissions each year and 251–300 deaths annually from fulminant hepatitis.

HBV infection is very common in Asia, China, Indonesia, the Amazon Basin, the Phillipines, sub–Saharan Africa, and the Middle East. These high prevalence areas have rates of HBV infection higher than 10 percent. The geographic distribution of hepatocellular carcinoma (HCC), the most common type of primary liver cancer, and the HBV carrier state are remarkably similar. Ethnic Chinese and black Africans have the highest rates (about 85 percent) of both HCC and HBV carriers [36].

Intermediate prevalence areas, with rates of 3–10 percent, include eastern and northern Europe, Japan, the Mediterranean basin, the Middle East, Latin and South America and central Asia.

Low prevalence areas, with HBV rates between 0.1 and 2.0 percent, include Canada, western Europe, North America, Australia and New Zealand.

HBV Infection

Epidemiology

The hepatitis B virus is responsible for approximately 28–44 percent of all cases of acute hepatitis in the United States, making it the most com-

monly reported cause of acute viral hepatitis. Data from the second and
third National Health and Nutrition Examination survey suggest that there
were 81,000 new HBV infections [15]in 2000; because many cases of HBV
are not diagnosed or reported, the CDC estimates as many as 200,000–
300,000 new cases annually [40].

Statistics for infection in children are difficult to obtain, because 90
percent of infected children do not show symptoms of disease. In perinatal infection, infants born to mothers who are HBeAg positive have a 70–90
percent risk of developing HBV infection by the time they're six months
old. However, many of these children never have follow-up tests. Up to 90
percent of these infected infants go on to develop chronic HBV infection.

HBV is the most common cause of chronic hepatitis worldwide, but
it is becoming less common in the United States due to the routine immunization of infants and children. HBV is considered endemic in areas that
contain 46 percent of the world's population [40]. Worldwide, approximately 461 million people are HBV carriers, causing about 1.5 million deaths
annually due to viral hepatitis-induced liver disease. In the United States,
about 1.25 million people are HBV carriers.

The incidence of HBV infection differs by race and ethnicity with
higher rates reported among blacks and Asians compared to Caucasians.
Rates are also higher among Hispanics than non–Hispanics. The highest
rates of new infection are seen in persons 20–40 years old.

Disease Course in HBV

Most adults and children older than 12 years infected with HBV develop
an acute disease phase that resolves within several months. In the early stage,
patients may develop right upper abdominal pain, nausea, headache, cough,
stuffy nose, and light sensitivity. About 5 percent of patients may develop
an enlarged spleen and enlarged lymph nodes. Younger children may not
develop symptoms of disease but are likely to develop chronic infection.

About 15 percent of infected persons, primarily children, go on to
harbor the HBV virus and develop chronic infection. About 5 to 10 percent
of adults develop chronic infection, whereas about 90 percent of children
younger than 2 years develop chronic disease. In 20–30 percent of cases,
chronic HBV infection may lead to cirrhosis. Of those who develop cirrhosis, many will go on to develop hepatocellular carcinoma (HCC). Worldwide, hepatitis B is the most common cause of HCC.

Phases of infection

There are two main phases of hepatitis B infection: an infective
(replicative) and an integrated phase. During the replicative phase the

patient's serum is positive for the hepatitis Be antigen (HBeAg), a protein found in the core of the hepatitis B virion, and also HBV DNA. During this period, the patient is highly infectious and there is rapid progression of hepatic inflammation.

After a variable period ranging from several months to several years, HBeAg disappears from the blood and HBe antibody is detected. During this phase, which is called the integrative phase, the viral genome becomes integrated into the host cells. The infected liver cells show evidence of viral DNA, and they can secrete surface antigen (HBsAg) but not core antigen. Clones of these integrated cells are suspected of causing the malignant transformation that eventually leads to hepatocellular carcinoma in some individuals [56].

The presence of HBeAb indicates low or absent HBV replication and presumably low viral activity with active disease resolution. However, in some patients infectivity persists and can be demonstrated by the continued presence of HBV DNA or hepatitis B core antigen in liver cell nuclei. In this case, infection is usually related to a pre-core mutant.

INCUBATION PERIOD

The incubation period for HBV ranges from 30–180 days with an average incubation period of 75 days from the initial exposure. Patients are

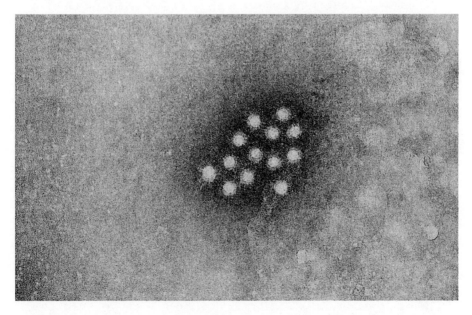

The Hepatitis B virus (Centers for Disease Control Public Health Imaging Library).

infectious during the incubation period although biochemical tests for HBV markers are usually negative.

Serologic evidence. The initial serologic response to HBV, which is demonstrated by the appearance of HbsAg, ranges from 2 to 26 weeks from the time of exposure. Hepatitis B DNA polymerase enzyme, hepatitis B DNA, and the hepatitis B surface antigen, HBsAg, may appear as early as six days after percutaneous exposure although HBsAg usually takes 6 weeks or longer to appear [38].

In most cases HBsAg appears about 2–8 weeks before biochemical evidence of liver damage or the onset of jaundice. Levels of HBV DNA can indicate how quickly viral replication is occurring, but this test is not routinely used. HBsAg persists until near the end of the acute clinical disease course. The hepatitis B e antigen, HBeAg, which is associated with infectivity, develops shortly after HBsAg although it only persists for several weeks. Following the incubation period, patients enter the prodromal phase of infection.

The immune response and serological markers. The immune system responds to infectious protein particles known as antigens by producing specific antibodies that are eventually able to neutralize the infectious agents. These antigens and antibodies can also be identified in the blood and used as markers of infection.

Viral marker terminology and viral markers in early infection. The term HB stands for hepatitis B, followed by s for surface, c for core, and e for the e unit of HB. These are followed by Ag for antigen and Ab for antibody. For example, the hepatitis B surface antibody is designated HBsAb. The addition of IgM represents the early immunoglobulin M antibodies seen in current infection, whereas IgG represents the immunoglobulin G antibodies, which generally persist for life. Most hepatitis antibody tests for viral markers indicate whether the test measures IgM, IgG, or total antibodies.

In acute HBV infection, HBV DNA and the enzyme HBV DNA polymerase appear within one week after infection. These are soon followed by the appearance of HBsAg. Shortly after the appearance of HBsAg, HBeAg also appears. The immune system responds to HBV infection initially by producing IgM antibodies to the HBV core antigen. These are known as HBcIgM or anti–HBc IgM and they appear around 8 weeks after HBV infection around the same time that levels of ALT and AST enzymes begin rising sharply.

Consequently, HBsAg, HBeAg, and HBcIgM and elevated AST and ALT levels are seen during acute infection. The hepatitis B core antigen (HBcAg) cannot be detected in the blood although it can be

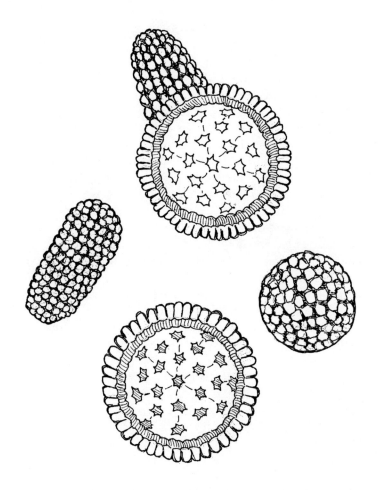

HEPATITIS B VIRUS AND SURFACE
ANTIGEN COMPONENTS

Hepatitis B virus and surface antigen components (Marvin G. Miller).

found in samples liver cells taken during biopsy of patients with acute infection.

THE WINDOW PERIOD

The period between the time HBsAg clears and HBsAb appears is known as the window period, a time when sero-conversion has not yet occurred. Thus, the blood is negative for both HBsAg and HBsAb, which can be misleading. Before HBV DNA tests became available for screening donor blood, the window period represented a time when HBV infections could easily be missed. In some cases, both HBsAg and HBsAb may co-exist, presumably when patients are infected with two strains of HBV. During the window period, antibodies to HBe and to HBcIgG are usually present but tests for these antibodies may not be ordered.

Because IgM antibodies occur early in infection and are followed by IgG antibody development, the blood test for HBc IgM is the only hepatitis antibody marker that can show current infection. Tests for viral DNA or DNA polymerase can also be used to determine active infection. The appearance of HBsAb antibodies directed against the HBV surface antigen usually indicates that infection has resolved and the patient has immunity or protection against re-infection. These antibodies also appear after a successful HBV vaccination.

Pre-core mutations. As DNA polymerase and HBeAg clear from the blood, antibodies to HBeAg, which are called HBeAb or anti–HBe, typically appear in the blood. Persistence of HBeAg for more than 3 months indicates chronic HBV infection [64].

Although the disappearance of HBeAg has been typically viewed as a sign of recovery and reduced infectivity, in about 10 percent of cases in the United States, HBV mutations in the pre-core region may prevent production of HBeAg. The presence of a mutant viral strain is associated with and may be involved in the development of fulminant hepatitis B and severe manifestations of chronic hepatitis B.

HBV Markers

Diagnostic Marker	Blood Test	Significance
HBV Surface Antigen	HBsAg	Current acute or chronic infection; HBV carrier
HBV e Antigen	HBeAg	Current infection with high infectivity; high titer HBV carrier
HBV DNA	NAT (nucleic acid amplification tests) for viral DNA	Current, active infection; test can be used as a quantitative measure of viremia.
HBV Surface Antibody	HBsAb or anti–HBs	Immunity to HBV from disease resolution or vaccine
HBV core antibody	HBcAb or anti–HBc	Past or present HBV infection
HBV IgM core antibody	HBc IgM Ab or anti–HBc IgM	Recent acute HBV infection
HBV e Antibody	HBeAb or anti–HBe	Reduced or diminished HBV replication, recovery phase; reduced infectivity in HBV carriers

Diagnostic Marker	Blood Test	Significance
HBV DNA polymerase	HBV DNA polymerase	Current infection; this test is rarely used since the development of NAT testing.

ACUTE PHASE OF HBV INFECTION

The acute phase of HBV infection is a self-limited period of infection lasting from several weeks to several months which may be 1) asymptomatic, causing few if any clinical symptoms although transaminase liver enzymes are typically elevated; 2) a mild to moderate disease characterized by liver tenderness, malaise and jaundice; or 3) in 0.5–1.0 percent of cases, a fulminant, potentially fatal, infection.

Patients who are asymptomatic may remain free of clinical symptoms but often develop weight loss and fatigue. The acute phase of HBV infection can be divided into a prodromal phase and a symptomatic or icteric phase followed by a recovery or convalescent phase.

Prodromal phase. The prodromal phase of acute hepatitis B infection is also known as the pre-icteric phase, before jaundice develops. Jaundice develops in about 30 percent of adults with HBV infection and it may last for a few days to several weeks. Early in infection, during the prodromal phase circulating Dane particles, HBsAg, HBeAg, HBV DNA, and DNA polymerase may be detected in the blood.

During the prodromal phase, about one week before jaundice develops, patients gradually develop a number of flu-like or serum sickness-like symptoms, including loss of appetite, malaise, aversion to greasy foods and cigarette smoke, fatigue, fever, and right upper quadrant pain. Fifteen percent of patients also experience fever, arthritis, arthralgias or a rash with hives. Serum sickness-like symptoms can also occur in chronic hepatitis B.

THE SYMPTOMATIC PHASE

In the symptomatic phase of acute HBV infection, most patients remain anicteric or free of jaundice. A smaller number, approximately 30 percent of patients, develop jaundice. Patients may have an enlarged, tender liver, low-grade fever and fatigue. In more severe cases, the urine darkens and stools become pale before jaundice of the eyes and skin becomes noticeable. Nausea, vomiting, aversion to food and skin itching may also occur during the symptomatic phase. Up to 15 percent of patients may have an enlarged spleen.

Skin changes. Rarely, patients develop palmar erythema, a condition of reddened palms, and spider nevi, which are broken blood vessels appearing on the face. Palmar erythema and spider nevi are more likely to appear in patients with chronic liver disease.

Patients with HBV, especially women, may also develop a flattened rash, hives, and itching during the early course of infection. After acute infection resolves, some patients may experience skin discoloration, particularly on the lower extremities. A condition of papular acrodermatitis, an inflammatory rash primarily affecting the extremities that is also known as Gianotti-Crosti syndrome, can also occur, usually in children with acute HBV infection.

Enzyme levels. The liver enzymes ALT and AST rise early in infection as they spill from damaged liver cells. At around the same time HBcIgM antibodies appear, the level of ALT starts to rise sharply. Levels may rise as high as 100 times the reference range, and ALT generally rises higher than AST. The ALT level is often used to indicate the severity of liver damage. However, severe damage can occur in the absence of marked ALT elevations. ALT levels begin to fall at about the same time HBeAg clears from the blood.

RECOVERY PHASE

During the symptomatic phase, the disease course is variable. Some patients experience a rapid recovery while others follow a prolonged course with a slow resolution of symptoms. Some patients may experience improvement and then relapse. In relapsing hepatitis, symptoms return and enzyme levels continue to rise. Relapsing hepatitis B can last for several weeks to several months.

About 95–99 percent of patients infected with HBV will eventually clear HBsAg from the blood and begin producing antibodies to the surface antibody of HBV, which is called HBsAb or anti–HBs. These antibodies are seen about two to four weeks after HBsAg clears. The persistence of HBsAg for six months after the onset of illness indicates chronic HBV infection.

Complications

A number of different complications can arise in hepatitis, including pancreatitis and a variety of inflammatory disorders. In addition immune complexes containing sandwiches of hepatitis B antigens and antibodies can cause complications.

PANCREATITIS

A rare complication associated with acute hepatitis B includes pancreatitis, an inflammation of the pancreas associated with elevated amylase levels. Elevated amylase levels are seen in up to 30 percent of people with acute infection and up to 51 percent of patients who develop fulminant infection.

INFLAMMATORY DISEASE

Other problems known to develop in association with acute hepatitis B include myocarditis (inflammation of the heart); pericarditis (inflammation of the heart lining); pleural effusion (abnormal appearance of fluid in the chest cavity); aplastic anemia (type of anemia resistant to treatment); transverse myelitis; atypical pneumonia; encephalitis (inflammation of the brain); and polyneuritis (inflammation of nerves).

IMMUNE COMPLEXES AND ACUTE SYMPTOMS

In about 10 percent of cases, immune complexes of HBV surface antigen and antibody may occur in the serum during the incubation period and acute phase of infection. Studies show the presence of these complexes in all patients who develop fulminant infection and in a small number of patients without fulminant infection.

These complexes are responsible for a serum sickness-like illness characterized by hives or a flattened rash and joint pain that typically affects the wrist, knees, elbows and ankles. The arthritis may affect different joints at different times and is often symmetrical, affecting both sides of the body. This arthritis may involve both large joints of the extremities and the small finger joints of the hands. These conditions are self-limiting and usually resolve before jaundice develops.

The presence of HBV immune complexes in chronic infection is also associated with the development of vasculitis (inflammation of blood vessels), the vascular disease polyarteritis nodosa, some forms of the kidney disease chronic glomerulonephritis, and the skin condition of infantile papular acrodermatitis.

FULMINANT INFECTION

Fulminant hepatitis B is a potentially reversible condition caused by a heightened immune response with massive liver cell destruction that can lead to acute liver failure. Fulminant hepatitis B is rare, occurring in only 0.5–1.0 percent of all cases of acute HBV infection in adults. However, hepatitis B is responsible for 51 percent of fulminant hepatitis cases.

Fulminant infection is defined by hepatic encephalopathy developing within 8 weeks of the onset of symptoms or within 2 weeks of the onset of jaundice. Patients with fulminant infection may develop cardiac abnormalities including arrhythmia, and pancreatitis is a common feature. Blood clotting abnormalities in fulminant infection may progress to diffuse intravascular coagulopathy (DIC), a general collapse of the body's blood coagulation system. Fulminant HBV infection is fatal in approximately 61 percent of all cases. However patients who survive fulminant HBV infection nearly always recover completely and rarely develop chronic or progressive liver disease.

Fulminant hepatitis B occurring within the first four weeks of infection is associated with a more rapid clearing of virus. Antibodies to surface antigen and e antigen increase, and levels of viral DNA decline. Hepatitis B surface antigen may be present at a low titer or it may be undetectable. In previously undiagnosed patients, the HBcIgM antibody is the only test that can reliably confirm acute infection in these patients.

Other infections and fulminant disease. Infection with another hepatitis virus, such as delta (hepatitis D) or HAV, can occur as a superinfection in hepatitis B carriers or in someone with mild HBV infection. This superinfection can cause a fulminant disease course.

SUBFULMINANT HEPATITIS

The term subfulminant or subacute hepatitis is used to describe conditions in which hepatic encephalopathy or hepatic coma occur with a slower onset, typically from 8 weeks to 6 months from the onset of symptoms.

Subacute hepatic necrosis is a condition of increasing severe disease symptoms evolving over a period of one to three months.

ACUTE LIVER FAILURE

In acute liver failure, the features of fulminant hepatitis occur along with coagulation defects, such as an elevated prothrombin time, that cause prolonged clotting. Hypoglycemia, a condition of low blood sugar, may also occur as the liver fails. Cerebral edema, an inflammation of the brain tissue, occurs in more than 75 percent of patients with fulminant hepatic failure.

The loss of liver cell function in acute liver failure initiates a multi-organ response in which death may occur even as liver function begins to improve. Acute liver failure is described more extensively in chapter 13.

RISK OF HEPATITIS D

Individuals with hepatitis B are at risk for developing hepatitis D. Hepatitis D can only occur in persons with HBV infection. Hepatitis D, which is described in chapter 8, can co-exist with HBV as a separate infection or it can occur as a superinfection, exacerbating symptoms in HBV.

MORTALITY RATE OF HBV

Mortality in acute hepatitis is usually due to the fulminant infection that affects up to one percent of patients with acute HBV infection. Mortality from fulminant HBV infection is about 61 percent. However, individuals who survive fulminant HBV infection seldom, if ever, develop progressive liver disease. Annually, about 1–2 million people worldwide and about 5,000 people in the United States die from HBV-related conditions. Of the 5,000 persons who die from HBV, 300 die from fulminant hepatitis; 3000–4100 from cirrhosis; and 610–1000 from primary hepatocellular carcinoma. In those with chronic HBV infection, mortality is estimated to be about 25 percent.

Chronic HBV Infection

Worldwide, HBV is the most common cause of chronic hepatitis. Chronic HBV infection is defined by the persistence of HBsAg, HBcAb and HBV DNA in the blood circulation for longer than 6 months. Chronic HBV infection occurs in approximately 5–10 percent of adults with HBV infection and in as many as 90 percent of infants and 30 percent of young children infected with HBV. In adults, the more severe and acute the original attack, the less likely it is that chronic HBV infection will develop. Chronic infection rarely develops in patients who survive fulminant infection.

Risk factors

Chronic HBV is found predominantly in males, and the very old and very young are at particular risk. Chronic HBV is most likely to develop in persons with immature or incompetent immune systems, such as neonates, homosexuals, patients with AIDS, leukemia, lepromatous leprosy, Down's syndrome, cancer or renal failure and in patients receiving medications that suppress their immune system. Other risk factors include having an ethnic origin from an area of high HBV prevalence or a high carrier rate, sexual relations with sexual contacts of infected individuals, occupations with exposure to human blood, and a history of organ transplant receipt, drug abuse and multiple transfusions of blood or blood products.

Disease course in chronic HBV

Chronic HBV infection may take one of two pathways:

1. chronic progressive disease with persistent mild to severe symptoms
2. the asymptomatic (absence of HBetg and symptoms) carrier state.

Chronic HBV and chronic HCV are major causes of hepatocellular carcinoma (HCC). The International Agency for Research on Cancer has classified both chronic HBV and HCV as carcinogenic to humans [40].

Chronic HBV disease

In the more severe form of chronic HBV, viral replication continues, causing a high plasma viral load and ongoing damage to liver cells, manifested by increased ALT and AST levels, usually in the range of 100–300 U/L. Changes to the liver tissue can range from very mild to severe and these changes can be categorized or staged with liver biopsy specimens.

In very mild cases, inflammation is limited to the portal tracts. In more progressive disease, a bridging necrosis with extensive liver cell destruction is seen. Depending on the cellular changes seen on biopsy, chronic hepatitis is staged or graded to indicate disease severity. These variations are described briefly here and more extensively in chapter fifteen.

In stage I, which used to be called chronic persistent hepatitis (CPH), inflammation is limited to the portal tracts and the liver tissue plate remains unaffected. In stage I, the virus may remain latent or undergo replication. Survival at five years is 97 percent compared to an 86 percent survival rate in patients with stage III.

Stage II is characterized by scarring that typically extends outside the portal tracts. The portal tracts contain the liver's blood vessels and are the first areas affected by inflammation.

Stage III, which used to be called chronic active hepatitis (CAH) is defined by piecemeal necrosis, that is, liver cell destruction and fibrosis that occurs throughout the liver. In the giant cell hepatitis variant of CAH giant cells with as many as 51 nuclei are seen. In giant cell hepatitis, the bile ducts may be involved and progression to cirrhosis can be rapid.

In stage IV fibrosis has progressed into cirrhosis and advanced scarring of the liver tissue. In this stage, which is technically called cirrhosis, many of the complications associated with advanced liver disease begin to develop.

SIGNS AND SYMPTOMS OF CHRONIC HEPATITIS

The course of chronic infection is highly variable. Some patients experience a waxing and waning of symptoms, where symptoms come and go, whereas others have continuous symptoms of hepatitis that vary in severity over time. Signs and symptoms in chronic hepatitis can range from a mild elevation of liver enzymes to progressive liver damage resulting in cirrhosis, liver failure and death.

The liver cancer hepatocellular carcinoma (HCC) is also a frequent legacy of HBV infection. Hepatitis B is second only to tobacco among the known human carcinogens [70]. In endemic areas, the risk of developing HCC among individuals with chronic HBV infection is 15 to 100 times that of non-infected persons [40].

Up to 30 percent of patients with chronic HBV infection may develop cirrhosis. Cirrhosis occurs when liver cells are destroyed and fibrous tissue replaces normal liver tissue. These fibrous deposits cause irreversible, progressive liver damage. Cirrhosis and advanced liver disease are described in chapter 13.

VIRAL LOAD

Viral load is a measure of the copies of viral DNA present in the blood. In chronic infection, the viral load test is used to determine if the virus is actively replicating. This determines infectivity as well as the need for treatment. Treatment for chronic HBV infection is usually reserved for patients with viral loads greater than 100,000 copies/ml.

HEPATITIS B CARRIERS

The HBV carrier state, a state in which HBsAg remains in the blood for more than six months after the onset of illness, is sometimes referred to as minimal hepatitis. In the chronic carrier state, viral DNA becomes integrated into the liver cell DNA. The viral load in the carrier's blood remains either very low in replicating carriers or in the case of nonreplicating carriers, the viral load is undetectable.

Chronic HBV carriers with normal ALT and AST levels usually do not have significant disease. They usually have a spontaneous remission rate of approximately 2–3 percent annually [62].

The HBeAg test was once used to determine viral replication. However, due to the prevalence of escape mutants (up to 15 percent of HBV infections in North America) that interfere with HBeAg production, a negative result cannot be interpreted to mean that replication is not occurring. In Asia, Africa and southern Europe these escape mutants are seen in up to half of all HBV infections.

In carriers, a positive serum HBV DNA test, the presence of IgM antibodies to the core antigen (HBcIgM Ab) and the hepatitis Be antigen (HBeAg) are indications of infectivity and ongoing disease.

Immune response in carriers. Individuals with HBV infection who fail to develop a complete immune response to the virus become carriers. Carriers who remain positive for HBeAg usually have circulating Dane particles and detectable DNA polymersase activity, making them highly infectious. These individuals are also more likely to develop significant liver disease, which resolves when HBeAg resolves and antibodies to the HBe antigen are produced through seroconversion. However, mutant strains incapable of producing HBeAg can develop during the course of infection. A viral load test is a better indicator of infectivity in carriers.

Chronic HBsAg carriers usually have very high titers of core antibodies, HBcAb (IgG), and they usually do not have surface antibodies (HBsAb). Some carriers may have both HBsAg and HBsAb with the surface antibodies directed against a different subtype of HBV. Most carriers are asymptomatic (without clinical symptoms) and show no evidence of significant liver disease; a minority has elevated serum aminotransferase enzyme levels. With liver biopsies these carriers may show varying degrees of liver cell inflammation and fibrosis. Over time, these lesions may progress to cirrhosis and liver failure.

Prevalence rates of carriers. The rates of HBV carriers in a population vary considerably worldwide. In the United States and England, the carrier rate is 0.1–0.2 percent; higher than 3 percent in Greece and Southern Italy; higher than 10–15 percent in Africa, the Amazon Basin and the Far East; and up to 46 percent in Alaskan Eskimos; and 85 percent in Australian Aborigines [56].

HBV in Children and in Pregnancy

HBV can be transmitted during childbirth. In the United States, tests for HBV are included in prenatal profiles, and children born to HBV positive mothers receive prophylactic treatment within hours of birth.

HBV in infants

Infants infected with HBV rarely show signs of infection. However, 70–90 percent of infants born to HBeAg positive mothers develop hepatitis. Of these, 90 percent develop chronic HBV. For infants born to mothers who are HBeAg negative, 10–41 percent develop HBV. Of these, 41–70 percent will become chronic carriers. Chronic infection with HBV acquired early in life is the major risk factor for the liver cancer hepatocellular carcinoma (CCC) in humans [36].

In the United States, up to 32,000 infants are born each year to mothers who are HBsAg positive. Post-exposure prophylactic vaccines are highly effective although up to 1,000 infants develop hepatitis annually due to failure to identify all HBsAg positive mothers and the failure to continue with the prophylactic vaccination protocol recommended for infants. Infants born to HBsAg positive mothers should receive their first HBV vaccination, receiving both active and passive vaccine, within the first 12 hours after birth.

HBV in pregnancy

The CDC recommends hepatitis B screening for all pregnant women. Women who test positive can receive appropriate treatment if indicated or be advised of their carrier status. If a pregnant woman is diagnosed with hepatitis B during her prenatal visits, she will receive HBIG, which provides passive vaccination and she will be advised to abstain from alcohol. Because alkaline phosphatase enzyme levels normally rise during pregnancy, the ALT enzyme test should be used to assess liver damage. Medications such as interferon should be discontinued during pregnancy since the effect on the fetus is unknown.

The children born to women who are positive for HBsAg can then be identified and promptly started on a series of vaccinations. In the United States, 15,000 women are positive for HBsAg. Normally, pregnancy does not affect the course of hepatitis although acute fatty liver of pregnancy can lead to severe liver disease. Hepatitis may contribute to a worsening of this condition.

Special Circumstances

Patients with HBV infection are at risk for other types of viral hepatitis and also HIV, the virus responsible for AIDS. In patients who abuse alcohol, a synergistic effect is seen, with the likelihood of severe liver disease.

HBV in AIDS (HIV infection)

In patients with co-existing HBV and HIV infections, the risk of developing chronic HBV infection is increased. Liver cell damage, which in HBV is primarily related to the immune system effects, is typically mild compared to chronic infection in persons who are HIV negative. In most cases, treatment benefits both conditions.

HBV with HAV

HAV infection can be severe and very dangerous in those who already have liver disease from chronic HBV infection.

HBV with HCV

Many risk factors for HBV infection are identical to those of HCV infection, particularly injection drug use, sexual activity and the use of multiple blood products.

HBV and alcohol abuse

Alcohol has been shown to accelerate the progression of liver disease in patients with HBV infection.

Diagnosis of HBV

Hepatitis is suspected in patients with elevated transaminase liver enzyme levels or jaundice. The various types of hepatitis, however, all cause similar symptoms. Blood tests for the viral markers of HBV are necessary to diagnose HBV infection.

Laboratory tests

Liver function tests are used to diagnose hepatitis and viral marker tests are used to diagnose HBV infection as its cause. Imaging and biopsy tests are used to eliminate obstructive causes and to help determine the degree of disease severity in chronic hepatitis. The diagnostic tests used for HBV are briefly described in this section and more extensively in chapters fourteen and fifteen.

Liver function tests

Liver enzymes are the key tests used to assess liver function. Acute hepatitis is associated with elevated levels of the enzymes alanine aminotransferase (ALT) and aspartate aminotransferaase (AST). These enzymes are usually elevated to levels of 1000–2000 IU/ml although values may be as high as 100 times the upper limit of the reference range. In acute HBV, the ALT level is usually higher than the AST level. Levels of the enzyme alkaline phosphatase may be elevated, but they are not usually elevated more than 3 times the upper limit of the reference range.

In chronic inactive HBV infection, patients may have normal enzyme levels although HBsAg persists in the serum. In chronic active infection patients continue to have mild to moderate ALT and AST levels and high levels of HBV DNA. If the AST levels rise higher than the ALT levels, cirrhosis should be suspected. In most cases, increases are less than four times the upper end of the reference range and often less than twice the upper end of the reference range [28].

Elevated gamma globulin levels may also be present in chronic active hepatitis, and patients may have slightly elevated titers of rheumatoid factor. Levels of albumin are often slightly decreased in acute hepatitis B, and serum iron levels may be elevated. In the prodromal period, the white blood cell (WBC) may be decreased and the erythrocyte sedimentation rate, a marker of inflammation, may be elevated. In severe acute hepatitis, the prothrombin time may be prolonged. Alpha-fetoprotein markers may also rise in acute HBV infection reaching levels as high as 8,000 ng/ml.

The prothrombin time test, which measures clotting time, is the best prognostic indicator in acute HBV infection. An elevated prothrombin time is indicative of a more severe progressive disease.

Viral markers

In acute HBV infection, HBV DNA, HBsAg, and HBeAg are the first markers to appear. The core antibody, HBc IgM, follows. Patients who recover show HBsAb and HBeAb. The persistence of HBsAg for longer than 6 months or HBeAg longer than 3 months following recovery is associated with chronic infection.

Tests for HBV DNA, which is the earliest indicator of infection, are primarily used to screen blood donors. They are also used to determine if patients are candidates for anti-viral therapy or if they are responding to treatment.

Stage of HBV Infection	*Positive laboratory tests and markers*
Acute infection, prodromal phase	+ HBV DNA, +HBV DNA polymerase, +HBsAg
Acute infection, symptomatic phase	+ HBV DNA, +HBV DNA polymerase, +HBsAg, +HBeAg, ↑ ALT, ↑ AST, +HBc IgM, -HBeAb, ± HBsAb
Convalescent or recovery phase; past infection	-HBsAg, -HBeAg, -HBcIgM, + HBsAb, +HBeAb, +HBcAb, +HBcIgG,
Chronic active infection	+HBsAg, +HBeAg, +HBV DNA, + HBsAb, ↑ ALT, ↑ AST
Chronic infection (carriers)	+HBsAg, -HBeAg, + HBsAb, +HBcAb, -HBcIgM, — HBV DNA, Normal ALT, AST
Vaccinated persons	+HBsAb, -HBcAb, -HBsAg

Imaging tests

Increased echogenicity of liver tissue may be seen in imaging tests during acute and chronic active hepatitis. In chronic hepatitis that has advanced to cirrhosis, coarse echogenicity of the liver may be accompanied by a nodular appearance. The primary benefit of imaging tests is to exclude other causes of jaundice such as obstruction.

Biopsy

Liver biopsy is not usually indicated for acute HBV infection because tests for viral markers are sufficient for diagnosis. In chronic HBV infection, infected liver cells typically have a ground-glass appearance, and stains can be used to identify the presence of HBsAg or HBcAg. In chronic disease, liver damage can be accessed and the severity of disease can be graded and classified into stages. These changes are described in chapter fifteen.

Complications of Chronic HBV

Complications of chronic HBV infection include vascular disorders, skin disorders, arthritic disorders such as polymyalgia rheumatica and Guillain-Barré syndrome, kidney diseases such as glomerulonephritis, cryoglobulinemia, cirrhosis and hepatocellular carcinoma. The vascular and rheumatic disorders seen in hepatitis are related to the development of immune complexes of HBsAg and HBsAb. These disorders are described in the following sections. Cirrhosis and hepatocellular carcinoma are described in chapters 13 and fifteen.

Vascular complications

Vascular complications of chronic HBV infection include vasculitis, an inflammatory disorder affecting blood vessels, and polyarteritis nodosa, which affects the blood vessels in multiple organs. All patients with vascular conditions related to HBV are reported to have circulating immune complexes. However, for reasons that are unclear, vascular disorders only develop in a small number of patients with immune complexes [70]. Besides being present in the blood circulation, deposits of these immune complexes have been found in hepatocytes.

Polyarteritis nodosa (PAN)

Polyarteritis nodosa (PAN) is a vascular disorder affecting small and medium-sized arteries and arterioles, which can cause a variety of different symptoms, including abdominal pain, renal insufficiency, heart disease, hypertension and arthritis. As many as 36–69 percent of people with PAN are positive for HBsAg, and circulating immune complexes are frequently seen. PAN develops early in the course of hepatitis and has a high prevalence in certain populations such as Alaskan Eskimos.

Symptoms of PAN in patients with chronic HBV include hypertension, abdominal pain, arthritis, peripheral neuropathy, and renal insufficiency, and their severity correlates with the severity of the liver disease and level of HBsAg [56]. Despite treatment, patients with PAN and chronic HBV have a 5-year mortality rate of 20–46 percent.

Cryoglobulinemia

Cryoglobulins are a class of immunoglobulin proteins which precipitate at temperatures below 31° C. Increased levels of mixed cryoglobulins cause a condition of mixed cryoglobulinemia, which causes vasculitis and nephritis (kidney inflammation). While mixed cryoglobulinemia is more commonly seen in chronic HCV infection, it can also occur in chronic HBV.

Glomerulonephritis (GMN)

Glomerulonephritis is an inflammatory disorder affecting the renal capillaries, the tiny blood vessels that provide circulation to the kidneys. This inflammation thickens the basement layer of the kidney's primary functional units, which are known as glomeruli. Glomeruli are capillary bundles that filter waste materials from the blood and pass it into urine, which is excreted. Ultimately, GMN causes a loss of protein and, in later stages, kidney failure.

Glomerulonephrtis primarily occurs in children with chronic HBV infection. However, infected adults that develop glomerulonephritis usually have a more severe form of the disease, which can lead to renal failure in about one third of all cases. Patients with chronic HBV and glomerulonephritis are usually positive for HBeAg, and immune complexes of the various HBV markers are often found in the kidney's glomerular and basement membranes.

In children, interferon treatment is often successful although the response to corticosteroids is reported to be poor. In children, glomerulonephritis often resolves spontaneously within 6 months to 2 years [56]. Adults do not respond well to interferon and the disease course is usually slowly progressive.

Skin disorders

Hepatitis B infection is associated with a number of skin disorders and lesions that are more often seen in women. The various rashes in hepatitis can cause periodic welts, itching and discolorations on the face and lower extremities. A condition of papular acrodermatitis, which is also called Gianotti-Crosti syndrome, that causes lesions on the extremities, is associated with acute HBV infection in children.

Prevention of HBV

Prevention measures for reducing the risk of HBV infection include vaccination, universal precautions for healthcare workers exposed to blood products, avoidance of injecting drug use, and safe sexual practices.

Vaccinations

Hepatitis B is one of the major infectious diseases that can be prevented with vaccination. Vaccines are recommended for all boys and girls up to age 18 years, a person whose sex partner has chronic hepatitis B, people with multiple sex partners, injection drug users, healthcare and emergency response personnel whose work involves occupational exposures, institutionalized patients, and people recently diagnosed with a sexually transmitted disease.

Two different recombinant hepatitis B vaccines are available in the United States. Passive immunization in the form of hepatitis B immunoglobulin (HBIG) is also available for patients exposed to HBV or at immediate risk of exposure.

ACTIVE IMMUNIZATION

Active immunizations involve the injection of treated non-infective hepatitis B antigens. These cause the immune system to respond as if the patient was exposed to HBV and the vaccinated person produces antibodies (HBsAb) to the hepatitis's B surface antigen. The first-generation HBV vaccines were prepared from treated non-infective HBsAg particles obtained from chronic HBV carriers. These were not popular among healthcare workers because of their suspected risk of transmitting other microorganisms.

RECOMBINANT VACCINES

These vaccines have been replaced with recombinant or genetically engineered vaccines. Recombinant vaccines are prepared from HBsAg produced in yeast cells. The hepatitis B vaccine is given in a series of 3 subcutaneous (directly under the skin) injections over a period of six months. This vaccine should be given in the deltoid muscle of the upper arm or the anterolateral (front side) of the thigh and not in the buttock. Vaccinations given in the buttock are associated with unexpectedly low antibody responses.

A series of 3 injections given in doses of 10 mcg causes HBsAb levels greater than 10 million IU/ml in approximately 95 percent of vaccinated persons. In individuals who do not show evidence of HBsAb three months after the series of vaccinations is complete, an additional vaccine dose should be given. Studies show that hepatitis B vaccines can protect against infection for at least 15 years. Individuals who showed a good initial vaccine response were most likely to remain protected after 15 years. Children who received vaccinations before 4 years of age showed the greatest declines in HBsAb titers.

In infants of mothers with HBeAg, recombinant vaccines administered immediately after birth are effective in 70 percent of cases. When HBIG is administered simultaneously, the vaccine is effective in 90 percent of cases.

Non-responders and low responders. About 10–15 percent of all persons do not produce hepatitis B surface antibodies following immunization.

Their peak levels of HBsAb are less than 1.0 IU/ml indicating that they do not have immunity. Low responders have peak antibody levels between 1–10 IU/ml and they have levels less than 1.0 IU/ml after 5–7 years. Good responders have peak antibody levels greater than 10.0 IU/ml.

Failure to respond to vaccines may be caused by injections given in the buttock rather than the deltoid region and vaccines that are stored frozen. Poor responses may also occur in the elderly and immunocompromised individuals, including persons infected with HIV. Poor responses are also seen in people with immune system markers that include the histocompatibility haplotypes HLA-B8, SC01, and DR3 [56]. In poor responders, a booster vaccine may be given or a dose of 20 mcg may be used [56].

PASSIVE IMMUNIZATION

Passive immunization is for persons who have not been vaccinated and who know they have been exposed to HBV.

Hepatitis B immunoglobulin (HBIG). HBIG is a special immune serum globulin protein containing a high titer of hepatitis B surface antibodies. HBIG is a passive form of vaccination and offers protection for several months, until the antibodies break down.

HBIG is usually given to persons exposed to HBV through occupational exposures, sexual assault victims of persons known to be infected with HBV, and to infants born to HBsAg positive mothers. In unvaccinated individuals exposed to hepatitis B, HBIG should ideally be administered within 24 hours of exposure and no later than 7 days following exposure. A repeat dose should be given 28–30 days later. HBIG has been found to prevent HBV infection in many, but not all, cases of exposure.

Universal precautions

Universal precautions, which were implemented to reduce the risk of blood-borne infections, involve handling all blood specimens as if they were potentially infectious. This includes wearing rubber gloves and protective clothing when working with blood or blood specimens, using needles with safety devices for medical procedures, disposing of contaminated medical waste properly, and cleaning up blood spills in a way that prevents accidental blood exposures.

SAFE SEX

Using latex condoms correctly can lower the risk of getting hepatitis B from persons infected with HBV. Persons with multiple sex partners or sexually transmitted diseases and men who have sex with men are at increased risk for hepatitis B.

GENERAL PRECAUTIONS

Don't share any items, including toothbrushes, razors, nail clippers or wash cloths, that could have an infected person's blood on them. Never share drugs, needles, syringes, or drug equipment. Only acquire tattoos or body piercings from certified artists.

Treatment of HBV

Until recently, no specific treatment has been available for individuals with acute HBV infection. However, the effectiveness of anti-retroviral agents in AIDS has influenced treatment protocols. The nucleoside analogues lamivudine (Epivir) or adefovir dipivoxil (Hepsera) are commonly used today along with interferon alpha (IFN-α) to help modulate the immune response. Other nucleoside analogues are being tested for HBV, with telbuvidine, a nucleoside analogue with specific anti–HBV activity, appearing to show great promise. The use of these compounds is further described in chapter 16.

For chronic HBV infection, interferon-alpha has been the mainstay of treatment since the mid-1980s. However, only 30–41 percent of patients respond to this treatment, and about 5–10 percent of these patients relapse after completion of treatment. In recent years the anti-retroviral nucleoside analogues lamivudine and adefovir have been added to the treatment protocol. In some protocols, Septra, a combination product containing trimethoprim and sulfamethoxazole, is used to increase the bioavailability of lamivudine.

The lifestyle recommendations and alternative medical treatments used in hepatitis B are described in chapter 17.

Economic impact

Each year, about 5,000 people in the United States die from complications associated with hepatitis B. Annual health care costs and lost wages associated with hepatitis B are estimated to be $700 million [64].

7

Hepatitis C

Discovered in 1988, the hepatitis C virus (HCV) is thought to have emerged in the United States after World War II. Since its discovery and the development of blood tests for its detection, researchers have learned a great deal about HCV, including its ability to mutate and remain undetected. However, many things about HCV, including its persistence, remain uncertain.

HCV is an insidious virus, in most cases causing no symptoms of acute disease. Its victims often have no idea they're infected until years later when the damage caused by chronic HCV infection is discovered. In about 20 percent of those who develop chronic disease, infection can progress to advanced liver disease, cirrhosis and liver cancer. Epidemiological studies show that the hepatitis C virus is responsible for the majority of chronic hepatitis in most of North America, Europe and Japan [28], However, with the development of blood tests for HCV and an awareness of its modes of transmission, the incidence of new HCV infections has declined significantly since 1990.

In this chapter readers will learn about the hepatitis C virus (HCV), its discovery, its replication, its genome and subtypes, its history, and its geographic distribution. Readers will also learn about the disease caused by HCV, including the incubation period, epidemiology, disease course, symptoms, diagnosis, treatment, risk factors, and disease progression.

The Hepatitis C Virus (HCV)

The hepatitis C virus (HCV), which accounts for most instances of what was once called non-A, non-B hepatitis (NANB), was first isolated in

1988, and the first rudimentary blood tests for detecting HCV antibodies became available in 1990. HCV is a spherical, enveloped, single-stranded RNA virus 30–61 nm in diameter belonging to the family *Flaviviridae*.

HCV's inclusion into the *Flaviviridae* family is based on several similarities in its genome organization, structure and replication to other flaviviruses, including the yellow fever and the dengue fever viruses. Like other flaviviruses, HCV is enveloped with two large glycoproteins incorporated into its viral envelope, similar to the E and NS1 proteins of flaviviruses, and it is defined by a single, large gene that encodes a polyprotein which is cleaved into functional proteins after synthesis. However, unlike the yellow fever virus and other flaviviruses, HCV is not transmitted by arthropod vectors. HCV is also unique in its propensity to cause a persistent chronic infection. In its peak, HCV has been shown to produce at least 10 trillion new viral particles daily.

HCV is also unusual in that it was discovered using molecular techniques to identify its genome instead of the usual approach of first isolating the virus and studying it directly. The genome of HCV resembles both pestiviruses and flaviviruses and has a high mutation rate. First seen microscopically in 1995, HCV primarily targets liver cells and on occasion it infects white blood cells known as monocytes.

The HCV genome

In the early 1980s it became apparent that injections of serum taken from patients with non-A, non-B (NANB) hepatitis could cause hepatitis in chimpanzees. The plasma from chimpanzees and infected patients were combined and the viral RNA extracted. This RNA was treated with enzymes to produce a DNA copy of the virus. By cloning this viral DNA into yeast, the genome of the HCV virus was finally identified in 1988 by a team of researchers from the National Institutes of Health and the Chiron Corporation.

The single-stranded RNA genome of the hepatitis C virus contains one large open reading frame. The structural proteins of HCV include the nucleocapsid protein, which remains within the cytoplasm; two envelope glycoproteins, E1 and E2; and a small membrane-associated protein, p7 or NS2A.

The HCV enzyme RNA polymerase, critical for replication, lacks proofreading capabilities. Thus, there are no systems in place to delete imperfect copies. Consequently, during replication, a number of mutant viruses known as quasispecies are formed. Several different quasispecies can occur in one individual. These different species can differ in their response to treatment and their ability to be recognized in analytical tests.

HCV types and subtypes

The hepatitis C virus consists of a family containing six major types with more than 51 subtypes characterized by alterations to the basic genome with variances in their nucleotide sequence as high as 30 percent. Worldwide, researchers have identified eleven types of HCV, but types 7–11 are commonly listed as subtypes of the first 6 types discovered. The ends of the genome that contain elements involved in virus replication and protein translation, and the initial coding region (the core gene) are identical in all of the subtypes.

The variations among the types and subtypes of HCV primarily occur in a specific portion of the viral envelope and in the polymerase coding region. The E1 and E2 genes coding for the envelope glycoproteins are highly variable, typically differing at more than 51 percent of sites between genotypes. Patients have been reported to be infected with more than one HCV subtype, and patients may have quasispecies consisting of multiple mutations. This typical variation makes it difficult to develop vaccines against HCV and may contribute to poor treatment responses.

CHARACTERISTICS OF HCV GENOTYPES AND SUBTYPES

The original species of HCV is genotype 1a and it accounts for 41–80 percent of all HCV isolates. From this initial strain, mutations have resulted primarily in the envelope (E2) and polymerase coding region (NS5) portions in the genome, resulting in a variety of different genotypes. Some HCV species, such as subtypes 1a and 1b, may be associated with higher viral loads and more aggressive disease although this view is not shared by all researchers. Disease progression may be a result of the likelihood of treatment failure with interferon seen in subtype 1 rather than a more progressive disease course. And because the original genotype of HCV is type 1, it could be that persons infected with subtype 1 have had longer periods of infection.

GEOGRAPHIC VARIATION OF HCV GENOTYPES

The HCV genotypes have an associated geographic variation. For instance, in the United States, the 1b genotype is a predominant type, and it often aggressively progresses to cirrhosis although it rarely causes hepatocellular carcinoma. However, in Japan where the 1b strain is also predominant, HCC is common. These findings suggest that environmental factors, such as diet and stress, affect the disease course.

Genotype 1 is the most common HCV genotype in the world, and genotypes 1, 2, and 3 are seen worldwide. Genotypes 2 and 3 respond well to 24 weeks of interferon treatment. With other genotypes, treatment is extended for 49 weeks and treatment response is poor. In genotypes other than 2 or 3 the viral load is checked every 12 weeks during treatment. If the viral load has fallen by less than two logs (see description of logs in viral load section in chapter 14), treatment success is unlikely and usually stopped.

The presence of numerous subtypes in some regions of the world such as Africa and Southeast Asia suggests that HCV may have been endemic in these areas for a long time. The limited diversity of subtypes seen in the United States and Europe could conversely suggest a recent introduction of these subtypes from endemic areas. The genotype of a particular strain is also helpful in that it helps in establishing a common source of infection in epidemics.

Table 7a. Geographic distribution of genotypes and subtypes

HCV Genotype/subtype	Geographic distribution	Characteristics
1a, 1b	Worldwide, most common genotypes in the United States and Europe; in Europe 1a and 1b are widely distributed, particularly in older age groups; 1b seen in 73% of cases in Japan	Genotype 1 is most resistant to treatment; 49 weeks of interferon are recommended compared to 24 weeks for other strains; 1a is associated with intravenous drug use, and 1b is seen more often in people who acquired HCV from transfusions of blood products.
2a, 2b	Relatively common in North America, Europe and Japan	
2c	Mostly found in northern Italy	
3a, 3b	3a is prevalent in intravenous drug abusers in Europe and the United States	3a and 3b reported to show a good treatment response to interferon
4	Prevalent in North Africa and the Middle East; most prevalent genotype in Egypt	
5	Mostly confined to South Africa	
6	Mostly confined to Southeast Asia, particularly in Hong Kong, Macao and Vietnam	

Table 7a (cont.)

HCV Genotype/ subtype	Geographic distribution	Characteristics
*7, 8, and 9	Only seen in Vietnamese patients	
*10	Only seen in patients from Indonesia	
*11	Only seen in patients from Indonesia	

* Investigators have proposed that genotypes 7, 8, 9, 10, and 11 be regarded as variants of genotype 6 [68].

QUASISPECIES

HCV circulates in the blood as a complex group of closely related but distinct molecules. This is thought to be related to the diversity in RNA polymerase enzymes used for replication. The consequences of this quasi-species swarm, as it is commonly called, include: the development of escape mutants; a generation of defective interfering viral particles; varieties in cell tropism or affinity for specific host cells; vaccine failure; and rapid development of drug resistance [41].

HCV surveillance

Hepatitis C is a reportable disease in all states. Between 1989 and 1998, the incidence of new HCV infections in the United States fell by more than 80 percent, from 230,000 to 36,000 new cases annually. However, according to the Third National Health and Nutrition Examination Survey (NHANES III) an estimated 3.9 million Americans (1.8 percent of the population) have been infected with HCV, most with chronic infection.

Population based studies show that 41 percent of chronic liver disease is caused by HCV infection. HCV is reported to cause from 8,000 to 10,000 deaths annually, and it is the most common cause of liver transplantation [19].

HCV viability

Studies show that HCV may survive on environmental surfaces at room temperature for at least 16 hours, but for no longer than 4 days. HCV is destroyed by solutions containing 10 percent sodium hypochlorite (household bleach). A process of heat inactivation can be used to destroy HCV in blood products.

HCV replication

HCV preferentially replicates in liver cells known as hepatocytes, and recent studies suggest that it can also replicate in monocytes, a type of white blood cell. HCV is not cytotoxic to liver cells, which means that HCV does not directly destroy the liver cells that it infects. Damage is primarily due to effects of the immune response. The benign effect of HCV itself on liver cells allows infection to persist. During acute infection HCV viral levels range from 105 to 107 genomes/ml of plasma. In chronic infection, HCV RNA levels vary in different individuals and generally fall in the range of 51,000 to 5 million. In chronic infection, without treatment intervention, levels stay remarkably stable.

SUSTAINED VIROLOGIC RESPONSE (SVR)

The goal of treatment in HCV is sustained virologic response (SVR), a condition characterized by negative blood tests for HCV RNA for 6 months after the end of treatment. However, recent studies indicate that in most patients HCV RNA can still be detected in various tissues, including liver tissue and white blood cells, several years after SVR is achieved.

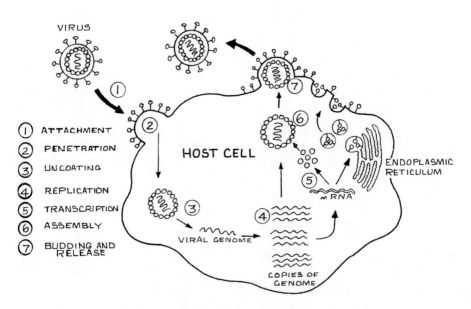

REPRODUCTIVE CYCLE OF A VIRUS

Viral Replication (Marvin G. Miller).

Discovery of HCV

In 1988, investigators headed by Daniel Bradley from the CDC and Michael Houghton from Chiron identified the hepatitis C virus through molecular genetic techniques. This was accomplished by extracting RNA from blood samples contaminated with the virus and cloning viral DNA into yeast cultures.

Origin of HCV

The oldest stored blood samples available for testing in the United States date from 1948, and a small number of these samples have tested positive for HCV antibodies. Without earlier samples, it is difficult to date when HCV first came into existence. Most experts suspect that the different subtypes of HCV originated about 200 years ago and that the six main genotypes of HCV originated in one common ancestor about 410 years ago. Most researchers think HCV was introduced in the U.S. following World War II.

Prevalence and incidence

Worldwide, 170 million people are infected with HCV, and more than one million new cases of HCV infection are reported each year. According to epidemiologists, HCV is suspected of being more prevalent than HBV [68].

In the United States, an estimated 1.8 percent of the population have antibodies to HCV, indicating past or current infection and approximately 4 million people are infected. Annually, in the United States, HCV is responsible for 8,000–10,000 deaths, 35,000 acute infections and approximately 230,000 newly reported infections. HCV is also the leading cause of liver transplants in the United States.

In industrialized countries, HCV accounts for 20–30 percent of acute hepatitis infections, 70 percent of chronic hepatitis, 41 percent of end-stage liver disease, 61 percent of hepatocellular carcinoma, and 30–41 percent of liver transplants.

Past or current infection with HCV is diagnosed by the presence of HCV antibodies. Patients with thallasemia and hemophilia are at highest risk of HCV infection because of multiple transfusions received before 1992. Thallasemics have a 10–51 percent prevalence of HCV antibodies. Hemophiliacs in the United States have a 51 percent prevalence of HCV antibodies. In the United Kingdom, the prevalence of HCV antibodies in hemophiliacs is 90 percent [56].

Transmission of HCV

HCV is primarily transmitted through blood and blood-contaminated body fluids. The most common causes of blood transmission are injection drug use, transfusion of blood and blood products, solid organ transplantation from infected donors, contaminated medical equipment including acupuncture needles, contaminated tattoo needles and dyes, razors, manicure and pedicure tools, and occupational exposure. Transmission can also rarely occur through vertical (childbirth) transmission and sexual transmission. High rates, from 15 to 51 percent prevalence, have also been seen in specific populations, including the homeless, incarcerated persons, and hemophiliacs.

In new HCV infections acquired after 1990, 61–70 percent are caused by injection drug use, less than 20 percent are acquired through sexual exposure, and 10 percent are due to other causes, including perinatal exposure, occupational exposure and hemodialysis.

Transmission via blood transfusions and blood products

Blood tests for HCV first became available in 1990 although it wasn't until 1992 that the more sensitive, second generation HCV antibody screening test still used today was developed. Since 1992 the risk of contracting HCV through blood transfusions is approximately .001 percent for each unit of blood transfused. Prior to the screening of blood products for HCV, as many as 300,000 Americans contracted hepatitis C through transfusions of blood and blood products.

Injection drug use

Since 1992, injection drug use has been the most significant mode of transmission for HBV. Injection drug use accounts for approximately 61–70 percent of all new HCV infections. HCV is more prevalent in larger cities where injection drug use is more common. Studies of injection drug users show an HCV prevalence ranging from 85 to 100 percent. Even a miniscule amount of infected blood can contain extremely high levels of the HCV virus. Contaminated straws and drug paraphernalia are known agents of HCV transmission.

Intranasal drug use (snorting) can also transmit the HCV virus. Blood vessels in the nose may break without apparent notice, transmitting HCV to straws, rolled-up dollars and other drug paraphernalia that are shared. The CDC reports that the majority of injection drug users with HCV acquired it relatively soon after they began injecting drugs. Within 5 years of beginning to inject drugs, 51–80 percent of injection drug users are infected with HCV.

Transmission via percutaneous exposure

Percutaneous exposure refers to skin entry and is typically caused by needles, tattoos and piercings. Contaminated equipment, including colonoscopy instruments, and solutions can transmit HCV. In Maryland, one hepatitis C related fatality was tracked to a contaminated solution of radioactive technetium used in a cardiac stress test [60]. The World Health Organization (WHO) estimates that 2.3–4.7 million cases of HCV occur each year in developing countries that are associated with the use of non-sterile and re-used needles. In Egypt approximately 7–15 million persons were infected with HCV because of non-sterile needles used in vaccinations against the liver fluke schistosoma.

Hepatitis can also be transmitted to hemodialysis patients from contaminated hemodialysis machines. Although risk still exists, the risk of HCV transmission during dialysis procedures has declined since the introduction of hemodialysis guidelines for preventing infection and the screening of blood products for HCV. Primarily due to exposures before 1992, in the United States, up to 30 percent of hemodialysis patients may be infected with HCV, either from blood transfusions or contaminated equipment. People with kidney failure are at higher risk for HCV infection.

One of the largest documented health-care associated outbreaks of HCV in the United States occurred in a Hematology/oncology clinic in eastern Nebraska in which 99 patients who visited the clinic from March 2000 through December 2001 became infected as a result of inadequate infection control procedures. As a consequence, this clinical voluntarily closed in 2002.

During this outbreak, transmission of HCV resulted from shared saline bags contaminated through syringe reuse, and all patients showed genotype 3a infection, which presumably originated from one patients. Shared saline bags were likely contaminated when syringes used to draw blood from venous catheters were reused to withdraw saline solution. Infection occurred in 77.1 percent of patients who received saline flushes at the clinic. No infections occurred in patients who were treated at the clinic but did not receive saline flushes [41].

Vertical transmission

The HCV virus can be transmitted during childbirth although the risk is low, occurring in an average of 3–7 percent of pregnancies in which the mother has HCV infection. HCV infection primarily occurs in infants born to mothers who have viral loads of HCV of 2 million IU/ml or higher during the third trimester or at the time of childbirth. The rate of newborn infection in mothers with viremia is reported to be 12.6 percent, compared to 1.5 percent in mothers with HCV who do not have viremia. Women co-infected with HCV and HIV are also more likely to transmit HCV, with maternal transmission rates as high as 20 percent [19].

Transmission via sexual practices

HCV may be transmitted sexually. Because of the high number of individuals chronically infected, sexual intercourse accounts for a significant number of infections. The risk of infection with a regular sex partner who is infected with HCV is 1–3 percent annually [64]. The possibility exists that HIV infection might increase the risk of HCV infection within a sexual partnership. In one study, the risk of developing HCV doubled in stable, heterogeneous partners of patients infected with HCV [38].

High risk groups and high risk factors

Certain groups are at high risk for HCV and should be tested for it even in the absence of symptoms. High risk groups include:

- Hemodialysis patients
- Anyone using blood, blood products, clotting factors or organ transplants before 1992
- Intravenous or injection drug users
- Healthcare including dental workers with exposure to blood and blood products
- Emergency response workers
- People who received tattoos or body-piercings at suspect places of business
- Sex partners of someone infected with HCV
- Household members of someone infected with HCV
- Prison inmates
- Persons with multiple sexual partners
- Veterans receiving Veterans Health Administration (VHA) health care. The prevalence of HCV is 5.4 percent in this group compared to a national prevalence of 1.8 in the United States. The highest rates of HCV were found among veterans who reported having used injection drugs, those who served in the Viet Nam era, those who had been incarcerated for more than 38 hours and those who had tattoos.

Any procedure or practice, even manicures, that can cause viral entry into the bloodstream is a risk factor for HCV infection. Any contaminated solution, including solutions used to clean barbering tools, tattoo dyes, and stock medical solutions and solvents can become contaminated with HCV. HCV can be contracted through contaminated electrolysis equipment, acupuncture needles and instruments used for tattooing or body piercing.

Geographic distribution

Some populations have particularly high incidences of HCV infection. In Egypt, the mean prevalence of persons with HCV antibodies is 22 percent. This is undoubtedly a result of the contaminated Schistosoma vaccines that were administered in Egypt. High incidence areas also include certain parts of Africa, Italy and Japan. The prevalence of HCV in Eastern Europe exceeds that of Western Europe. Practices of skin-piercing with non-sterilized instruments and the use of non-sterilized needles are thought to be responsible for the high incidence in these areas.

HCV Infection

HCV typically causes a mild acute infection. Many people do not develop symptoms, and jaundice occurs in only 20–25 percent of acute infections. However, up to 80 percent of all HBV infections persist and progress to chronic disease. Rarely, HCV can cause fulminant hepatitis. Approximately 20 percent of patients infected with HCV will progress to severe forms of hepatitis, which can progress to cirrhosis and hepatocellular carcinoma (HCC), a type of primary liver cancer, over a period of 14 to 28 years [64].

Epidemiology

HCV occurs in all parts of the world, although its prevalence varies in different regions. In blood donors, the prevalence of antibodies to HCV ranges from .02 to 1.25 percent. In the United States, at least 1.8 percent of the population shows signs of infection. Higher rates have been found in southern Italy, Spain, central Europe, Japan and parts of the Middle East. Worldwide about 170 million people are infected.

In the United States, almost 4 million people are infected, and hepatitis C accounts for about 20–30 percent of all cases of acute hepatitis [64].

In the United States, persons aged 30 to 50 years have the highest rates of HCV infection, and infection is more common among minority populations such as African-American and Hispanic persons. In the United

States, genotype 1 is more prevalent in African-Americans than in other racial groups.

Disease Course in HCV

The disease course in HCV is variable. In most cases the acute disease course persists for several weeks to several months. One of the most striking features of HCV infection is that up to 85 percent of patients develop chronic disease.

Acute HVC infection

Most HCV acute infections cause no or minimal symptoms. For this reasons, the incidence of acute HCV is probably under-reported. Only 25 percent of patients with acute HCV infection develop jaundice and most patients have no symptoms. Although treatment of acute infection can be effective in preventing chronic hepatitis, in 75 percent of patients, acute infection is usually not recognized [62]. In a small minority of patients, acute infection may be self-limited and viral persistence may not be established. The clinical outcome in acute HCV infection is related to the immune system's response to the virus. This, in turn, may be dependent on the amount of virus in the contact source, the genotype of the virus, and the patient's general health.

INCUBATION PERIOD

The incubation period for HCV infection, the time between exposure and the onset of symptoms, is 5–12 weeks, although it can be as short as two weeks and as long as 5 months. The highest peak of viral replication in the blood or viremia occurs shortly after infection. During this period the viral load is at its highest. With the appearance of HCV antibodies the viral load begins to decline. In most persons the viral load remains constant at a relatively fixed level for many years without the intervention of treatment.

SIGNS AND SYMPTOMS

From 61–75 percent of patients with acute HCV remain asymptomatic. Of those who develop symptoms, only 20–30 percent become jaundiced. Symptoms, which only occur in 25–41 percent of patients, include fatigue, malaise, weakness, an enlarged liver, anorexia, and jaundice. Rarely, patients develop a rash or muscle and joint pain. Symptoms subside after several weeks as enzyme levels fall. Disease severity may be related to the virulence of the strain or the amount of viral particles present in the initial exposure dose.

In one report of a 79-year-old man who died after being infected with HCV through contaminated technetium tracer used in a diagnostic procedure, the level of contamination in the tracer was considered to be a contributing factor. All of the patients who received tracer from the same vial showed evidence of HCV infection [60].

Enzyme levels and bilirubin levels are used to monitor acute disease activity and predict remission. Levels of viral RNA are used to confirm diagnosis and response to treatment. However, on occasion RNA levels are negative early in infection and rise many months later.

ENZYME LEVELS

Within 2–8 weeks of exposure to HCV, serum ALT and AST levels usually rise 10 to 15 fold, indicating liver cell injury. However, the rise in enzyme levels may occur as early as two weeks after infection or as long as 26 weeks later. The normal ranges for ALT and AST are usually 0–46 IU/L although this can vary with different laboratories. Approximately 25 percent of patients reach a plateau level where ALT levels remain below 46 IU/L for many months. In others, ALT levels can normalize, suggesting recovery, and then flare again after many months to years.

Biochemical recovery. A continued decline in liver enzyme levels called a biochemical recovery does not mean that levels of HCV RNA have also declined. Likewise, patients who continue to have elevated enzyme levels are not always chronically infected with HCV. Complete resolution of HCV infection is defined as both the absence of HCV RNA and a normal ALT level.

If ALT and AST enzyme levels remain elevated or rise after a period of being normal over the course of 6 months, progression to chronic HCV is likely. Levels of the cholestatic liver enzymes alkaline phosphatase and gamma GT usually only show mild elevations in acute HCV infection.

BILIRUBIN LEVELS

In patients who develop jaundice, peak total bilirubin levels are usually less than 12 mg/dl. Levels typically return to normal in less than four weeks. Patients who develop jaundice are most likely to successfully clear the virus and least likely to develop chronic disease.

SEROLOGIC MARKERS

After exposure to HCV, the HCV RNA can be detected in blood specimens of infected persons in 1–3 weeks. HCV RNA is usually present at the onset of symptoms although antibodies to HCV (HCVAb), using enzyme (EIA) and chemiluminescence immunoassays (CIA), are only seen in 51 to 70 percent of patients. Studies show that in most patients HCV antibodies can be detected 41–51 days after infection. Three months after exposure to HCV, up to 90 percent of infected persons show evidence of HCVAb. Rarely, antibodies may not be detected for up to one year after infection. The use of tests for HCV RNA and HCV antibodies are described further in chapter fourteen.

In some cases, the HCV RNA level is negative early in infection and rises many months after sero-conversion. This suggests that the disease course in HCV requires several follow-ups and can't be monitored with a single HCV RNA test.

About 20 percent of patients develop symptoms before they seroconvert and begin producing HCV antibodies. The presence of HCV antibodies does not indicate immunity. Rather, it indicates HCV infection. The average time from exposure to seroconversion is approximately 51 days although it can take up to 12 months. HCV antibodies do not neutralize HCV, although they may inhibit the binding of HCV virus-like particles to target cells. The presence of HCV antibodies indicates HCV infection.

Fulminant HCV infection

Although acute infection in HCV can be severe, HCV rarely causes fulminant hepatitis. Because superinfection with other hepatitis viruses, particularly HAV, can cause fulminant disease, in the United States it's recommended that patients with chronic liver disease receive vaccinations for HAV and HBV.

Patients with HCV who acquire superinfection with HAV have a substantial risk for fulminant hepatic failure. In one large study, HAV superinfection in persons infected with HCV who have certain HLA markers, including A1, B8 and DR3, are most likely to develop fulminant infection. Patients with HCV who are also co-infected with the hepatitis G virus (HGV) also tend to develop fulminant infection when they develop superinfection with HAV [63].

Chronic HCV Infection

Chronic HCV infection refers to the presence of HCV RNA in the blood, using either qualitative or quantitative tests, for a period of six months or longer. Persistence of HCV appears to be related to the virus's ability to mutate when the immune system launches a defense against it. The virus is also able to down-regulate its replication, remaining latent within the liver in order to escape detection by the immune system.

RISK FACTORS

Males are more likely than females to develop chronic infection, and older people are more likely to develop chronic infection than younger individuals. In the United States, African-American men are most likely to develop chronic HCV infection. Persons who abuse drugs are also more likely to develop HCV.

DISEASE COURSE IN CHRONIC HCV

Because many people with acute HCV infection do not have symptoms and do not realize they're infected for many years, there are no long-term studies that accurately describe the disease course in chronic HCV infection. In addition, many people with recognized chronic infection receive early treatment or make lifestyle changes that alter the disease course.

Overall, studies show that approximately 20–30 percent of individuals with chronic hepatitis C will go on to develop progressive liver disease. Of these, about 41 percent may develop advanced liver disease. Individuals with HCV antibodies who have normal ALT levels and who tests persistently negative for viral RNA are at the lowest risk for significant liver disease.

However, there is no accurate clinical correlation between laboratory results, including viral load, and the extent of fibrosis or the development of cirrhosis. Many patients with advanced cirrhosis have no obvious biochemical abnormalities [38].

Data suggest that during the first two decades following chronic infection, mild symptoms are related to relatively low mortality and morbidity. However, cirrhosis has been reported as occurring within as little as 61 months following HCV infection. Certain strains or quasispecies of HCV are more predictive of advanced disease and this may explain why the rates of progressive disease are higher in Japan than in the United States. This increased prevalence of advanced liver disease is not seen when Japanese people infected with HCV migrate to other countries.

SIGNS AND SYMPTOMS OF CHRONIC HCV

Studies show that approximately 10–15 percent of HCV carriers have persistently normal liver enzyme levels, although in most cases these individuals have mild liver lesions seen on biopsy. Short-term, chronic HCV is generally benign. Studies of blood donors whose infections were diagnosed years after they were infected indicate that fatigue and liver enlargement are the most common early symptoms of chronic disease. Other symptoms include jaundice, pruritis or itching, which is related to excess bile salts, edema or fluid retention, and nausea. A number of extrahepatic manifestations of chronic HCV may also occur. These are described in a separate section later in this chapter.

The clinical course is more serious in patients with elevated liver enzyme levels. In individuals with fluctuating liver enzyme elevations, progression of liver fibrosis can occur after 5–7 years. Alcohol has a synergistic effect on HCV infection and accelerates the liver cell damage. Cellular damage in HCV is primarily caused by the toxic effects of immune system cells that target infected liver cells and from the immune system chemicals produced during the inflammatory process.

In patients with fluctuating levels, ALT levels frequently fluctuate between normal and increased, and it is not unusual for a person to have five to 10 normal ALT values separating elevated levels. In most cases progression towards severe fibrosis and cirrhosis is minimal at 10–15 years in carriers with normal enzyme levels and in 5–10 percent of patients with elevated enzyme levels. Up to 30–41 percent of patients with elevated enzymes and early signs of fibrosis on biopsy will show progress toward severe fibrosis and cirrhosis at 10–15 years.

Hepatic steatosis and insulin resistance. Chronic HCV infection is associated with symptoms caused by the liver's inability to carry out its normal metabolic functions. Studies show that hepatitic steatosis and insulin resistance can result. These factors need to be considered when assessing disease outcome and management.

Steatosis refers to abnormal fat accumulations in liver cells. Steatosis is associated with both alcoholic and non-alcoholic fatty liver disease. The incidence of steatosis in chronic HCV infection varies, with some studies showing rates as high as 30–70 percent and others showing a lower incidence than that of the general population. These discrepancies are related to diet, general health, and ethnicity. Caucasians are more likely to have steatosis than Hispanics or African Americans. Alcohol abuse and obesity are both associated with higher incidences of steatosis. Steatosis is also more prevalent in patients with co-existing HIV and HCV infection. This may be related to immune suppression. Steatosis contributes to fibrosis and to insulin resistance.

Insulin resistance is a condition of impaired glucose metabolism. In this condition, the body's cells become unresponsive to the normal glucose-lowering effects of insulin and blood sugar levels rise. Chronic HCV infection is associated with a higher incidence of insulin resistance even in lean patients. Insulin resistance in chronic HCV is suspected of impeding the response to interferon therapy.

PROGRESSIVE DISEASE SYMPTOMS

Symptoms of advanced or progressive disease include ascites, jaundice, encephalopathy, severe bacterial infection and gastrointestinal hemorrhage. About 20–30 percent of patients with chronic hepatitis go on to develop cirrhosis. Of those with cirrhosis, approximately 3–5 percent develop hepatocellular cancer (HCC) annually [28]. In the United States, deaths from HCC have nearly doubled since 1980 and they are expected to double again by 2025. Fibrosis and HCC are described further with advanced and decompensated liver disease in chapter thirteen.

Mortality rate in chronic HCV

In the United States, mortality in HCV infection is most often caused by end-stage liver disease rather than hepatocellular carcinoma. Studies estimate mortality of HCV in the United States ranges from 1.6 to 6.0 percent. Blood donor studies of persons with HCV also show a higher mortality rate among heavy drinkers [55]. Studies also indicate that the mortality risk is approximately 4 percent in the first two decades after infection, and that the risk increases over time in those who do not succumb to other events.

Progression in chronic infection is also more likely to occur in patients who are immunosuppressed, have elevated liver iron levels, and older age at the time of infection. Co-infection with either HIV, which causes AIDS, and hepatitis B are associated with increased mortality.

In the United States, the number of deaths resulting from HCV complications has increased from fewer than 10,000 in 1992 to nearly 15,000 in 1999. This number is expected to increase due to the large number of individuals with chronic HCV infection.

RISK OF DEVELOPING PROGRESSIVE LIVER DISEASE

Risk factors for developing progressive liver disease include infection with subtypes 1b HCV, older age at the time of infection, male gender, an immunosuppressed (weakened immune system) state such as HIV infections or immunosuppressant drug treatment, co-infection with HBV, alcohol use, iron overload, nonalcoholic fatty liver disease, certain hepatotoxic medications such as acetaminophen, and environmental contaminants. Co-infection with HIV has been shown in hemophiliacs to increase HCV RNA levels and to worsen the disease course [55].

Extrahepatic Manifestations of HCV

The term extrahepatic, which means away from the liver, refers to other organs and systems besides the liver. Chronic HCV infection is related to a number of different extrahepatic symptoms and conditions. The most common of these include the kidney disease glomerulonephritis and type II mixed cryoglobulinemia associated with vasculitis.

Other HCV associated diseases include porphyria cutanea tarda, sicca syndrome, vasculitis, spontaneous bacterial peritonintis, an inflammation of the peritoneum membrane covering the abdomen; hypertrophic cardiomyopathy, which causes an enlargement and thickening of the heart muscle and its valves; pancreatitis, which is an inflammation of the pancreas; the metabolic bone disease osteodystrophy, which causes bone softening; peripheral neuropathy, a condition of nerve cell damage; gall bladder disease, which is more likely to occur in males; and several autoimmune conditions, including thyroid disorders.

Blood disorders and malignancies

Blood disorders associated with chronic HCV include autoimmune hemolytic anemia, a condition of anemia in which red blood cells are destroyed by the immune system; thrombocytopenia, a condition of low platelets associated with bruising and abnormal bleeding.

Cancers associated with chronic HCV include cholangiocarcinoma, a malignant growth in one of the bile ducts that carries bile from the liver to the small intestine; head and neck squamous-cell carcinoma, a malignant tumor affecting the middle layer of the skin, which may result as a consequence of lichen planus; multiple myeloma, a cancer of plasma cells, which are produced in the bone marrow, that can destroy bone and interfere with the production of red and white blood cells; Burkitt's or B-cell lymphoma, a non–Hodgkin's type of lymph gland tumor that can affect multiple organs; verrucous cell carcinoma of the tongue and mouth; and liver cancer, which is described in chapter fourteen.

Pain syndromes

Patients with chronic hepatitis C often experience pain, particularly pain in the liver area, muscle pains and headaches. Because hepatitis impairs the liver's ability to process medications appropriately, analgesics may not have their usual effects. The drug acetaminophen is widely used for pain in hepatitis, but it should only be taken under the directions of a physician and the dose should not exceed 2,000 mg (2 grams) daily.

FIBROMYALGIA

Fibromyalgia is a condition of widespread muscle aches, pain, stiffness and fatigue. Although its causes are still unclear it's generally considered a disorder or miscommunication between the endocrine and nervous systems. Some researchers suggest that fibromyalgia is caused by an abnormal sensory processing or defect in the central nervous system that causes pain impulses to be amplified, whereas other researchers attribute it to low serotonin levels, impaired deep sleep, or viral injury. Patients infected with HCV, especially women, have a higher incidence of fibromyalgia than the general population.

Pain in fibromyalgia, which is described as aching, throbbing, twitching, stabbing and shooting pain in the deep muscles, usually arises in the neck, shoulders, back and hips. Unlike the pain of arthritis, which typically affects the joints, pain in fibromyalgia extends to muscles and ligaments. Symptoms are generally worse in the morning and may be accompanied by sensations of numbness and tingling in nerve endings. Sleep disorders, headaches, restless legs syndrome, impaired memory, rashes, dry eyes, depression, and impaired coordination can also occur in fibromyalgia.

The American College of Rheumatology has developed specific criteria for diagnosing fibromyalgia. These include: 1) widespread pain in combination with tenderness in at least 11 of 18 specific tender point sites, and 2) widespread pain in all four quadrants of the body for at least three months duration.

Patients with fibromyalgia are prescribed treatment protocols that include a combination of medications, exercise, physical therapy, heat and massage. While there are no specific medications for fibromyalgia, symptoms are alleviated with a combination of one or more of the following: analgesics, antidepressants, interferon alpha, benzodiazepine tranquilizers and muscle relaxants.

Immune complex disorders

The immune system responds to HCV by producing antibodies that target and attempt to destroy HCV. In the process, HCV antibodies latch on to the surface of HCV molecules or antigens forming an immune complex. These complexes, which resemble a lattice, can lodge in blood vessels or between cells, potentially causing other disorders.

GLOMERULONEPHRITIS

Immune complexes can clog the filtering process within the basement layer of the kidney. Immune complexes along with increased levels of the immune system chemical known as complement factor C3 can also trigger kidney inflammation. Over time, these immune systems mechanisms can cause a kidney disorder known as membrano-proliferative glomerulonephritis (MGN). MGN, which is often accompanied by a condition of cryoglobulinemia, improves with interferon therapy and with ribavirin monotherapy (used alone without interferon).

CYROGLOBULINEMIA

Cryoglobulinemia is a condition characterized by increased levels of cryoglobulin protein. Cryoglobulins are immunoglobulin proteins, a type of protein from which antibodies are derived, that precipitate or clump together in the cold and dissolve when re-warmed. Normally, immunoglobulin levels rise during the immune response.

Three basic types of cyroglobulins exist: Type I, Type II and Type III. Increased levels of these proteins are associated with specific conditions. Disorders also arise from elevations of more than one type of cryoglobulin, causing conditions known as essential mixed cryoglobulinemia.

Common symptoms of cryoglobulinemia include vasculitis, which is an inflammation of blood vessels, and purpura. Purpura is characterized by small purple discolorations on the skin surface that are caused by ruptured vessels. Other symptoms associated with cryoglobulinemia include hives, skin ulcerations, arthritic disorders, kidney disorders, nerve pain, abdominal pain, bleeding disorders, enlarged liver, and pulmonary insufficiency.

Table 7.1 Cryoglobulin disorders

Cryoglobulin	Elevations seen in	Associated diseases, symptoms of elevated levels
Type I	Lymphoma, multiple myeloma, Waldenstrom's macroglobulinemia	Type I cryoglobulinemia; increased thickness or viscosity of blood
Type II	Rheumatic diseases, chronic infections	Vasculitis, purpura, kidney disease, nerve inflammation (peripheral neuropathy)
Type III	Rheumatic diseases, chronic infections	Vasculitis, purpura, kidney disease, nerve inflammation (peripheral neuropathy)
Type II or III essential mixed cryoglobulinemia (EMC)	Chronic infections, especially HCV infection	Leukocytoclastic (associated with white blood cell infiltration) vasculitis involving the smaller blood vessels of the skin, kidneys and gastrointestinal tract, causing raised purpura, ulcerations, hyperpigmentation, muscle pain, itching, arthritic symptoms and fatigue.

Autoimmune and inflammatory disorders

Autoimmune disorders occur when the immune system attacks the body's own (self) tissues. Autoimmune disorders are caused by a combination of genetic and environmental factors. Patients with certain immune system genes are predisposed to developing autoimmune diseases when they're exposed to certain environmental triggers, including viruses. Most autoimmune conditions are characterized by periods of variable symptoms interspersed with periods of remission.

Besides the immune complex disorders, HCV is associated with several different autoimmune disorders, including systemic lupus erythematosus, the clotting disorder antiphospholipid syndrome which can cause vascular destruction, celiac disease (gluten sensitivity), rheumatoid arthritis, hemolytic anemia, and several other disorders which are described in the following sections.

BEHCET'S DISEASE

Behcet's disease is a system chronic inflammatory disorder characterized by recurrent ulcers in the mouth, genitals and eyes. Patients with Behcet's disease may also develop skin lesions, arthritis, bowel inflammation, meningitis (central nervous system inflammation) and cranial nerve palsies capable of causing memory loss, impaired speech, and gait disturbances.

SJOGREN'S SYNDROME/SICCA SYNDROME

Sjogren's disease is an autoimmune condition affecting the glandular system. It primarily destroys the glands that produce tears and saliva, resulting in a condition of sicca syndrome characterized by dryness of the mouth and eyes. In chronic HCV, dry mouth without dry eyes is a common feature. Sjogren's disease can also become systemic, affecting the glands in the vagina and stomach as well as the kidneys, blood vessels, lungs, liver, pancreas and brain.

VASCULITIS

Vasculitis is a condition of inflammation of the blood vessels. Blood vessels include arteries, veins, and the tiny tributaries of veins known as capillaries. When small blood vessels become inflamed, they can break and bleed into the surrounding tissues, causing small red dots or purple spots known as purpura. Larger blood vessels that become inflamed may swell, causing the internal vessel to narrow. This can result in clots that can block blood flow, resulting in tissue death or necrosis. Vasculitis can also cause an aneurysm, which is a weakening or bulging in a large blood vessel. Aneurysms can rupture and bleed.

Vasculitis can primarily affect the skin in a condition called cutaneous vasculitis, which can caused raised purple lesions, broken capillaries, and purpura. When vasculitis prevents blood flow to tissues, causing tissue death, it is described as necrotizing. Vasculitis can also affect blood vessels in different organs including the brain (cerebral vasculitis). Common types of vasculitis that can occur in HCV infection include cerebral vasculitis, cutaneous vasculitis, and polyarteritis nodosa, which is described in chapter six, with complications of hepatitis B infection.

Skin changes in chronic HCV

Besides the skin lesions associated with vasculitis, HCV can cause several different inflammatory and autoimmune and skin disorders. These are primarily caused by direct infection of HCV in the skin, lymphocytes, dermal (skin) cells, and blood vessels. HCV-RNA particles have been found in the epidermal (outer layer of skin) cells in patients infected with HCV [5].

Cutaneous or skin changes that occur in HCV include pruritis, an itching sensation; urticaria, a skin rash; acral necrolytic erythema, a blistering reddened rash found on the extremities of the body; erythema multiforme, a hypersensitivity reaction causing bull's-eye lesions that can itch or burn, oral and anal ulcers, and widespread hives; palmar eythema, a reddening of the palms of the hands and soles of the feet and systemic involvement. Other skin changes prominently associated with HCV are described in the following sections.

Porphyria cutanea tarda. Porphyria cutanea tarda is a skin condition characterized by blisters, eruptions and flat bumps usually seen on the outer surface of the extremities, especially the tops of the hands. Porphyria cutanea tarda, which can also occur as a familial disorder, is seen in chronic HCV infection, iron overload, in chemical or toxic exposures and in alcoholism.

LICHEN PLANUS

Lichen planus is a skin disorder that causes a recurrent, itchy, scaly, inflammatory rash or plaque-like lesion affecting the skin, mouth, lip, tongue, nails, scalp and genitals. Some lesions are purple-red with an angled appearance. Skin lesions are typically seen on the inner wrist, legs, torso, genitals and nail ridges. Lichen planus is also associated with dry mouth, a metallic taste, and hair loss.

MOOREN'S CORNEAL ULCER

Mooren's ulcer is a chronic superficial ulcer of the cornea that is often painful and progressive. The ulcer is suspected of being caused by the reaction of corneal proteins with HCV envelope proteins. Mooren's ulcer may result in vision loss.

SPIDER ANGIOMA AND NEVI

Spider angioma refers to an abnormal collection of blood vessels near the surface of the skin resembling a small spider web. Spider angioma lesions or nevi typically have a red dot in the center with reddish extensions. In liver disease, spider angiomas can occur anywhere but usually appear on the face and trunk and are common manifestations of cirrhosis.

HCV in Infants and in Pregnancy

HCV in Infants

Neonatal HCV infection occurs in 3–12 percent of infants born to mothers infected with HCV. Infection usually occurs at birth, and there is no preventive treatment available. Most infants infected with HCV remain free of symptoms throughout childhood, and studies show that children are more likely to clear HCV.

Infants born to HCV-infected mothers can have passive transfer of HCV antibodies for up to 18 months, causing false positive results. Infants can be tested for HCV after one to two months with tests for viral RNA or after 18 months with tests for HCV antibodies. Infants with positive tests for viral RNA should have two confirmatory repeat tests three to four months apart from each other.

HCV in Pregnancy

Pregnant women with HCV should not be treated with interferon or ribavirin until after delivery. Both of these medications have been linked to birth defects. As long as the liver disease is stable, pregnancy is usually uneventful in women with HCV. In women co-infected with HIV, aggressive treatment of HIV prior to pregnancy can reduce the chance of HCV transmission.

HCV can be transmitted in breast milk although there are no reports of HCV being transmitted during breastfeeding. Breastfeeding is considered safe unless the nipples are cracked, chafed, or bleeding.

Special Circumstances

HCV in AIDS

The HCV and HIV virus, which is responsible for AIDS, are remarkably similar. Both are transmitted by exposure to infected blood, and both viruses are able to easily mutate. Both viruses are frequently transmitted in injecting drug users. The CDC reports that 51–90 percent of injection drug users with HIV also have HCV infection.

In persons with HCV who are co-infected with HIV the disease course in AIDS remains the same. However, HCV infection progresses faster. Studies show that co-infected persons have higher viral loads of HCV RNA than in patients who are HIV-negative. In addition, they have a more progressive form of chronic disease and have an increased risk for cirrhosis and liver cancer. Liver disease from HCV is the leading non-AIDS cause of death in the U.S. in persons co-infected with HIV and HCV.

Treatment for both HIV and HCV involves long-term therapy with multiple drugs. However, while interferon alone offers benefits, the addition of ribavirin is associated with severe complications including death. Studies show that co-infected persons who stop injecting drugs and abstain from alcohol have response rates similar to those who do not inject drugs.

Co-infection of HCV and type 1 HIV, the predominant type in the U.S., appears to increase the risk of both sexual and maternal-fetal transmission of HCV.

Co-infection with HBV and HAV

Studies show that patients with HCV that develop co-infections with HBV have an increased risk of developing advanced liver disease and cirrhosis. Fulminant HCV infection has been reported in patients co-infected with HAV.

Diagnosis of HCV

Because patients with hepatitis C do not usually have symptoms in early infection, diagnosis is often made when patients have blood tests for HCV antibodies during routine physicals or in screening tests for blood donors. Patients who have received blood transfusions prior to 1992, and in some cases prior to 1990, may also have been diagnosed through Look-Back procedures implemented in 1998. However only about 2 percent of blood recipients notified through Look-Back have been diagnosed with HCV infection [52]. Many patients with HCV infection are not diagnosed until they develop symptoms associated with chronic liver disease.

Laboratory tests

Tests for detecting antibody to HCV were first licensed in 1990. Since that time, new versions of these tests with greater sensitivity and specificity (greater than 99 percent) have been introduced. Approved screening tests for HCV include either enzyme immunoassays (EIA) or enhanced chemiluminescence (CIA) assays. Results are reported as negative, positive or indeterminate. Positive results include the signal/cutoff result, which compares the test reading to a positive standard. Higher signal/cutoff ratios are more likely to be true positives.

In populations with a low prevalence of HCV infection, even test specificities greater than 99 percent cannot ensure total accuracy. For this reason, the CDC recommends that it is important to not exclusively rely on HCV antibody screening tests to determine if a person is infected with HCV.

The CDC recommends that positive results be confirmed with an independent supplemental test. Approved supplemental tests include the strip immunoblot assay (RIBA) for HCV antibodies and nucleic acid amplification (NAT) testing for HCV RNA. Negative confirmatory RIBA results indicate that the initial test was a false positive. Indeterminate RIBA results can occur in infected persons who are in the process of seroconversion and occasionally in patients with chronic infection. Indeterminate results might also indicate a false-positive screening result, and it is recommended that indeterminate results be repeated in two weeks to one month.

False negative HCV results can occur during the first weeks after infection before antibody is produced. HCV RNA, however, can be detected as early as 1–2 weeks after exposure to the virus. In the United States, Blood Banks use NAT testing to screen blood donors for HCV. Although it is a more expensive test, it has greatly reduced the risks for HCV in blood products [13]. With NAT testing, the risk of a unit of blood containing HCV has fallen from about 1:103,000 units using serological tests to close to 1 in 2 million units [52].Other laboratory tests used for the diagnosis and monitoring of HCV infection are described in chapter fourteen.

The U. S. Preventive Services Task Force in a March 2004 press release recommends against routine screening for HCV in asymptomatic adults who are not at increased risk for infection. The rationale is that the prevalence of HCV in the general population is low and most people infected with HCV do not develop cirrhosis or other major negative health outcomes. And although treatment, which is expensive and can cause undesirable side effects, can reduce viremia, there is no evidence that such treatment improves long-term health outcomes.

Imaging tests

Imaging tests are not needed to diagnose HCV infection but they may be used if signs of liver disease are present. Sonograms are typically used in evaluating chronic hepatitis C, especially when liver enzymes are elevated. MRI or CT scans can also be used to detect nodules, ascites, and varices if advanced liver disease is suspected.

Biopsy

Biopsy of liver tissue is a useful tool for staging HCV infection and determining if fibrosis or cirrhosis have developed. Biopsy results and limitations are described in chapter 15.

Complications of HCV

Complications of HCV infection include the extrahepatic manifestations of infection, such as cryoglobulinemia, described earlier in this chapter and progression to advanced liver disease. Potential complications of progressive disease include cirrhosis and hepatocellular cancer, which are described in chapter thirteen.

Prevention of HCV

Because vaccinations for HCV are not yet available, primary prevention activities that reduce risk for HCV infection and secondary prevention activities that reduce the risk of liver disease in HCV infected persons are the key steps in HCV prevention programs.

Primary prevention activities include: screening and testing of blood, plasma, organ, tissue and semen donors; heat inactivation of plasma-derived products; risk-reduction counseling and services; infection control practices and universal precautions for healthcare workers. Universal precautions include the use of latex gloves, proper disposal of blood and contaminated items and similar approaches when exposure to blood or blood products is possible.

Secondary prevention activities include: identifying, counseling and testing of persons at risk; and medical management of infected persons. Other prevention recommendations include professional and public education, and surveillance programs that identify risk factors [19].

Treatment of HCV

Because many of the treatments used for HBV and HCV infection are the same, conventional and complementary treatment options are described in chapters sixteen and seventeen respectively. In chapter eighteen, lifestyle influences such as diet are described.

The primary medications approved for the treatment of HCV infection are interferon alpha-2b (Intron A), interferon alpha-2a (Roferon A), interferon alphacon-1 or consensus interferon (Amgen) and ribavirin. Pegylated interferon-alpha (Peg-Intron or PEGASYS), which is a longer acting form of interferon, used in combination with ribavirin results in a sustained response rate of approximately 51 percent.

Economic impact

Medical care costs related to HCV infection in the United States are estimated to be more than $610 million annually. Most of this money is spent on medical care for patients with end-stage chronic liver disease.

8

Hepatitis D, Delta Virus

The hepatitis D virus (HDV), a defective virus also known as the delta virus, is unique among the hepatitis viruses in that it requires hepatitis B viral particles to replicate and infect other hosts. On its own, the hepatitis D virus does not infect man. In this chapter readers will learn about the hepatitis D virus, its discovery, its replication, and its geographic distribution. Readers will also learn about the diseases caused by HDV, including their incubation period, epidemiology, disease course in superinfection and co-infection, symptoms, diagnosis, treatment, risk factors, and complications.

The Hepatitis D Virus (HDV)

Hepatitis D virus (HDV) is a very small (36 nm) single-stranded circular antisense RNA virus coated with hepatitis B surface antigen (HBsAg). HDV has no structural relationship to hepatitis A, B, or C viruses. HDV cannot replicate on its own. It is only capable of infection when activated by the presence of the hepatitis B viruses. HDV resembles satellite viruses of plants which cannot replicate without another specific virus.

HDV is also unique in that is has an unusual secondary structure similar to that previously seen in disease-causing plant viroids, satellite RNAs, and satellite viruses. Electron microscopy shows that HDV RNA is circular although under physiologic conditions it assumes a rod-shaped form. Analysis of the nucleotide sequence shows that up to 70 percent of the bases are paired to form a double-stranded rod-like structure.

Interaction with HBV

The interaction between HBV and HDV is very complex. Synthesis of delta virus may reduce the appearance of hepatitis B viral markers in infected cells. HDV synthesis can also eliminate active hepatitis B viral replication. HDV is very infectious and can induce hepatitis in an HBsAg positive carrier host. In studies, HDV has been successfully transmitted to chimpanzee HBV carriers [56].

HDV genotypes

Three known HDV genotypes with seven distinct subtypes or clades have been described. Genotype 1 has a worldwide distribution. Genotype 2 has been discovered in Taiwan, Japan, and northern Asia. Genotype 3 is found in South America.

Replication

HDV can replicate within liver cells independently but it requires hepatitis B surface antigen for propogation. Replication of HDV RNA is thought to occur by a "rolling circle" mechanism under the direction of a cellular polymerase enzyme. The formed RNA particles are capable of cleaving away and acting independently. This propagation is similar to that of plant satellite viruses or viroids. Viral replication is totally dependent on the helper function of HBV. Consequently, HDV infection doe not outlast the duration of HBV infection.

Discovery of HDV

Delta virus was discovered in 1977 by Rizzetto and colleagues while they were studying liver biopsies of patients with hepatitis B surface antigen (HBsAg) positive chronic liver disease. HBsAg is seen in patients with acute HBV and in hepatitis B carriers. Rizzetto observed that antibodies to hepatitis B core antigen (HBcAb) reacted with tissue containing core antigen (HBcAg) and also with tissue negative for core antigen. Curious, these researchers set out to discover the source of viral protein in the specimens negative for HBcAg. Their research led to the discovery of the delta antigen.

Soon after, tests for detecting delta antigen (HDVAg) and delta antibody (HDVAb) were developed, and it soon became apparent that HDVAb were only seen in patients who were HBsAg positive. These early studies also characterized the differences between delta co-infections and delta superinfections.

Transmission

Delta virus is a bloodborne pathogen and is transmitted in the same manner as HBV although HDV transmission is more likely among certain groups. Transmission occurs through person-to-person contact involving parenteral exposure to blood or body fluids. In the United States, the highest incidence of HDV infection is seen in intravenous drug users and hemophiliacs who received concentrated clotting factors, especially prior to 1983. However, HDV is not transmitted as readily as HBV in institutionalized patients, hemodialysis patients or homosexual men.

Perinatal transmission of HDV occurs although it is less likely to occur than HBV transmission. HDV has been shown to be transmitted through the following mechanisms:

1. Direct percutaneous exposure to contaminated blood via intravenous drug use or blood products; rare perinatal transmission
2. Horizontal, nonparenteral (other than through skin punctures) transmission of HBV among siblings
3. Sexual contact
4. Unapparent transmission through open skin wounds or environmental contact

High risk group and high risk factors

In the United States HDV infection occurs more often in adults than children. Hepatitis D appears to be primarily confined to certain high-risk groups. The highest rates of HDV infectivity are seen in intravenous drug users, in persons from the Mediterranean basin, and hemophiliacs who received clotting factors prior to 1983. Other groups at high risk for HBV, such as homosexual men and hemodialysis patients, have increased risk for HDV infection, but the risk isn't as high as it is for HBV.

Outbreaks have occurred and have been primarily related to transmission occurring through open skin lesions, overcrowding, sexual contact, and inapparent percutaneous exposure, for example human bites. High risk groups include:

• Injection drug users
• Men who have sex with men
• Hemodialysis patients
• Sex contacts of infected persons
• Healthcare and public safety workers
• Infants born to infected mothers

Geographic distribution

Delta virus is found worldwide, with greatest prevalence in Southern Europe, the Balkans, Middle East, South India, and parts of Africa. It is rarely seen in the Far East, Brazil, Chile, and Argentina although epidemics of delta infection have been reported from the Amazon Basin, Brazil (where it causes Labrea fever), Colombia (where it causes Santa Marta hepatitis), Venezuela, and Equatorial Africa. In these areas children of the indigent population are affected and mortality is high.

In the United States, HDV infection is strongly associated with illicit injection drug use, hemophilia, or a history of multiple transfusions. HDV is not a reportable disease in the United States, but the CDC estimates that approximately 7510 infections occur each year. Studies indicate that approximately 4 percent of all new HBV cases are thought to involve co-infection with HDV. In studies of HBsAg positive drug addicts, up to 42 percent have evidence of HDV infection [12].Worldwide, hepatitis D has caused more than 10 million infections in people infected with HBV.

HDV Infection

HDV infection may occur as a co-infection with acute hepatitis B in someone who was previously susceptible to HBV or it may occur as a super-infection in an HBV carrier. HDV is not a new infection. Analysis of stored blood specimens shows evidence of HDV among American army troops in 1948, in Los Angles residents since 1968, and in liver specimens from 1930s Brazil [56]. HDV has direct cytotoxic effects and can directly injure liver cells. And like the other hepatitis viruses, HDV can evoke an immune system response that damages liver cells. Of the seven clades or subtypes of HDV that have been discovered to date, the South American genotype 3 is associated with a high frequency of fulminant hepatitis.

Epidemiology

The epidemiology of HDV infection is similar to that of HBV. Worldwide, there are approximately 300 million HBV carriers, and more than 5 percent of carriers (15 million people) are infected with HDV. Epidemiologic studies suggest that although HDV dates back to the 1940s, the current epidemic started when HDV was introduced into Europe in the mid–1970s. The exact number of people infected with HDV isn't known because patients with HBV may not be tested for HDV. Transmission is similar to that of HBV.

Areas of high endemicity, in which HDV is above 20 percent in asymptomatic carriers and above 61 percent in patients with chronic HBV, include southern Italy, North Africa, the Middle East, the Amazon Basin, the American South Pacific islands of Samoa, Hauru, and Hiue, and South America. In highly endemic areas, transmission is largely from person-to-person contact.

Areas of low endemicity (in which HDV prevalence is 3–9 percent in asymptomatic carriers and 10–25 percent in patients with chronic HBV) include the United States, China and Japan. In low endemic areas, transmission is limited to groups with frequent percutaneous exposure to blood, such as intravenous drug users and hemophiliacs.

In highly endemic areas, HDV prevalence varies widely. For instance prevalence is high in northern Kenya, the Central African Republic and low in Ethiopa, Liberia and South Africa. In areas of very low endemicity (less than 2 percent of asymptomatic carriers), such as China, Japan and Southeast Asia, there can be isolated groups with high prevalence. For instance high levels of HDV infection have been found in up to 84 percent of intravenous drug users in Taiwan and in approximately 20 percent of Taiwanese prostitutes. The high prevalence of HDV in some isolated Pacific island populations suggests that HDV spreads rapidly when it is introduced into a population.

In the United States, the prevalence of HDV infection is low. In studies of blood donors, prevalence varies widely, from 1.4 percent in one southeastern region to 12.4 percent in Southern California.

Disease Course in HDV

The disease course varies, causing superinfection in hepatitis B carriers and causing co-infection in patients with simultaneous HBV infection. In co-infection up to 90 percent of patients experience complete clinical recovery and clearance of both HBV and HDV, with less than 5 percent of patients developing chronic infection with both HBV and HDV. Fulminant hepatic failure occurs in less than 10 percent of cases of acute HBV/HDV co-infection. In superinfection, 80–90 percent of patients become chronic carriers of HDV as well as HDV, and 5–20 percent of cases of superinfection may progress to fulminant liver failure.

Incubation Period

The incubation period for HDV is 21–46 days, with an average of 35 days although it can be shorter in cases of superinfection.

Superinfection

In patients with superinfection, the acute attack may be severe and even fulminant or it may merely cause a transient rise in serum transaminase enzyme levels. The determining factor appears to be the HBV infection, with abundant HBsAg levels associated with more severe infection.

Delta infection is suspected when hepatitis B carriers who have remained stable show signs of relapse. Superinfection causes acute hepatitis in approximately 51–70 percent of HBV carriers who become infected. Asymptomatic infection can also occur.

Delta infection reduces active synthesis of HBV and patients usually are also HBeAg negative and HBV DNA negative. Up to ten percent of patients with superinfection show a resolution of the HBV carrier state and end up having negative HBsAg titers after superinfection. However, in 70–80 percent of cases of superinfection, patients develop chronic delta infection along with chronic HBV infection and this results in an accelerated move towards cirrhosis. Overall, superinfection of healthy HBV carriers causes liver disease to be more severe. Superinfection also has a higher rate of fulminant infection than seen in acute HBV infection.

Long-term, as many as 70–80 percent of individuals who become both HBV and HDV carriers have evidence of chronic liver disease with cirrhosis, compared to only 15–30 percent of patients with chronic HBV alone. Hepatocellular carcinoma is reported to be less common in carriers of both HBV and HDV. This may be due to HDV's inhibitory effects on HBV.

RELAPSE IN SUPERINFECTION

The delta virus can reactivate causing high viral titers of delta DNA. If HBV viremia also persists, the outcome is worse because this facilitates the spread of delta virus to more liver cells, increasing cellular damage. Hepatocellular cancer appears to be less common in HBsAg carriers with chronic delta infection. This may be due to the inhibiting effect of delta on HBV or rapid disease progression, causing the patient to die before cancer develops. However, in cases of hepatocellular cancer with chronic delta infection, HDV does not seem to influence survival.

Co-infection

In co-infection, acute infection is usually self-limited as the delta virus cannot persist after patients stop producing HBsAg. In co-infection the long-term outlook is good, and the clinical picture is the same as in HBV infection except that ALT enzyme levels often rise and peak twice. The first peak is caused by HBV and is followed several weeks later by a rise in ALT related to delta. After this second peak, delta IgM antibodies and HBsAg both begin to clear.

However, the disease course may be more severe in cases where the disease course progresses to chronic co-infection. Up to one-third of patients with chronic co-infection may go on to develop fulminant hepatitis [12].

Symptoms of HDV

In up to 90 percent of patients, Hepatitis D causes no symptoms. Patients who develop symptoms develop symptoms similar to those of hepatitis B, including jaundice, fatigue, abdominal pain, confusion, bruising, loss of appetite, nausea, vomiting and joint pain. In addition, HDV can severely worsen the disease course in HBV infection, and it can cause fulminant infection in apparently healthy HBV carriers.

Biopsy studies show that tissue damage is greater in delta-positive patients compared to HBV carriers without superinfection. Inflammatory activity and necrosis are more apparent. In the South American and Equatorial African epidemics, patients showed evidence of microvesicular fat deposits in hepatocytes, intense necrosis and large amounts of delta antigen within the liver. These changes have also been seen in New York intravenous drug users with delta infection.

Fulminant infection

About one third of the cases of fulminant HBV infection are related to delta infection. There are marked geographic differences in severity. Fulminant infection in one child in the Northern Brazil epidemic resulted in mortality after three days of symptoms [56].

Mortality rate of HDV

In co-infection, 1–4 percent of all cases progress to a chronic state. In superinfection, chronic infection occurs in more than 80 percent of cases. The mortality rate in HDV is high, particularly in cases of superinfection, and ranges from 2–20 percent.

Diagnosis of HDV

Hepatitis D is diagnosed with blood tests for HDV IgM and IgG antibodies (anti-HD IgM and IgG), HDV antigen and for HDV DNA. These blood tests are used to diagnose concurrent HDV infection in patients newly diagnosed with HBV, patients with known chronic HBV who are experiencing acute hepatitis symptoms, and in patients with fulminant HBV infection.

HDV markers in co-infection

Co-infection is diagnosed by finding Delta IgM antibodies in patients with high titers of hepatitis B core IgM antibodies (HBc IgM). Delta IgM antibodies appear after one week and persist for 5–6 weeks although they may be present as long as 12 weeks. When IgM delta antibodies disappear, IgG delta antibodies appear.

There may be a window period between the disappearance of IgM and the appearance of IgG. If HDV is suspected and antibody tests are negative, blood tests for HDV Ag or HDV RNA can be used although these tests are not widely available.

Loss of IgM delta antibodies confirms resolution of infection, whereas persistence of IgM HD antibodies predicts chronic infection. Note: both HBsAG and Hepatitis B IgM core antibodies are suppressed by acute delta infection. Unless delta markers are also tested, infection with HDV and HBV may be misdiagnosed.

In co-infection, 20 percent of patients test positive for HDV antigen and 90 percent of patients test positive for HDV RNA. HDV IgM antibodies are positive early in infection and then become positive for HDV IgG antibodies. Liver enzyme tests show ALT and AST elevations greater than 510 IU/L. A Prothrombin time test greater than 17 seconds or a PT ratio greater than 1.5 are considered early indicators of fulminant liver failure.

HDV markers in superinfection

Superinfection occurs in hepatitis B carriers who become infected with HDV. High levels of HBsAg in these patients allow rapid replication of HDV and establishment of both acute and chronic infection. Superinfection is marked by the early presence of IgM delta antibodies, usually at the same time delta IgG antibodies develop. Both IgM and IgG delta antibodies persist in superinfection along with HBsAg and HBc IgG antibodies. In superinfection, HBc IgM is usually negative but patients may have low titers of this antibody. HDV Ag and HDV RNA are also seen in superinfection.

Patients with superinfection are likely to become HDV as well as HBV carriers. Patients with both chronic delta infection and chronic HBV infection have an increased risk for progressing to cirrhosis. Patients with chronic HBV and HDV who develop active cirrhosis usually have a persistently positive HD IgM antibody test. Assays for HDV Ag are not always reliable because HDV antigen tends to be encapsulated by HBsAg or complexed with Hepatitis D antibodies.

Imaging studies

Imaging tests can be used to assess disease severity and evaluate the liver for signs of biliary obstruction or liver cancer.

Complications of HDV

The extrahepatic (other than liver) conditions that can develop in HBV infection are not as likely to occur in HDV superinfection or co-infection. However, several researchers have described neurological complications, including Guillain-Barré syndrome, a disorder in which the myelin sheath covering nerves is destroyed affecting muscle coordination, and seventh-nerve paralysis with myokomia.

Prevention of HDV

Hepatitis B vaccinations provide protection against hepatitis B and hepatitis D. Vaccinated individuals are immune to both hepatitis B and delta virus. Persons with active HBV or who are HBV carriers are at risk for co-infection or superinfection with the delta virus. These individuals should receive counseling to reduce high-risk behaviors.

Treatment of HDV

There are no effective treatments for delta infection. Interferon is only able to suppress delta virus transiently although studies using 9 million units of interferon three times weekly for one year yielded better results. Relapse after extended treatment is likely. Patients receiving liver transplants and HBIG to prevent HBV recurrence have been shown to develop recurrence of HDV infection without evidence of HBV recurrence and no signs of clinical liver disease. Conventional and alternative treatment options for hepatitis are described in chapters sixteen and seventeen, and lifestyle recommendations are described in chapter eighteen.

9

Hepatitis E, F, G/GB, and NANE Virus

Chapter nine describes the hepatitis E virus (HEV), the hepatitis F virus (HFV), the hepatitis G/GB viruses (HGV, HGBV) as well as several possible candidates for non-A-E (NANE) hepatitis. The discovery, incidence and replication of these viruses is described, along with what's currently known about the diseases they cause, including the incubation period, epidemiology, disease course, symptoms, diagnosis, treatment, risk factors, and complications.

The Hepatitis E Virus (HEV)

The hepatitis E virus (HEV) is a 34 nm, single-stranded, un-enveloped RNA virus belonging to the *Caliciviridae* family, which includes viruses seen in swine and rabbits, hemorrhagic disease virus and Norwalk-like viruses. The Norwalk virus was associated with gastrointestinal ailments occurring on cruise ships in 2004. Because HEV has similar biological properties to some of these viruses but has a genome that resembles the rubella virus, it may eventually be reclassified. The hepatitis E virus is similar to the hepatitis A virus in that it is enterically transmitted. Most outbreaks of HEV occur in developing countries. Hepatitis E infection was first documented in the United States in 1997 in a patient with no history of travel.

Discovery of HEV

Before its discovery in an infected volunteer in 1983, hepatitis E was long known and commonly referred to as enterically transmitted non-A,

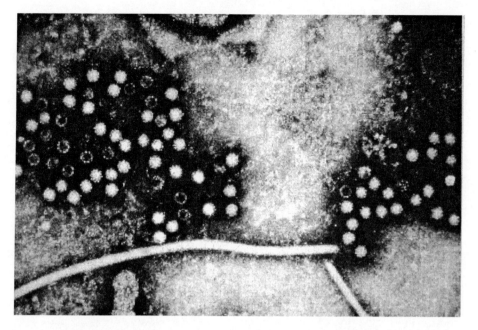

Hepatitis E (Centers for Disease Control Public Health Imaging Library).

non-B hepatitis (ET-NANBH). In 1983 the name was changed to the hepatitis E virus (HEV).

Transmission of HEV

The hepatitis E virus is primarily transmitted by the fecal-oral route, with fecally contaminated water the most common means of transmission. Transmission by person-to-person contact has also been documented. The potential also exists for food borne transmission.

HEV strains identical to those seen in the United Kingdom have been found in a pig herd in the United Kingdom and in pig and deer meat found in retail outlets in Japan. HEV was discovered in pigs in 1997 although there is evidence that it had been present since the early 1990s. In Japan, HEV infection has been linked to eating grilled or undercooked pork [3].

HIGH RISK FACTORS

Risk factors include travel to endemic areas, eating or drinking contaminated food and water, and participating in outdoor recreational activities in contaminated waters.

GEOGRAPHIC DISTRIBUTION

Hepatitis E is primarily seen in tropical and subtropical countries. Outbreaks have occurred in Asia and North and East Africa. In the United States the prevalence rate of anti–HEV antibodies is less than two percent. The route of exposure in these instances isn't well known but presumed to be a result of travel to endemic areas.

HEV is seen worldwide although it is most prevalent in tropical areas and in areas of inadequate sanitation. It occurs most often in developing countries near the equator in both the Eastern and Western hemispheres. Outbreaks are associated with rainy seasons, floods and overcrowding. The largest outbreak was reported in northeast China, affecting 100,000 people between 1986 and 1988. The origin or reservoir of HEV is unknown but it is suspected of being transmitted by animals.

HEV Infection

HEV causes a disease similar to HAV primarily causing gastrointestinal symptoms. And like HAV, the hepatitis E virus typically infects young people and is not associated with chronic infection. Infection is most often seen in young to middle-aged adults (15–41 years).

EPIDEMIOLOGY

The highest incidence of HEV is seen in tropical and subtropical countries. Hepatitis E has only rarely been reported in the western hemisphere, and in these cases most infected persons had traveled to HEV endemic areas. Waterborne epidemics have been reported in India in 1956 and 1975–1976; in the USSR (1995–1996); in Nepal (1973); Burma (1976–1977)l Algeria (1980–1981), Ivory Coast (1983–1984); and Borneo (1987). Tsunami survivors experienced sporadic HEV infection in 2004.

Disease Course in HEV

The hepatitis E virus is the primary cause of enteric hepatitis not caused by hepatitis A or hepatitis B. HEV usually causes an acute self-limited disorder similar to HAV infection but of shorter duration, usually resolving within two weeks. HEV has not been found to cause chronic infection. However, it can cause fulminant infection in up to 10 percent of cases. In women who are pregnant HEV infection is particularly virulent and has a case fatality rate of 20–25 percent in the second and third trimesters of pregnancy.

Hepatitis E has a prodromal and an icteric phase. During the prodromal phase symptoms can develop with the most common symptoms being abdominal pain, malaise, nausea and enlarged liver. During the icteric phase jaundice can develop, affecting the skin and eyes. An associated dark urine and pale stools are also seen. Patients can also develop rash and diarrhea.

INCUBATION PERIOD

The incubation period for HEV is 15–61 days with an average of 46 days.

SYMPTOMS OF HEV

Symptoms in the prodromal phase of HEV infection include malaise, loss of appetite, abdominal pain, arthralgia (joint pain), weight loss (average 8 lbs), muscle pain, nausea, vomiting, dehydration, right upper quadrant pain, and fever. During the icteric phase, symptoms include jaundice and itching.

Diagnosis of HEV

Diagnosis of HEV is sometimes based on the epidemiological characteristics of the outbreak and by excluding HAV and HBV with serological tests. HEV can be identified by immune electron microscopic examinations of feces.

Although serology tests for HEV are not performed at most local laboratories, specimens can be sent to reference laboratories for analysis. The hepatitis E virus can be detected in stool and serum using a reverse transcription polymerase chain reaction (PCR) method for HEV RNA. An ELISA method is also available for detecting IgM and IgG antibodies to HEV antigen. HEV IgM antibodies are present in acute infection and persist for up to six months. HEV IgG antibodies are seen in resolving or past HEV infections and appear to cause HEV immunity.

ENZYME AND BILIRUBIN LEVELS

In HEV infection, serum ALT and AST levels begin to rise a few days before the onset of symptoms and usually peak within 4–6 weeks from the onset of symptoms and gradually fall, decreasing to normal within 1–2 months. Total and direct bilirubin levels rise moderately and take longer to return to normal than ALT levels.

Treatment of HEV

Treatment for HEV infection is generally supportive to prevent dehydration. Hospitalization is only indicated for patients unable to maintain oral intake.

The Hepatitis F Virus

Hepatitis F was first reported in India in 1983. In 1994 French researchers also found this virus in the stool of patients with NANE hepatitis. Injection of viral particles from the stool of these patients into Indian rhesus monkeys was reported to cause symptoms of hepatitis although this has not been confirmed and hepatitis F has not been universally accepted. Technically, hepatitis F is considered a nonexistent virus although this is still a matter of debate.

Hepatitis F is described as a double-stranded DNA virus causing elevation of liver enzymes after an average of 20 days. According to several scattered reports in Great Britain, Italy, India and France, the F hepatitis virus, like the hepatitis A and E viruses, is enterically transmitted. In infected individuals, the clinical picture is that of acute hepatitis with a 20 percent fatality rate. Hepatitis F is generally not considered capable of causing significant disease although in Great Britain sporadic fulminant cases of hepatitis F have been reported [71].

The Hepatitis G/GB Virus

The hepatitis G virus (HGV) is a positive-stranded RNA virus belonging to a group called GB viruses in the family *Flaviviridae*. The GB viruses are named after the initials of a Chicago surgeon who contracted acute non-A-E hepatitis in 1995. Inoculations of his serum to tamarin monkeys were shown to induce acute hepatitis. However, there is no clear evidence that HGV causes hepatitis in humans either during infection or after long-term carriage of the virus. Most patients infected with HGV show persistent evidence of HGV RNA. Although HGV is detected with varying frequency in patients with various forms of chronic liver disease, no clear-cut association with the virus has been determined.

Hepatitis G is also referred to as hepatitis GB, hepatitis GB-A, and hepatitis GB-C. Hepatitis G has been found to cause both acute and chronic hepatitis, which are usually mild and only affect about 30 percent of infected patients. Recent studies in the United States and Germany suggest that the hepatitis G virus prolongs survival of people infected with HIV, the virus that causes AIDS.

Discovery of Hepatitis G/GB

The hepatitis G/GB virus was discovered simultaneously in 1995 by the viral group at Abbott Laboratory in Chicago and at Genelabs. Since the discovery of the hepatitis C virus, researchers had realized that there was likely yet another cause of transfusion-related hepatitis and community-based hepatitis, which is commonly referred to as the non-A-E or NANE virus. Whether HGV is this virus, is still a matter of debate. Studies show that hepatitis G is transmitted through blood, and that it causes viral hepatitis, but most researchers feel that HGV is not associated with any significant disease.

Transmission of HGV

Hepatitis G is found in about 1–1.5 percent of volunteer blood donors with normal ALT levels, and in about 4 percent of blood donors with elevated ALT values. Hepatitis G is suspected of being transmitted through blood transfusions, intravenous drug use and other percutaneous exposures although there is not enough study data to confirm this. Hepatitis G is found in 15 percent of intravenous drug users and 13 percent of paid plasma donors.

GEOGRAPHIC DISTRIBUTION

Hepatitis G is found worldwide with evidence of active or past infection ranging from 5–15 percent. HGV is found in highly isolated populations such as indigenous tribes people in Papua New Guinea, sub–Saharan Africa and Central/South America. The highest prevalence (18 percent) of HGV is found in West Africa.

HGV Infection

EPIDEMIOLOGY

Hepatitis G/GB is found worldwide and is seen in 1.0–1.5 percent of blood donors in the United States and United Kingdom. In various populations studied, the prevalence of HGV ranges from 5–15 percent. In blood donors with elevated ALT enzyme levels, the incidence of HGV is about 4 percent, and in paid plasma donors, the incidence is 13 percent. In intravenous drug users the incidence of HGV is 15 percent. About 20 percent of patients with acute or chronic hepatitis C infection are reported to be positive for HGV.

Disease Course in HGV

Hepatitis G has been studied in patients who received blood from infected donors. Up to 65 percent of patients remain asymptomatic after infection. In about 30 percent of patients, after an incubation period of about 30 days, hepatitis G causes mild elevations of ALT, AST, nausea and malaise followed by an icteric phase. These patients are likely to have persistent infection, usually asymptomatic, for a period of three to nine years.

Co-infection with HCV and HGV does not appear to worsen the disease course in HCV. The clinical significance of HGV has not been fully established and is still a matter of debate.

INCUBATION PERIOD

In studies of infected tamarin monkeys, the incubation period was approximately 30 days with a range of 20–47 days.

The Nane Virus (Non-A-E Virus)

The NANE virus is a term used to describe the causative agent in the approximately 20–40 percent of instances of viral hepatitis that cannot be attributed to hepatitis viruses A-E. This condition is sometimes also referred to as hepatitis X. Patients with NANE hepatitis are reported as being less likely to be jaundiced, have lower peak ALT levels and a lower frequence of chronic hepatitis compared to patients with hepatitis C infection. However, a small number of fulminant hepatitis cases are suspected of being caused by the NANE virus.

Potential NANE candidates

Potential candidates include the hepatitis F and G viruses, the Sen-V virus, and Transfusion transmitted virus (TTV). Studies indicate that hepatitis viruses F and G do not cause significant infection making them the least likely cause of NANE hepatitis. The Sen-V virus is present in 16 percent of the normal population, 22.1 percent of patients with NANE hepatitis, and 36.2 percent of cirrhosis patients. Because of its high prevalence in the general population, the Sen-V virus is not considered to be the cause of NANE hepatitis although more studies are needed.

TTV was first reported by Japanese researchers in 1997. TTV is a single-stranded DNA virus lacking an outer envelope that was named after the initials of the first patient in which it was discovered. Six distinct genotypes of TTV have been identified. TTV has been demonstrated following blood transfusions in patients in the United States, United Kingdom, Japan, Thailand and Germany.

Risk factors include hepatitis B infection and Mediterranean origin. TTV causes a mild asymptomatic form of hepatitis, which has been confirmed by biopsy studies. It does not contribute to liver damage in patients co-infected with HCV, and it does not contribute to the development of cirrhosis or liver cancer. TTV can be detected by blood tests for viral DNA.

10

Autoimmune Hepatitis

The Autoimmune Hepatitis (AIH) Condition

Autoimmune hepatitis (AIH) is a chronic condition of hepatitis that originates in the immune system. AIH develops when the immune system launches an inappropriate immune response that targets the body's liver cells. AIH is characterized by liver cell inflammation, increased blood levels of gamma globulins, autoantibodies that target the liver, and a favorable response to immunosuppressive treatment such as corticosteroids.

The inflammatory reaction in AIH is directed against the liver's cells and, in some instances, against the bile ducts. Similar to other autoimmune disorders, this condition primarily affects young women although it can affect both men and women of all ages. The direct cause of AIH is unknown although several environmental factors, including the hepatitis viruses A, B, and C, and the antibiotic minocycline, have been implicated.

Subtypes of AIH

Autoimmune hepatitis has three general subtypes, type I, type II, and type III. In addition, AIH may also occur as a variant accompanied by other autoimmune liver diseases. Rarely, AIH may also occur as part of a genetic polyendocrine disorder. AIH affects nearly eight times as many women as men and it primarily targets two age groups: 1) young people between the ages of 10 and 20 years and 2) people older than 55 years.

Discovery of AIH

In 1950 Doctor Waldenstrom first described autoimmune hepatitis after noticing an increased incidence of chronic hepatitis occurring in young people, especially women. He reported patients with this condition having features of cirrhosis, liver inflammation and increased blood gamma globulin levels.

Other researchers in the 1950s also noticed this condition and described affected patients in greater detail. Some patients were reported to have an enlarged spleen, jaundice, acne, puffy facial features, hirsutism (increased facial hair), obesity, pigmented abdominal striae (stretch marks), and amenorrhea (scant or absent menstrual periods).

Early laboratory results

In 1955, laboratory scientists noted that many of these patients also had positive LE cell preps. The LE cell prep test, now considered obsolete, was a rudimentary blood test used to diagnose systemic lupus erythematosus (SLE) based on changes that occurred when blood cells were treated with various chemicals. Because of the positive LE prep results seen in patients with AIH, the researcher Mackay and his associates called this newly recognized form of hepatitis "lupoid hepatitis," a term that is no longer used.

In the 1970s, with the introduction of more sophisticated immunological tests for diagnosing lupus disorders, it became clear that autoimmune hepatitis had no similarities to lupus other than the fact that they both have an autoimmune origin. In 1992, an international panel codified the diagnostic criteria and selected the name autoimmune hepatitis to replace older terms such as autoimmune liver disease, lupoid hepatitis, and autoimmune chronic active hepatitis.

Epidemiology

Autoimmune hepatitis is found worldwide. Approximately 100,000–200,000 cases occur in the United States at any given time, accounting for about 11–23 percent of all chronic liver disease. AIH is known to develop in a minority of patients who recover from viral hepatitis.

Worldwide, AIH accounts for about 10–20 percent of all cases of chronic hepatitis with the highest prevalence among northern European/Caucasian groups with a high frequency of HLA-DR3 and HLA-DR4 markers. In Japan, where HLA-DR3 frequencies are low, AIH is only associated with HLA-DR4. The frequency of AIH seems to be decreasing, and this may the result of newer blood tests that make it easier to diagnose viral hepatitis with greater accuracy [56].

Autoimmune Diseases

Autoimmune disorders include more than 100 separate diseases, such as systemic lupus erythematosus (SLE) and multiple sclerosis (MS) that are caused by a destructive immune system reaction that targets the body's own organs and cells. Autoimmune disorders develop in persons with certain immune system genes that predispose them to developing autoimmune diseases when they're exposed to certain environmental triggers.

Autoantibodies

Autoimmune diseases develop when the immune system is weakened by the constant response to environmental triggers. Over time, the weakened immune system becomes ineffective and responds erratically and inappropriately, producing autoantibodies.

Most autoimmune diseases are associated with the development of specific autoantibodies. Autoantibodies are antibodies that react with the body's own proteins and cells. Patients with AIH have been found to have several different autoantibodies, both antibodies that target the liver and antibodies that target other tissue cells. Tests for these antibodies, which are described later in this chapter, can be used to help diagnose autoimmune liver disorders.

Autoantibodies in AIH

A number of different autoantibodies are seen in AIH including:

- Antinuclear antibody (ANA) with a homogenous pattern primarily seen in subtype I
- Antibodies to double-stranded DNA (anti-dsDNA)
- Anti-smooth muscle antibody (anti-SMA) primarily seen in type I
- Anti-liver-kidney microsomal antibody (anti-LKM-1), primarily seen in type II
- Anti-soluble liver antigen (anti-SKA) directed against cytokeratins type 8 and 18 primarily seen in type III AIH.
- Antibodies to liver-specific asialoglycoprotein receptor or hepatic lectin
- Antimitochondrial antibodies, which are primarily seen in primary biliary cirrhosis (PBC) and may occur in overlap syndromes with AIH
- Rheumatoid factor
- Antiphospholipid antibodies

Autoimmune disease associations in AIH

Patients with AIH frequently have other autoimmune disorders. Disorders most often seen with AIH include autoimmune thyroid disease (both Graves' disease and Hashimoto's thyroiditis), insulin-dependent diabetes mellitus (IDDM), vitiligo, primary biliary cirrhosis (PBC), rheumatoid arthritis, celiac disease (gluten sensitivity enteropathy), myasthenia gravis, Sjogren's syndrome and autoimmune hemolytic anemia. Vitiligo, IDDM, and thyroiditis are most commonly seen in subtype II AIH.

ADULT GIANT CELL HEPATITIS

Giant cell hepatitis, a type of hepatitis associated with specific cellular changes, is usually seen in children. However, it can also occur in association with autoimmune diseases, the use of certain medications, paramyovirus infection, and after liver transplants. Adult giant cell hepatitis typically causes a fulminant, rapidly progressive disease with a disease course resembling that of viral hepatitis that has been reported to respond to the anti-viral drug ribavirin. Several incidences of giant cell hepatitis have also been reported in patients with both primary sclerosing cholangitis and autoimmune hepatitis. These patients showed a good response to immuno-suppressant medications and ursodeoxychlic acid.

Genetic Influences in AIH

Several different genes, including the HLA genes that regulate the immune system and genes that regulate specific organs, are associated with AIH development.

Human leukocyte antigens (HLA system)

The major histocompatibility complex (MHC) refers to a system of genes that regulate the immune system, directing what substances the immune system will react to and orchestrating the severity of these reactions. In humans the MHC is known as the human leukocyte antigen (HLA) system. These genetic markers code for proteins expressed on the cell surface of all the body's nucleated cells.

HLA markers include HLA-A, HLA-B, HLA-C, and HLA-D, and a subset of D markers known as HLA-DR, HLA-DP, and HLA DQ. Each marker has a subset of Class I, Class II, or Class III antigens, and antigens from different classes have different functions. For instance, Class II antigens are found on macrophages, B-lymphocytes, endothelial or tissue cells and activated (responsive) T lymphocytes. The presence of Class II antigens on target organs in patients with autoimmune disease indicates an autoimmune process.

Most autoimmune diseases are associated with more than one HLA antigen. And each antigen may be associated with more than one autoimmune disease. Certain HLA markers can also offer protection against specific diseases. In different races, different antigens can be associated with different autoimmune disorders [56].

HLA markers in AIH

Autoimmune hepatitis is associated with several markers including HLA-DR3. HLA-DR3 markers are associated with a decreased number of lymphocytes known as T suppressor cells. A decline in these cells, cells that would keep T cells from reacting with and producing autoantibodies against our own tissue, contributes to the development of autoimmune disease.

In autoimmune hepatitis, various HLA markers, such as HLA-A2, HLA-B8, HLA-DR3, HLA-Dw3, and HLA-DR4 are expressed as Class II antigens on hepatocyte cell membranes, making these cells more susceptible to destruction by the autoantibodies seen in AIH. A self-perpetuating antigen-antibody reaction in AIH leads to the production of cytotoxic (capable of destroying cells) lymphocytes and cytokines that contribute to chronic liver disease.

Organ-specific genes

A number of organ-specific genes are also associated with autoimmune disease development. For instance, polyglandular syndrome, a disorder that affects multiple endocrine organs, which can include autoimmune hepatitis and autoimmune polyendocrinopathy-candidiasis-ectodermal dystrophy (APECED), is associated with the APECED gene found on the long arm of chromosome 21.

Environmental Triggers in AIH

Certain environmental triggers are known to stimulate the immune system and trigger autoimmune disease in genetically susceptible individuals. These triggers include stress, chemical overload, infectious agents, sugar and saturated fats, aspartame, vaccines, and allergens. Continuous exposure to these triggers is not necessary for the disease to persist, but their continued presence often exacerbates or worsens the disease course.

The frequent reports of AIH developing after infection with the hepatitis viruses A, B, and C suggests that they act as specific triggers for AIH disease development. Other suspected triggers include the Epstein-Barr virus (EBV) and the measles virus; the bacteria *Salmonella* species and *Escherichia coli*; and the medications halothane, interferon, minocycline, melatonin, alpha methyldopa, oxyphenisatin, and nitrofurantoin; and the herbs black cohosh and Dai-saiko-to. Latent autoimmune hepatitis has been found to occasionally emerge during interferon therapy for chronic hepatitis C.

Disease Course in AIH

The disease course in autoimmune hepatitis is variable. The majority of AIH patients have subtype I AIH, which usually has a milder disease course than subtype II. About 10 percent of AIH patients, especially patients in subtype I, have mild symptoms that wax and wane and spontaneously resolve. A smaller number of patients may have a subclinical course with mild or absent symptoms. Most patients have a chronic fluctuating course with variable symptoms and severity.

Disease onset

The onset of AIH is usually insidious with patients noticing vague symptoms such as fatigue, malaise, fever, joint pain, fluctuating periods of jaundice, right upper quadrant pain, or lethargy. Some patients have abnormal laboratory test results, including elevated liver enzymes and a low platelet count (thrombocytopenia), but no clinical symptoms. A small number of patients may present with severe symptoms resembling those of fulminant viral hepatitis that have a sudden onset.

Chronic disease

Overall, most patients develop chronic disease with continuing liver cell inflammation and necrosis, which often progresses to cirrhosis if left untreated. The most severe course tends to occur in young girls with type II AIH. Overall, up to 70 percent of patients show a good response to continuous treatment with steroids (prednisone or prednisolone) and azathioprine (Imuran).

Autoimmune hepatitis can be categorized into three basic subtypes that are useful in helping to determine optimal treatment and to predict the disease course. In addition, AIH can occur as part of a syndrome in association with other diseases. The changes seen in the various subtypes and syndromes are described in the following sections.

TYPE I AIH

Type I AIH, the most common form of AIH, is primarily seen in two age groups: 1) age 10–20 years and 2) 45–70 years, and the female to male ratio is 8:1. Up to 40 percent of subtype I patients have a concurrent autoimmune disorder and most patients show a favorable response to steroid medications. Associated HLA markers include B8, DR3, and DR4. About 45 percent of patients eventually progress to cirrhosis. Patients in this subtype usually have markedly elevated gamma globulin levels, smooth muscle antibodies (SMA), anti-nuclear antibodies (ANA), dsDNA antibodies, perinuclear anti-neutrophil cytoplasmic antibodies (p-ANCA), and anti-asialoglycoprotein receptor antibodies (anti-ASGPR).

TYPE II AIH

Subtype II AIH, which accounts for about 4 percent of AIH cases in the United States, primarily affects children between the ages of 2–14 years and is rarely seen in adults. Subtype II AIH is seen frequently in Europe. The female to male ratio is 9:1 and the response to steroids is poor compared to subtypes I and III. About 82 percent of patients progress to cirrhosis. About 35 percent of patients have a concurrent autoimmune disease, and patients typically have anti-LKM type 1 or 3 antibodies without ANA or SMA. HLA associations include B14, DR3, and C4AQO.

Patients of subtype II who have antibodies to cytochrome P450 1ID6 and who do not show evidence of HCV infection are sometimes classified as belonging to subtype II a. These patients, usually children, generally respond to steroid therapy although remission does not occur when steroids are withdrawn.

A subgroup of subtype II, known as type II b occurs in older men and is associated with HCV infection. In this subgroup, serum globulin levels are typically normal and patients respond to interferon treatment. Patients with subtype II b are most likely to show evidence of hepatitis C infection, and they are more likely to have severe symptoms. These patients typically have symptoms primarily associated with chronic HCV infection and they usually do not have antibodies to cytochrome P450 1ID6. They are also likely to respond to treatment with interferon

TYPE III AIH

Subtype III, which is sometimes referred to as a subgroup of subtype I, accounts for less than 5 percent of AIH cases in the United States. It primarily affects adults aged 30–50 years and the female to male ratio is 9:1. About 55–60 percent of patients have a concurrent autoimmune disease and about 70 percent of patients show a good response to steroid therapy. However, about 75 percent of patients eventually progress to cirrhosis.

Patients in this subset usually have no liver antibodies although some patients have antibodies to soluble liver kidney antigen cytokeratins 8 and 18 (anti-SKA) or antibodies to soluble liver antigen/liver pancreas (anti-SLA or anti-SLP). The HLA associations for subtype III have not yet been determined.

Polyglandular syndromes

Autoimmune polyendocrinopathy or polyglandular syndromes are disorders in which patients have several autoimmune glandular diseases, for instance, thyroid and adrenal disorders.

AUTOIMMUNE POLYENDOCRINOPATHY-CANDIDIASIS-ECTODERMAL DYSTROPHY SYNDROME (APECED)

Patients with autoimmune polyendocrinopathy-candidiasis-ectodermal dystrophy (APECED) syndrome have several concurrent autoimmune conditions, including autoimmune hepatitis, hypoparathyroidism (parathyroid gland deficiency), adrenal insufficiency and candida infection (candidiasis). In this syndrome, patients with hepatitis have liver microsome antibodies (anti-LM) that target cytochrome P450 1A2.

APECED is associated with mutations of the autoimmune regulator gene (AIRE) and predominantly affects young patients with a Sardinian, Finnish, or Iranian Jewish ancestry. Treatment consists of hormones to correct the glandular insufficiencies, immunosuppressive therapy for AIH, and ameliorative therapies such as analgesics used to reduce symptoms.

AIH Overlap Syndrome Variants

Up to 20 percent of patients with AIH are reported to have overlap syndromes. In the overlap syndromes, patients have subtype I AIH along with a second autoimmune liver disease, such as primary biliary cirrhosis (PBC), autoimmune cholangitis, or primarily sclerosing cholangitis (PSC). Patients with overlap syndromes typically have an enlarged liver, jaundice and features of cirrhosis, such as spider angiomata and occasionally ascites. Patients with features of PBC, which primarily affects the bile ducts, have a positive test for antimitochondrial antibodies (AMA) and increased stores of liver copper. Patients with features of PBC usually show a favorable response to ursodeoxycholic acid.

Patients with features of PSC usually have symptoms of concurrent inflammatory bowel disease and duct injury is seen on liver biopsy. Antineutrophil cytoplasmic antibodies (ANCA) are seen in 65 percent of patients with PSC and 50 percent of patients with AIH. These antibodies are only rarely seen in PBC.

Patients with AIH may also have coexisting conditions of autoimmune cholangitis. Although tests for AMA are negative in this group, these patients have positive ANA and ASMA tests and biopsy results that show bile duct destruction similar to that seen in PBC.

DIAGNOSIS OF OVERLAP SYNDROMES

The International Autoimmune Hepatitis Group has developed a scoring system to help diagnosis the overlap disorders in patients with subtype I AIH. Patients with overlap syndromes must show evidence of cholestatic (disruption of bile flow) disease, and specific biopsy changes . In addition, patients with overlapping PBC typically have positive anti-mitochondrial antibody (AMA) titers and patients with autoimmune cholangitis have negative AMA titers. A positive response to steroid therapy is also used to confirm the diagnosis of overlap syndrome. Remission in overlap syndromes was most often seen in patients with only modest elevations of alkaline phosphatase (values not elevated more than twice the reference range).

Patients with PBC overlap syndrome are reported to have lower serum levels of immunoglobulin G (IgG) and higher levels of immunoglobulin M (IgM). They are also less likely to have smooth muscle antibodies. Patients with AIH and PBC are usually middle-aged females, similar to most patients who only have PBC.

Patients with PSC overlap syndrome are reported to more likely to also have an additional concurrent autoimmune disorder, usually inflammatory bowel disease and are less likely to achieve remission than patients with AIH alone or AIH and PBC. Patients with PSC overlap are more likely to have positive ANA and smooth muscle antibody (SMA) titers.

Features seen in patients with AIH and autoimmune cholangitis overlap syndrome include a lower AST and a higher alkaline phosphatase level than is seen in most patients with AIH alone. In addition, these patients only rarely have concurrent inflammatory bowel disease.

AIH in Pregnancy

Women with AIH are able to become pregnant and deliver healthy babies especially if they are in remission or their symptoms are well controlled with treatment. These women are often able to reduce or stop prednisone treatment during the second half of pregnancy when the immune system slows down its activities, although if they continue to have flares of symptoms prednisone should be continued.

Women with active disease are much less fertile and are more likely to have complications during pregnancy. Women with active disease or who have already developed cirrhosis as a consequence of AIH have a higher risk of premature delivery and fetal death. However, the babies born to these women are normal.

Mortality rate of AIH

Without treatment, mortality is high with a 50 percent 5-year survival rate. With treatment hepatic fibrosis and cirrhosis may be reversible, and up to 70 percent of patients can achieve remission or be maintained on a low-dose of corticosteroids. In patients treated prior to the onset of cirrhosis, the 10-year survival rate is 90 percent. In patients treated after the onset of cirrhosis, the 10-year survival rate is 65 percent [56].

Symptoms and Signs of AIH

Symptoms and signs in AIH are similar to those seen in viral hepatitis. Similar to viral hepatitis, signs and symptoms can vary depending on the stage of disease. Patients may present as acute hepatitis, fulminant hepatitis, chronic hepatitis or well-established hepatitis with progression to cirrhosis.

About one-third of patients initially present with acute symptoms, including fever, liver tenderness, and jaundice. Of these, a small number may present with fulminant disease. About 20 percent of patients initially present with end-stage cirrhosis, and the remainder show symptoms of chronic hepatitis. Symptoms range from mild liver enzyme elevations to fulminant disease. Abnormal coagulation function tests indicate advanced disease.

Common symptoms of AIH

- Fatigue
- Upper abdominal pain
- Pruritis (itching)
- Myalgia (muscle pain)
- Diarrhea
- Edema or swelling
- Joint pain
- Skin rashes, including acne
- Hirsutism
- Amenorrhea (scant or absent menstrual periods)
- Chest pain from pleuritis
- Weight loss
- Ascites and mental confusion in advanced disease

Signs of AIH

- Jaundice
- Low platelet count (thrombocytopenia)

- Spider angiomatas
- Enlarged liver or spleen
- Elevated liver enzymes
- Elevated serum immunoglobulin levels
- Positive tests for liver autoantibodies, ANA

Diagnosis of AIH

Diagnosis of AIH is made by ruling out other viral or toxic causes of hepatitis and by finding certain abnormal changes on blood test and biopsy results. According to the diagnostic criteria established for AIH, symptoms do not need to be present for six months to diagnose AIH as a chronic condition, certain immunological or serological changes (presence of autoantibodies) must be detected in blood tests, and specific histology changes must be seen on liver biopsy (see chapter fifteen).

Table 10.1 Autoantibodies seen in AIH

- antinuclear antibodies (ANA)—50–80 percent of type 1; not seen in type 2
- anti-smooth muscle antibody (SMA)—50–70 percent of type 1; not seen in type 2
- antiasialoglycoprotein receptor antibody (anti-ASGPR)—80 percent of type 1
- anti-liver-kidney microsomal antibody type 1 (LKM-1)—primarily seen in type 2
- anti-liver cytosol 1 antigen (LC1)
- anti-neutrophil cytoplasmic antibodies (ANCA)
- anti-soluble liver antigen (cytokeratin)
- anti-soluble liver antigens or liver pancreas (SLA/LP)
- anti-liver microsomal antibodies (LM)
- anti-liver specific proteins (LSP)—found in AIH and HAV infection
- anti-mitochrondrial antibodies (AMA)—low titer in 20 percent of type 1 AIH and high titers seen in nearly all patients with PBC.

The presence of anti-ASGPR is associated with relapse, and patients with anti-actin-specific smooth muscle antibodies are younger and tend to have more aggressive disease. Antibodies to LKM1 primarily occur in subtype 2 and are directed against components of cytochrome P450 1A2.

Enzyme and protein changes in AIH

The transaminase liver enzymes ALT and AST are generally increased two to ten times the upper limit of normal. Serum gamma globulin levels can be increased as much as two times normal and generally fall within the range of 3–5 mg/dl.

Liver antibody changes

Occasionally, the immune response in viral hepatitis also induces the production of liver antibodies. Up to 40 percent of patients with chronic HBV and HCV may have low liver antibody titers, generally less than 1:160 of SMA or LKM antibodies. Because steroid treatment for AIH can worsen symptoms of viral hepatitis by promoting viral replication, and interferon treatment for viral hepatitis can worsen AIH, it's important to run both liver antibody and viral marker tests in patients with suspected hepatitis to determine the definitive cause. In the rare event that both chronic viral hepatitis and AIH are present, steroid treatment is usually effective [45].

Simultaneous autoimmune conditions

Up to seventeen percent of patients with AIH are reported to have a second autoimmune disorder, predominantly autoimmune thyroid disease. Other autoimmune disorders seen in association with AIH include pernicious anemia, autoimmune hemolytic anemia, rheumatoid arthritis, ulcerative colitis, myasthenia gravis, Sjogren's syndrome, glomerulonephritis, Hashimoto's thyroiditis, Graves' disease, gluten sensitivity enteropathy (celiac disease), vitiligo, and type I diabetes. These disorders, like AIH, are associated with certain HLA markers, particularly HLA-B8, HLA-DR3 and HLA-DR4 although the incidence of HLA markers can vary among different ethnic groups.

Liver biopsy in AIH

Liver biopsies are used to help diagnose AIH and evaluate the extent of liver damage. Liver biopsies in AIH show a characteristic periportal inflammation with piecemeal necrosis and prominent plasma cell infiltration of the portal tracts. Liver biopsy is the only test that can determine the extent of inflammation and tissue damage present. Liver biopsy changes in AIH are described further in chapter fifteen.

Definite or probable AIH

Because elevated liver enzymes or autoantibody tests can be seen in other disorders, diagnosis of AIH has been subject to various pitfalls. To aid in diagnosing AIH, international experts have developed a weighting system. According to criteria designated in 1999, patients are diagnosed as either having definite or probable AIH depending on certain weighted factors. The cumulative scores are used to determine if AIH is definite or probable (high scores), whereas very low scores rule out a diagnosis of AIH. Definite and probable scores indicate that treatment should be recommended.

Table 10.2 Positive weighting factors for AIH diagnosis

- Female
- High AST and ALT; low ALP
- Elevated gamma globulin levels
- ANA, SMA or LKM antibodies
- Negative HBV and HCV viral markers
- Negative drug history
- Low alcohol use
- Liver biopsy results suggestive of AIH
- Concurrent autoimmune disease or family history
- Positive for relevant HLA markers
- Positive corticosteroid treatment response

Table 10.3 Negative weighting factors for AIH diagnosis

- High ALP and low AST and ALT
- AMA positive (suggesting primary biliary cirrhosis)
- History of drug abuse
- Alcohol abuse
- Liver biopsy inconsistent with AIH

Risk Factors for AIH

Autoimmune hepatitis often occurs following infection with the hepatitis A, B, C, and D viruses. AIH development also frequently occurs in patients who have been treated with interferon therapy, particularly female patients with chronic hepatitis C. The use of interferon is suspected of triggering latent AIH.

AIH may also occur after withdrawal of prednisone in patients who have had liver transplants. In this case, the incidence of AIH development increases over time as immunosuppressant therapy is reduced.

Treatment of AIH

Most patients with AIH are treated with immunosuppressant drugs that slow down the immune response. However, patients who are free of symptoms but have abnormal blood test results at presentation have a good prognosis and may not require specific treatments.

Corticosteroids such as prednisone, which also have anti-inflammatory properties, are usually used in AIH for extended periods. In addition, the immunosuppressant medications azathioprine, 6-mercaptopurine, cyclosporine, mycophenylate mofetil, tacrolimus, and similar medications may also be used in conjunction with corticosteroids or as the sole therapy. Several studies have established that the non-steroid therapies listed, which may have fewer side effects compared to steroids, can effectively decrease symptoms and signs of fatigue, loss of appetite and fever and improve biochemical markers such as liver enzymes.

Patients with AIH may also be treated with ursodeoxycholic acid (UDCA), a compound primarily used for patients with primary biliary cirrhosis. UDCA can reduce liver inflammation and liver damage and reduce symptoms associated with high bilirubin levels, such as itching and rash. UDCA is essentially free of side effects and at a dosage of 500 mg used twice daily it can be used long-term.

Treatment response

The response to treatment can be evaluated by monitoring liver enzyme and gamma globulin levels. Usually, treatment must be continued indefinitely. However, in about one-third of patients immunosuppressant medications may be gradually tapered and withdrawn as liver enzyme and gamma globulin levels return to normal.

In about 70 percent of patients, the disease goes into remission with a lessening of severity of symptoms within two years of starting treatment. Some of these people will experience relapse within three years and therapy must then be continued. The use of interferon has been found to worsen the disease course in AIH.

Immunosuppressant medications can cause serious side effects that must also be managed. Usually, side effects are dose-related and may not develop until after prolonged use of these compounds. Possible side effects include weight gain, anxiety, nausea, low white blood cell count (leukopenia), confusion, thinning of bones, thinning of hair and skin, hypertension, diabetes, cataracts and glaucoma.

Liver transplants are often recommended at earlier stages of disease to prevent severe complications from developing. However, although its incidence is low, a recurrence of AIH can occur in the graft tissue. Transplantation has a 1-year survival rate of 90 percent, and a 5-year survival rate of 70 to 80 percent.

11

Alcohol, Drugs & Toxins

Physicians have long known that drugs and chemicals react differently in different people. All substances can act as toxins. With considerable variation between different individuals, a certain dose can make the difference between a poison and a remedy. Toxins include numerous chemicals that damage the body's cells and organs and interfere with their functions. Some toxins are indiscriminate, affecting any of the body's cells that they encounter. Other toxins target specific organs, primarily those which they have most contact with. Because chemicals that enter the body ultimately travel to the liver, the liver is the organ most often affected by these substances.

Hepatotoxins are substances with the propensity to injure or destroy the liver and its cells. Hepatotoxins include alcohol, environmental chemicals, more than one thousand medications, herbal preparations, recreational drugs, and chemicals known as endotoxins that are produced and released by bacteria during the course of infection.

Chapter eleven serves as an introduction to toxic hepatitis, including hepatitis caused by drugs, alcohol, supplements and environmental chemicals. In this chapter readers will learn about the various plant-derived and synthetic chemicals capable of injuring the liver, and they'll learn about other factors that influence the development of toxic hepatitis. In addition, this chapter includes a description of the various types of liver damage caused by hepatotoxins.

The Liver and Detoxification

The liver normally detoxifies or breaks down (metabolizes) chemical substances that enter the body, especially substances administered orally. Normally, the liver is able to remove these chemicals from the blood circulation and, through a process of biotransformation, transform them into chemical metabolites that can be eliminated from the body through bile or urine.

Although the process of drug metabolism is usually uneventful, many serious reactions occur each year. Some of these reactions cause hepatitis and other forms of liver disease. In some cases, damage to the liver results in fatality. About 2 percent of all cases of jaundice in hospitalized patients are drug induced [56]. About 25 percent of fulminant hepatic failure in the United States is related to drug toxicity.

Physiologic Effects of Drugs and Chemicals

Drugs have chemical properties that allow them to react with the cells of living organisms. As drugs react with these cells, they cause specific effects. For instance, drugs known as analgesics can block the chemical messages that cause impulses of pain. Antibiotic and anti-viral molecules destroy the cell walls of certain bacteria and viruses or interfere with their replication cycles.

To achieve their intended effects, drugs must be absorbed by the body and then transported and distributed to certain sites in the body. Drugs also have a property of fate. That is, drugs are effective for specific periods of time before they're transported to the liver, metabolized, and excreted.

Pharmacology and pharmacodynamics

Pharmacology is a science that studies drugs and their properties. Before the 20th century, most drugs were derived from plants, and the extracted drugs retained the botanical properties of these plants. For example, digitalis, still used today, is a chemical compound derived from the foxglove plant that affects the conduction of heart muscle.

Today, in the United States, most drugs are synthetic (chemically manufactured). Whether they are derived from plants or manufactured, drugs are formulated into compounds with specific drug concentrations that usually have predictable effects.

Pharmacodynamics is the scientific study of the action of specific drugs on living organisms. It focuses on the physiological responses of drugs, and their absorption, fate, metabolism by the liver, and excretion.

Toxicology

Toxicology is the scientific study of the noxious effects of drugs and chemicals. Toxic effects can be caused directly by chemicals as they interact with the body's cells and indirectly by the intermediate compounds or

ALCOHOL DISRUPTS METABOLISM BY INTERFERING WITH THE NAD / NADH RATIOS

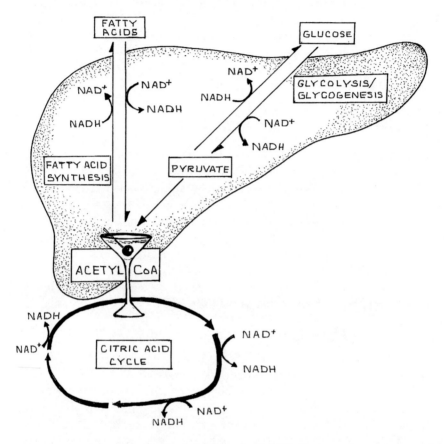

Alcohol toxicity (Marvin G. Miller).

metabolites produced as the drug is processed by the liver. Toxicity can also be cause by immune system cells and chemicals reacting to drugs and their metabolites. Toxic effects can also occur when drug metabolism is impaired and drugs and their metabolites accumulate in the liver.

Drug Metabolism

Drugs entering the liver are either eliminated unchanged or they are transformed into compounds that can be dissolved in water (made water soluble). This change or biotransformation facilitates the elimination of drug molecules through urine or bile. The biotransformation of drugs occurs in two separate steps known as phase I and phase II reactions. Some drugs only require one of these reactions for metabolism.

Cytochrome P450 (CYP) genes and enzymes

Cytochrome P450 (CYP 450) is a superfamily of three genes, P450 I, P450 II, and P 450 III, with nearly 300 subtypes. A person's ability to metabolize drugs varies, depending on their CYP 450 genes.

These genes control the 50 or more CYP P450 enzymes that are essential for phase I drug metabolism. These enzymes are found primarily in the liver, within the smooth endoplasmic reticulum component of liver cells and in lesser amounts in the cells of the gastrointestinal tract, kidneys, brain, and other tissues.

FUNCTION OF CYP 450 ENZYMES

Cytochrome P450 enzymes are proteins that cause specific chemical reactions that alter the chemical structure of drugs. For instance, CYP 450 enzymes can shift oxygen molecules from cellular energy and link these molecules to the chemical molecules present in drugs. In this manner, CYP 450 enzymes alter the chemical properties of the drug and transform or convert it into new compounds known as metabolites. Each CYP 450 enzyme reacts with specific chemical molecules. Consequently, each enzyme can react with one or more, but not all, drugs.

The CYP 450 genes also control the rate of the drug's chemical reaction. This causes some people to metabolize specific drugs quickly and other people to have an idiosyncratic untoward reaction caused by faulty metabolism of the drug.

ENZYME INDUCTION

Certain compounds are known to induce or increase production of specific CYP 450 enzymes. Enzyme induction can increase the production of toxic metabolites. For instance, alcohol induces the induction of P450-II-E1 enzymes. These enzymes are known to produce toxic acetaminophen metabolites when acetaminophen is ingested. Thus, the toxicity of acetaminophen is increased when it's taken together with alcohol.

The metabolic process

Drug metabolism is a process in which drugs are detoxified and transformed into compounds that can be excreted. Drug metabolism occurs in several steps, including phase I and II reactions and also through metabolism of the antioxidant glutathione.

PHASE I REACTIONS

In phase I reactions, drugs are transformed by specific CYP 450 and related enzymes into structurally similar polar (water soluble) compounds known as metabolites that they can be excreted in urine. Drugs that induce phase I enzymes include barbiturates, alcohol, and several drugs used to reduce glucose levels in diabetics and several drugs used to reduce seizure activity (anticonvulsants).

During phase I reactions, alcohol is transformed into a chemical known as acetaldehyde by the enzyme alcohol dehydrogenase. Genetic differences in alcohol dehydrogenase levels impair this process and contribute to liver damage in alcohol abuse. This is why people have different tolerances for alcohol.

PHASE II REACTIONS

In phase II reactions the transformed drug molecules or metabolites are linked to a naturally occurring attachment of chemicals, for instance, a sulfate group. This reaction or chemical process transforms drug metabolites into compounds with even greater polarity. These transformed molecules react with other molecules that facilitate their transport from the liver into urine or bile.

Certain compounds undergo chemical processes known as glucuronidation (attachment of a combined oxygen and hydrogen molecule) before they can be excreted. Examples of these compounds include acetaminophen (Tylenol and related products), morphine, and the diuretic furosemide. Phase II reactions can occasionally lead to toxic byproducts or carcinogenic (cancer causing) byproducts.

Electrophilic metabolites

During drug metabolism, enzymes can cause the production of electrophilic metabolites, which are chemical byproducts that seek out and bind with the amino acid glutathione. When glutathione levels are low, levels of electrophilic metabolites are high. Excess electrophilic metabolites injure liver cells, interfering with their function and causing necrosis. This is the underlying mechanism in acetaminophen toxicity.

Drug metabolites can also release destructive free radicals (unattached chemical molecules). The free radicals can attach to proteins found on the surface of liver cells. This causes a condition of lipid peroxidation, which damages the liver cell membrane causing necrosis. Free radicals are known to cause the greatest necrosis in zone 3 of the liver, where drug metabolizing enzymes are found in the highest concentration.

GLUTATHIONE METABOLISM

Glutathione is a naturally occurring antioxidant compound rich in sulfur. Glutathione levels are typically decreased in illness, especially disorders associated with wasting such as AIDS. Glutathione is not absorbed from food or supplements although it can be converted from dietary sulfur compounds and cysteine-containing drugs such as N-acetylcysteine (NAC).

Glutathione molecules attach to potentially harmful electrophilic compounds produced during drug metabolism, including those produced during acetaminophen overdoses. As glutathione stores are depleted, these toxic compounds accumulate. Glutathione can also be depleted by alcohol ingestion and fasting. Both conditions contribute to drug toxicity. The compound NAC is an effective treatment for acetaminophen toxicity if administered early in the disease course.

Development of hepatocellular necrosis

Necrosis is a term describing cell death. Hepatocellular necrosis, which is liver cell death, is characterized by cell swelling and rupture or lysis. In contrast to apoptosis, which is a programmed cell death that can be accelerated by some toxins, necrosis is associated with disintegration of the cell membrane. The cellular contents, including normal components and toxins, are thereby released, causing inflammation and contributing to toxicity.

Intrinsic toxins, idiosyncratic toxins, depleted stores of glutathione, the immune system response to toxic drug molecules, and the production of electrophilic metabolites all cause hepatocellular necrosis. As the liver cells are destroyed, functional liver tissue becomes depleted and hepatitis develops. Other organs, especially the kidneys, are also affected in drug toxicity.

Hepatic necrosis is usually dose-dependent, although some drugs cause zone 3 necrosis in a small number of people even when low doses are given. In mild cases, jaundice may be slight and transient. In overdoses, cellular destruction is rapid, causing marked rises in transaminase enzymes and prothrombin levels.

Metabolic influences

Drug bioavailabilty, or the amount of drug available to the body's cells before being transported to the liver, depends on several factors. These include hepatic blood flow and the efficiency of liver cells to remove drugs from the blood circulation.

Drug metabolism in liver disease

When liver cell function is impaired because of liver disease, drug metabolism is affected. In liver disease drug metabolism slows down and toxic compounds and drug metabolites can accumulate within the liver.

Development of Liver Toxicity

Hepatotoxins are capable of causing injury, but many hepatotoxins only affect a small number of people. In these people, toxicity is caused by rare idiosyncratic or unpredictable effects. This explains why drugs deemed safe in clinical trials involving thousands of patients are later found to have toxic effects after being introduced into the general population. In some cases, hepatotoxins only cause injury when high doses are used. Certain factors are known to promote the development of toxic hepatitis.

Table 11.1. Factors influencing the development of toxic hepatitis

- Individuals with genetic alterations of metabolic CYP 450 enzymes
- Enzyme induction by other drugs or chemicals, such as alcohol and cigarettes
- The dose or amount of toxin ingested
- Simultaneous ingestion of other hepatotoxins or drugs that alter drug metabolism
- General health; kidney and liver diseases can impair drug metabolism
- Glutathione depletion by fasting and alcohol ingestion
- Age, with drug toxicity more likely to occur in persons older than 50 years; children rarely develop drug toxicity except in the case of accidental overdoses and valproic acid toxicity. Elderly persons experience decreased disposition of drugs undergoing phase 1 but not phase 2 biotransformation caused by diminished hepatic volume and reduced liver blood flow.

Drug-Induced Hepatitis

Drug-induced hepatitis is a condition of liver inflammation and injury caused by many different drugs and chemical toxins. Drug-induced hepatitis occurs in approximately eight of every 10,000 people. Women are affected twice as often as men, and older people are more likely to be affected because their bodies lack the restorative properties of younger people.

All drugs have the potential to cause toxicity, and nearly every drug manufactured has been implicated in causing hepatic toxicity. Some drugs such as acetaminophen are well known for their hepatotoxic potential. Most toxic liver injury results from the reaction of drugs or their metabolites with cell proteins or DNA. If reactive compounds accumulate in the liver, they interfere with cellular oxidation and ultimately destroy cells.

Alternately, certain drugs can induce the production of intermediate compounds and free radicals that contribute to cellular injury. Hepatotoxins may cause liver cell damage, arrested bile flow, or both of these symptoms. Liver cell injury is caused by three different primary physiological responses: direct and indirect toxicity by intrinsic hepatotoxins; idiosyncratic reactions; and by immune system effects.

Intrinsic hepatotoxins — direct and indirect toxicity

Direct toxicity is considered a predictable side effect of certain drugs and chemicals. These chemicals can act as intrinsic hepatotoxins after sufficient bodily exposure. Intrinsic hepatotoxins are recognized by the high incidence of hepatic injury they cause in persons exposed to them and by similar reactions observed in animals under experimental conditions. In the past, occupational chemical exposures caused most intrinsic liver damage, whereas today medications are the primary cause.

Examples of direct toxins include cleaning solvents, *Amanita* mushrooms, carbon tetrachloride, the anticonvulsant valproic acid (Depakene), the cardiac drug amiodarone, the chemotherapeutic agent methotrexate, the anesthetic agent halothane, oral contraceptives, and the analgesic acetaminophen. Intrinsic hepatotoxins can cause necrosis, fibrosis, cholestasis, circulatory problems, angiosarcoma (tumors of blood vessels and tissue), and fatty liver disease.

Indirect toxicity is caused by intrinsic hepatotoxins when they interfere with specific metabolic pathways rather than directly injuring liver cells.

Idiosyncratic reactions

Idiosyncratic reactions are unpredictable responses that occur in a very small number of exposed individuals. Idiosyncratic reactions, which are sometimes called hypersensitivity reactions, are primarily caused by genetic changes affecting the metabolism of specific chemical compounds and immune system reactions, and they do not seem to be related to drug dosage.

Idiosyncratic hepatotoxins can cause hepatitis, cholestasis, and granuloma (type of tumor) formation. Drugs causing idiosyncratic reactions include the anti-tuberculosis drug isoniazid, the tranquilizer chlorpromazine (Thorazine), and the anti-inflammatory agent phenylbutazone. Idiosyncratic reactions typically develop after a fixed incubation period of 1–5 weeks and they recur quickly when the offending drug is re-administered (challenge). Idiosyncratic reactions may be accompanied by fever, rash, elevated counts of eosinophilic white blood cells, a type of cell also increased in allergic reactions.

Immune system effects

In some people the immune system responds to noxious substances by launching an idiosyncratic immune response. As a result, white blood cells produce and secrete cytotoxic chemicals that contribute to liver cell injury and inflammation. This response is seen in less than .01 percent of the population and occurs twice as frequently in women.

Multiple medications — polydrug syndrome

Multiple drugs taken at about the same time compete for enzyme binding sites in the body. This causes the drug with lower affinity for absorption to be metabolized more slowly. This prolongs its action and causes the active drug to stay in the blood circulation longer. With multiple doses, drug concentrations can rise to toxic levels.

Incidence of Toxic Hepatitis

Hepatotoxins can cause liver injury resembling every type of naturally occurring liver disease, including hepatitis, steatosis (fatty liver), cholestasis (impaired bile flow), vascular liver injury, and liver tumors. About 10 percent of all cases of hepatitis are due to toxins, and most toxic hepatitis today results from adverse drug reactions [71]. In persons older than 50 years, adverse drug effects are responsible for about 40 percent of all hepatitis cases. Up to 25 percent of cases of fulminant hepatic failure may be attributed to adverse medicinal reactions.

Effects of Hepatotoxins

Specific hepatotoxins are associated with a specific type of liver injury. For instance the industrial chemical carbon tetrachloride causes severe zone 3 necrosis and fatty infiltration. Yellow phosphorus compounds produce zone 1 liver damage, and *Amanita* mushrooms causes a fatal hemorrhagic form of necrosis. Biopsy results help pinpoint the responsible hepatotoxin based on its known cellular effects.

Acute hepatitis

Toxic hepatitis occurs in only a very small proportion of persons taking a particular drug. With the exception of overdoses, the drug reaction in acute hepatitis is more likely to occur after multiple exposures. In acute toxicity, symptoms typically occur about one week after exposure. Most toxic hepatitis occurs as an acute inflammatory process that resolves when the drug is withdrawn.

Acute hepatitis is usually caused by toxic metabolites that either injure the liver or evoke a destructive immune response. An individual drug can cause more than one type of reaction and symptoms of acute hepatitis, cholestatic disease, and hypersensitivity reactions may overlap.

Fulminant hepatitis

Some cases of acute hepatitis, particularly those occurring in older women, emerge as fulminant reactions with a high mortality rate. About a quarter of all cases of fulminant hepatitis are caused by adverse drug reactions. Patients with acute, fulminant drug-related liver failure often require liver transplants for survival.

Liver failure

Liver failure can occur as a result of fulminant hepatitis caused by drugs and bacterial endotoxins. An example of a bacterial toxin is that produced by *Staphylococcus aureus* in cases of septic shock syndrome, which can cause liver failure.

Chronic hepatitis

Although most drug-related hepatitis causes acute hepatitis, certain drugs can cause a chronic form of hepatitis even after the drug is withdrawn. One example is chlorpromazine, a tranquilizer that rarely causes chronic liver disease. Similar reactions have been reported with tricyclic antidepressants such as amitriptyline, the antibiotic erythromycin estolate, and several other drugs.

Isoniazid, methyldopa, clometacin, and nitrofurantoin can all cause ongoing liver damage and chronic hepatitis. A chronic form of hepatitis with scarring and fibrosis can also occur in patients using long-term low doses of acetaminophen. This is more likely to occur in patients who abuse alcohol. The heart medication amiodarone can cause chronic hepatitis that causes liver tissue changes similar to those seen in alcoholism, such as the presence of Mallory bodies in biopsy specimens.

A sclerosing form of hepatitis can occur in patients receiving intra-arterial infusions of certain chemotherapeutic agents, especially floxuri-dine, and it has been reported in patients following liver transplants. Long-term methotrexate therapy for arthritis or psoriasis is known to cause chronic liver fibrosis. The clinical picture in chronic disease is similar to that of autoimmune hepatitis. However, in drug induced chronic hepati-tis, improvement usually occurs when the drug is withdrawn.

Alcohol and Acetaminophen

Alcohol and acetaminophen are both intrinsic hepatotoxins capable of causing hepatitis ranging from mild disease to fatal injury depending on the circumstances. These two compounds are responsible for the majority of drug-induced liver disease. Their contributions to liver disease are described in the following sections.

Alcohol and the liver

Ethyl alcohol or ethanol is an intrinsic hepatotoxin. Alcoholic liver disease (ALD) is one of the major medical complications of alcohol abuse. ALD can result in alcoholic hepatitis, fatty infiltration of the liver, cirrho-sis, accelerated progression of other liver diseases, a higher incidence of liver cancer, and liver failure. Approximately 90–100 percent of heavy drinkers show evidence of fatty liver, and transient episodes of fatty liver can occur after binge drinking. About 10–35 percent of heavy drinkers develop alcoholic hepatitis, and 8–20 percent develop cirrhosis.

The safe limits for alcohol intake are controversial and likely depend somewhat on the individual's genetic makeup, size, diet, and other factors. In general, 210 grams of alcohol in men and 140 grams of alcohol in women each week are considered safe amounts. The average intake in patients who develop cirrhosis is 160 grams/day for approximately 8 years. Symp-toms of ALD range from asymptomatic to behavioral changes and the incidental findings of elevated liver enzymes. In overt disease, patients may have jaundice, ascites, spider veins, palmar erythema, testicular atro-phy, and gynecomastia (enlarged breasts in males due to increased estro-gen levels).

Studies show that alcohol only injures the liver in the presence of polyunsaturated fatty acids, and carbohydrates have a protective effect on alcohol-induced liver injury. If polyunsaturated fats are absent from the diet, the liver is not injured [31]. However, diseases related to fatty acid deficiency can occur, and alcohol ingestion increases the dietary require-ments for specific nutrients, particularly B vitamins.

Table 11.2. Risk factors that
increase susceptibility to ALD

Female gender
Lifetime intake of alcohol
Genetic factors
Drinking without eating
Binge drinking
High concentration alcoholic drinks
Consuming multiple types of alcohol

ALCOHOLIC STEATOSIS

Steatosis, a condition of fatty liver, is the most prevalent type of alcoholic liver disease. Steatosis invariably occurs when alcohol intake exceeds 80 grams/day. In steatosis, the liver cell cytoplasm is displaced by triglycerides. Liver function can remain normal until steatosis impairs liver function. With abstinence, steatosis is reversible.

ALCOHOLIC HEPATITIS

Alcoholic hepatitis typically occurs after 15–20 years of excessive drinking although it can occur much sooner. Factors influencing disease development include the quantity of alcohol consumed, the individual's nutritional status, and genetic and metabolic traits. It tends to be more severe in females and in Northern European descendants. Alcoholic hepatitis is characterized by hepatocellular necrosis, fibrosis, and inflammation, frequently accompanied by cholestasis. Fatty change is usual but it is not invariably present. The mortality rate is 30–60 percent, and patients often deteriorate after diagnosis, even if they abstain from alcohol. Alcoholic hepatitis is considered the first step in the development of alcoholic cirrhosis.

The major physiological cause of liver damage in ALD is cellular toxicity and necrosis caused by acetaldehyde, the primary metabolite of alcohol. Ethanol is oxidized to acetaldehyde inside liver cell mitochondria by the enzyme alcohol dehydrogenase. Acetaldehyde is then oxidized and transformed into acetate by the enzyme acetaldehyde dehydrogenase. These metabolites alter liver cell metabolism and promote fatty accumulations. Malnutrition and nutrient deficiencies also contribute to the disease process. Free radicals directly injure liver cells and invoke a cellular immune response, which also contributes to liver injury.

ALCOHOL AND VIRAL HEPATITIS

Epidemiologic data show that the hepatitis B virus (HBV) and the hepatitis C virus (HCV) are important factors in the development of ALD. Evidence of HBV, including the presence of HBsAg, is more prevalent in patients with ALD than in the general population. This suggests a higher than expected incidence of HBV infection in heavy drinkers. Infection with HBV or HCV in patients with ALD is associated with accelerated liver damage and lower survival rates compared with uninfected patients [7].

Studies suggest that the risk of alcoholic hepatitis proceeding to alcoholic cirrhosis varies from 10–20 percent. Patients who progress to cirrhosis are more likely to have HBV or HCV markers, and patients with ALD who have these markers are also more likely to develop hepatocellular carcinoma (HCC) at a younger age than people without evidence of viral hepatitis [7].

Synergism refers to effects that are greater when two factors are combined than if the individual effects of each factor were combined. The apparent synergistic effects of alcohol and viral hepatitis are also demonstrated by the fact that infected ALD patients are more likely to develop complications of liver disease, such as hepatic encephalopathy.

Acetaminophen and the liver

Acetaminophen is a safe analgesic, even in patients with liver disease, when used in recommended amounts, typically 2 grams daily or less. Taken as an overdose or as a therapeutic misadventure in which excessive doses are used, acetaminophen is the most common drug-induced cause of liver failure.

Normally, acetaminophen is efficiently metabolized. In the phase I reaction, about 90–95 percent of the drug is converted by glucuronide and sulfate pathways into inactive metabolites, and about 10 percent is converted into an intermediate, highly reactive, electrophilic metabolite known as N-acetyl-p-benzoquinone amine (NABQI). In the phase II reaction, NABQI is detoxified by glutathione substrate, converted into a nontoxic compound (mercapturic acid) and excreted.

ACETAMINOPHEN TOXICITY

In overdoses, high levels of acetaminophen deplete the glucuronide and sulfate pathways. This causes more of the drug to be converted into the toxic NABQI. Levels of NABQI quickly deplete glutathione. In the absence of glutathione, NABQI react with the thiol groups of liver proteins, injuring the cells and causing necrosis. When alcohol or other enzyme inducers are ingested and during periods of starvation, there is even less available glutathione and cellular necrosis is accelerated.

The reaction of toxic acetaminophen metabolites with liver proteins causes a diffuse type of necrosis. When large amounts of acetaminophen are ingested, massive necrosis occurs and leads to complete liver failure. Other effects of acetaminophen toxicity include acute tubular necrosis (kidney tissue destruction), pancreatitis, and myocardial necrosis (heart muscle destruction).

Studies show that at therapeutic doses as low as 150 mg daily, gene changes can occur that increase susceptibility to liver injury when higher doses or other hepatotoxins are consumed. The usual adult dose of acetaminophen is 1,000 mg (one gram) taken every 4 hours. Doses as high as 4 grams daily are generally considered safe although people with liver disease or who abuse alcohol are advised to limit daily use to 2 grams.

Viral hepatitis, and other drugs besides alcohol that induce cytochrome P450 enzymes can predispose individuals to acetaminophen toxicity. These drugs include barbiturates, phenytoin, carbamazepine, rifampin, isoniazid, Phenobarbital and omeprazole.

SUICIDAL OVERDOSE AND THERAPEUTIC MISADVENTURES

In fatal intentional overdoses and accidental therapeutic misadventures, the dose of acetaminophen usually ranges from 7 to 70 grams. The extent of injury is usually dose-related. In some cases, biochemical changes indicating toxicity do not occur until 24–36 hours after ingestion. Toxicity usually occurs in 4 phases.

Table 11.3. Phases of acetaminophen toxicity in overdoses

Phase 1) within 2–24 hours after ingestion, symptoms of nausea, vomiting, and loss of appetite occur; patients with acetaminophen concentrations higher than 300 mg/dl at 4 hours post ingestion, and higher than 15 mg/dl at 15 hours post ingestion, have a 90 percent risk of developing serious or fatal liver damage.

Phase 2) within 24–48 hours after ingestion, symptoms improve, but evidence of hepatic injury develops with transaminase enzyme, bilirubin, and prothrombin levels beginning to increase; right upper quadrant pain and liver enlargement may occur and urine output may increase;

Phase 3) within 72–96 hours after ingestion, nauseas and vomiting may recur or worsen and be accompanied by malaise, jaundice, and mental changes, including confusion, sedation, and coma; liver function declines and enzyme levels peak, with AST often exceeding 10,000 IU/L;

Phase 4) within 6–7 days after ingestion, resolution of hepatic damage occurs, and liver function tests return to normal. About 1–2 percent of patients, especially those who do not receive treatment, fail to show signs of recovery and usually progress to liver failure.

Acetaminophen levels. Risk of hepatotoxicity is typically assessed in suspected overdoses using a Rumack-Matthew nomogram that relates the blood acetaminophen level to hours passed since ingestion. For instance, an acetaminophen level of 150 mg/dl 2 hours after ingestion indicates toxicity. The nomogram is helpful for assessing toxicity, but it presumes a known time of dosage, no concomitant risk factors for liver disease, and it assumes that only a single dose of acetaminophen and no other drugs were ingested.

Treatment of acetaminophen toxicity. The primary treatment for acetaminophen toxicity is N-acetylcysteine (NAC), an amino acid that restores glutathione levels. Better results are observed the earlier that treatment is started. Optimal treatment should begin within 24–30 hours after drug ingestion, using 150 mg/kg NAC intravenously. The dose is reduced the second day, using 100 mg/kg over 16 hours until the patient has three consecutive normal prothrombin time levels.

Other treatments used in overdoses include charcoal lavage, which binds and absorbs acetaminophen that is still in the stomach, ventilators as supportive therapy, hemodialysis, plasmapheresis to rapidly dilute and reduce blood levels, and nutritional supplements.

Mortality in acetaminophen overdoses. Studies show that patients with acetaminophen-induced liver injury who have higher levels of the liver protein alpha fetoprotein (AFP) are more likely to survive the injury without undergoing liver transplants. AFP levels less than 3.9 ug/L 24 hours after overdose are highly predictive of death. Prothrombin levels with an INR ratio greater than 2.4 at 24 hours post exposure are also highly predictive of mortality.

Hepatotoxins and Types of Liver Injury

Hepatotoxins are often classified according to their status as intrinsic or idiosyncratic toxins. However, because most toxins cause a specific type of liver injury, some systems of classification group toxins together according to the primary type of liver injury they induce.

Direct and idiosyncratic effects

Usually, although there are notable exceptions, intrinsic hepatotoxins cause zonal necrosis (liver cell destruction occurring in specific regions of the liver). Unlike the necrosis seen in viral hepatitis, drug-induced necrosis is usually accompanied by only slight inflammation.

Idiosyncratic toxins are similar to hepatitis viruses in their ability to cause diffuse and, in severe cases, massive necrosis. In cases of massive necrosis, the liver tissue suffers complete diffuse cellular destruction with complete tissue collapse.

Steatosis

Some drugs cause abnormal accumulations of liver fat, causing a condition of steatosis. Steatosis may be characterized by small microvesicular or large macrovesicular fat droplets. In some cases, abnormal accumulations of phospholipid fats are found in the liver, causing conditions of phospholipidiosis.

Vascular liver injury

The liver's vascular system (veins, arteries, sinusoids, capillaries) may be damaged in drug toxicity. Blood vessels may be dilated and stretched, or occluded and blocked by scar tissue. For example, anabolic and contraceptive steroids can cause focal dilation of zone 1 sinusoids, a condition causing enlarged liver, abdominal pain, and liver enzyme elevations. The condition improves when the hormones are stopped. In contrast, azathioprine administered after renal transplants may result in fibrosis and cirrhosis 1–3 years later.

PELIOSIS HEPATITIS

Peliosis hepatitis is characterized by large blood-filled cavities that may be lined with random distributions of sinusoidal cells. Red blood cells can pass through these cavities and, over time, fibrosis can develop. Peliosis has been reported in patients taking oral contraceptives, androgenic and anabolic steroids, and tamoxifen.

VENO-OCCLUSIVE DISEASE (VOC)

The earliest reports of VOC came from Jamaica and were caused by toxic injury to small hepatic veins by pyrrolidizine alkaloids taken as senecio in medicinal bush teas. Later instances, some of which were related to contaminated wheat, have been reported in India, Israel, Egypt and Arizona.

Rhabdomyolysis

Rhabdomyolysis is a condition of muscle fiber breakdown caused by injury from toxins, shock, and burns, and it may occur as a complication of hyperthermia (heat stroke). In up to 10 percent of patients with hyperthermia, liver damage contributes to death. Liver damage is characterized by microvesicular fat deposits, congestion, necrosis, cholestasis, and blocked or occluded blood vessels.

COCAINE

Cocaine toxicity is caused by production of a hepatotoxic metabolite, norcocaine nitroxide. This highly reactive metabolite causes liver injury by peroxidation, free radical formation, and by binding to hepatic proteins. Up to 59 percent of patients with cocaine intoxication that develop rhabdomyolysis show evidence of liver damage. Changes include necrosis in zones 1,2, or 3 and accumulations of microvesicular fat in zone 1 [56].

Granulomas

Up to 60 different drugs, including penicillin, ampicillin, sulfasalazine, cotrimoxazole (Septrin), and pyrimethamine-sulfadoxine (Fansidar), may also cause granulomas, which are tumors composed of inflammatory tissue and white blood cells [71]. In the following lists, drugs and environmental chemicals that cause similar types of liver injury are grouped together.

Table 11.4. Hepatotoxins that cause toxic hepatitis

Acebutalol	Mephenytoin
Acetaminophen	Methyldopa
Allopurinol	Metoprolol
Amitriptyline	Naproxen
Anabolic steroids	Nifedipine
Atenolol	Oral contraceptives
Carbamazepine (Tegretol)	Oxyphenisatin laxatives
Chloramphenicol	Penicillamine
Chlorpropamide	Phenytoin (Dilantin)
Chlorzoxazone	Phenacemide
Cincophen	Phenobarbital
Cocaine	Piroxicam
Colchicine	Pirprofen
Dantrolene	Retinoids
Diclofenac	Rifampin
Ecstacy (MDMA)	Salicylates (aspirin)
Erythromycin	Statins (cholesterol-lowering)
Etretinate	Sulfa compounds
Fenoprofen	Sulindac
Gold compounds	Trichloroethylene (found in glue)
Halothane	Urethane
Ibuprofen	Valproic acid
Indomethacin	Vitamin A
Isoniazid	Zidovudine
Ketoconazole	

Table 11.5. Hepatotoxins that produce hepatic necrosis without steatosis

Acetaminophen
Aniline dyes
Beryllium compounds
Dioxin
Ferrous sulphate (iron supplements)
Manganese compounds
Selenium
Urethane
Yellow phosphorus

Table 11.6. Hepatotoxins that produce hepatic necrosis and steatosis

Aflatoxins
Amanita mushrooms
Carbon tetrachloride
Chlorinated diphenyls
Chloroform
DDT insecticide
Dinitrotoluene
Ethylene dichloride
Galactosamine
Halothane
Iodoform
Naphthalene
Tannic acid

Table 11.7. Hepatotoxins that cause steatosis

Alcohol
Antimony
Barium salts
Chromates
Hydrazine
Methotrexate
Phosphorus
Tetracycline
Thallium compounds
Uranium compounds
Warfarin (coumadin)

Table 11.8. Hepatotoxins that cause microvesicular steatosis

Cocaine
Tetracycline

Table 11.9. Hepatotoxins that cause macrovascular steatosis

Alcohol
Corticosteroids
Methotrexate

Table 11.10. Hepatotoxins that produce Mallory bodies and phospholipid accumulations

Alcohol	Perhexilene maleate
Amiodarone	
Corticosteroids	Thioridazine (Mellaril)
Nifedipine	Stilboestrol

Table 11.11. Hepatotoxins that can cause hepatic granulomas

Allopurinol	Penicllin
Aspirin	Phenylbutazone
Carbamazepine	Phenytoin
Cephalexin	Procainamide
Chlorpromazine	Quinidine
Contraceptive steroids	Quinine
Dapsone	
Diazepam	Ranitidine
Gold compounds	Sulphadiazine
Halothane	Sulphamethoxazole-trimethoprim
Isoniazid	Sulphathiazole
Mineral oil	Tocainide
Nitrofurantoin	Tolbutamide
Oxacillin	

Table 11.12. Hepatotoxins that can lead to chronic hepatitis

Acetaminophen	Nitrofurantoin
Dantrolene	Oxyphenisatin laxatives
Diclofenac	Papaverine
Isoniazid	Pemoline
Methyldopa	

Clinical Trials and Drug-Induced Liver Injury

During a drug's development, before it is released to the public, manufacturers conduct animal tests that assess the drug's effects on liver function. Additionally, liver function testing is conducted on humans, and in many cases, the results keep the drug from entering the market. Liver failure, due to a new drug, is a rare event, and, unfortunately, it may not show up until after a drug has been approved.

Why do adverse drug effects occur after a drug has been approved? Most clinical trials involve 3,000 subjects. Rare adverse drug effects including liver failure may only show up in one per 50,000 exposures. In addition, genetic variations cause individuals to metabolize drugs differently, and individuals may be taking more than one drug.

New drug scrutiny

The FDA also monitors newly reduced drugs for adverse effects. In March 2000, the FDA asked Parke-Davis/Warner Lambert to voluntarily withdraw the diabetes drug Rezulin (troglitazone) because it appeared to cause greater liver toxicity than similar drugs on the market. The FDA also asked Wyeth-Ayerst Laboratories to voluntarily remove the analgesic Duract (bromfenac) from the market after receiving reports of liver failure when the drug was used for longer than the 10 days specified in the labeling.

Sometimes drugs that are reported to cause liver toxicity may be kept on the market if there are no other effective drugs in their category. In this case, changes in labeling are often recommended or their use is restricted to hospitalized patients. The FDA has also developed a web page on drug-induced liver toxicity at www.fda.gov/cder/livertox.

The FDA also advises consumers to follow dosing requirements and study labels for adverse effects. In addition, consumer should learn to recognize the signs of liver disease, which can include nausea, dark urine, jaundice, and mental confusion.

Drugs with Limitations

The FDA lists the following drugs as having limitations on their use due to potential liver problems (warnings, dose restrictions, monitoring):

Table 11.13. Drugs with potential to cause liver problems

Niaspan Extended Release Tablets (niacin)
Dantrium (dantrolene)
Tylenol (acetaminophen)

Table 11.13. (cont.)

Normodyne (labetalol)
Cylert (pemoline)
Felbtol (Felbamate)
Zylo (zileuton)
Tasmar (tolcapone)
Trovan (trovafloxacin, alatrofloxacin)
Source: U.S. Food and Drug Administration,
FDA Consumer Magazine, May-June, 2001.

Environmental and Plant Toxins

Numerous plants and chemicals have the potential to injure the liver
and cause acute and chronic hepatitis. Some of these toxins are described
in the following sections.

Plants and household chemicals

Amanita mushrooms cause hepatitis and liver injury in some parts of
the world, outside of the United States. Aflatoxin molds cause severe liver
disease and liver cancer in many undeveloped countries. In the United
States, liver injury is rarely linked to aflatoxin consumption although there
are reports of aflatoxin being present in contaminated peanuts and peanut
products.

Food products can contain toxic preservatives or they may be accidentally contaminated with toxic chemicals. Flour contaminated with the
chemical methylene dianaline caused cholestatic jaundice and a condition
of Epping jaundice in hundreds of customers at a bakery in Epping,
England.

Insecticides often contain toxic chemicals such as DDT that can persist in the body for decades, possibly causing liver damage years later. Carbon tetrachloride, a chemical once widely used for dry cleaning, can cause
neurological symptoms, hepatitis, liver failure and kidney failure. Phosphorus, once widely used in the manufacture of matches and firecrackers,
can cause fulminant hepatitis and liver disease.

Herbs

Numerous herbs can damage the liver and cause hepatitis as a result
of direct toxicity or idiosyncratic reactions. However, because herbal use
is not always suspected in cases of hepatitis, cases of hepatitis may go unrec-
ognized. The compounds listed in table 11.14 have been reported to cause

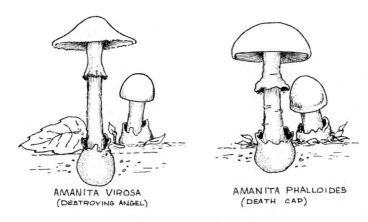

AMANITA VIROSA
(DESTROYING ANGEL)

AMANITA PHALLOIDES
(DEATH CAP)

Amanita species (Marvin G. Miller).

toxic hepatitis although in some reports high doses, much higher than the recommended amounts, were used before toxicity developed, and, in some cases, other medications and supplements were used simultaneously.

In addition to those listed, some herbal products, such as St. John's Wort, that are not hepatotoxins, can affect the metabolism of other drugs. Others have been found to be contaminated with bacteria. When using herbal medicine, it is important to buy products from reputable manufacturers that have labels documenting the authenticity of the ingredients. Side effects and drug interactions with herbal products can be found by consulting the *PDR for Herbal Medicine* and Mark Blumenthal's *The Complete German Commission E Monographs* listed in the resource section.

Table 11.14 Herbs and supplements reported to cause hepatitis/liver injury

Amanita species	Jin bu huan
Asafetida	Kalms tablets
Atractylis gummifera	Kava-kava (*Piper methysticum*)
Black cohosh	Kombucha
Buckthorn (*Rhamnus cathartica*)	Lobelia
Bush tea	Ma huang
Cascara sagrada	Mate
Celandine	Mistletoe
Chaparral	Nicotinic acid (niacin, Nicolar)
Coltsfoot	Noni (*Morinda citrifolia*)
Comfrey (*Symphytum*)	Nutmeg
Crotalaria	Pau d'arco
Echinacea	Pennyroyal oil (*Mentha pulegium*)

Gentian	Pyrrolizidine alkaloids, especially comfrey
Germander (*Teucrium chamaedrys*)	Senna
Groundsel (*Senecio vulgaris*)	Skullcap (*Scutellaria gaericulata*)
Impila (*Callilepsis laureola*)	Valerian
Irish tea	Vitamin A
Iron supplements	

Dietary supplements

Dietary supplements can cause hepatitis in overdoses, in idiosyncratic reactions, and in individuals with impaired liver function. Some of the most well known hepatotoxic supplements include vitamin A and extended-release formulations of niacin.

VITAMIN A

Excessive doses of vitamin A used for extended periods can cause chronic hepatitis. Symptoms include headache, appetite loss, weight loss, fatigue, itching, dry skin and loss of body hair. Clinical signs include enlarged liver and spleen, ascites, and, occasionally, jaundice. Liver biopsies show zone 3 fibrosis, chronic hepatitis, cirrhosis, peliosis hepatitis, and occlusive disease. Toxicity has occurred in people taking 20 times the recommended dose and in people using recommended doses daily for many years.

Vitamin A derivatives, a class of drugs known as retinoids, may also damage the liver. Similar to vitamin A, these compounds can cause cirrhosis and chronic hepatitis.

NIACIN

Niacin or vitamin B3 is known to lower cholesterol levels. Low doses of niacin can cause an unpleasant flush. To reduce severe flush in people requiring doses sufficient to lower cholesterol levels, manufacturers have developed high-dose, time-release (extended release) niacin preparations. Extended release preparations containing more than 500 mg of niacin are hepatotoxic and can cause both acute and chronic hepatitis.

Bacterial toxins

During bacterial infections, many bacteria release potent enterotoxins and endotoxins and other extracellular proteins such as urease that contribute to the symptoms seen in infection. In severe infections, such as toxic shock syndrome, which is caused by *Staphylococcus aureus*, the toxins that they release, exotoxin C and enterotoxin F, can contribute to hepatic failure. Another cause of toxic shock syndrome, *Streptococcus pyogenes*, also produces exotoxins that can cause hepatitis.

REYE'S SYNDROME

Reye's syndrome, a potentially fatal condition of hepatitis and coma, occurs in children with viral infections. A higher incidence of Reye's occurs in children with viral infection who are treated with low doses of aspirin. Although the link with aspirin has not been confirmed, numerous studies have strongly implicated aspirin as a causative agent.

Environmental hepatotoxins

Environmental toxins include chemicals used in the munitions industry, rocket assembly, plastics, pharmaceutical, cosmetic and chemical industries, and agriculture. Today environmental agents rarely cause hepatitis. However, because injury develops over a long period of time, the offending agent may not be implicated.

ARSENIC

Organic arsenic compounds, such as arsenic trioxide (Fowler's solution) used for extended periods to treat psoriasis, can cause portal hypertension. Acute arsenic poisoning can cause fibrosis and vascular occlusive liver disease. In some regions arsenic is found in drinking water and in folk remedies or locally prepared (native) drugs.

VINYL CHLORIDE

Workers exposed to vinyl chloride for many years develop hepatotoxicity. Early changes include sclerosis or scarring in zone 1, enlarged spleen, and portal hypertension. Later changes include peliosis hepatitis and angiosarcoma.

Radiation

Radiation treatments using 35 Gy over time or 3000–6000 rads to the upper abdomen leads to a hepatic lesion and a syndrome termed radiation hepatitis. Symptoms, which typically develop within 2–12 weeks after treatment, include ascites, enlarged liver, enlarged spleen, jaundice and abdominal pain. Liver biopsy shows sinusoidal congestion, zone 3 necrosis and hemorrhage, and fibrotic occlusions of hepatic veins [71]. Venous occlusion may be a transient condition or a fatal disease caused by liver failure.

Disease Course In Toxic Hepatitis

Drug reactions may be immediate in acute overdoses. In reactions that occur over a prolonged course of treatment, disease development may be subtle. Some drugs, such as sulphonamides, phenytoin, and dapsone, may also cause an idiosyncratic hypersensitivity syndrome resembling mononucleosis with fever and rash.

In idiosyncratic reactions, symptoms may occur within a few weeks of drug use. In some cases, they develop on the second course of drug treatment after a period of sustained drug withdrawal. In most intrinsic and idiosyncratic drug-induced liver injuries, symptoms of liver toxicity improve after the drug is withdrawn. Some drugs, such as halothane, cause a mixed intrinsic/idiosyncratic reaction.

Halothane hepatitis

With the anesthetic halothane, liver injury typically occurs after multiple exposures although it may occur after the first exposure. Obese, elderly females are at particular risk for halothane toxicity although children can also be affected.

Symptoms that occur after the first exposure usually develop more than 7 days (range 8–13 days) later and include fever, usually with rigors, malaise, and upper right quadrant pain. Jaundice usually develops after 10–28 days. After several exposures to halothane, the temperature rise occurs 1–11 days after surgical use, and jaundice develops within 3–17 days [56].

Bilirubin levels are typically very high especially in fatal cases. Transaminase levels are similar to those seen in viral hepatitis although alkaline phosphatase levels can occasionally be markedly elevated. In patients who develop jaundice mortality is high, especially if the prothrombin time rises markedly even when vitamin K is administered. Halothane administration should not be repeated in patients who even show a very mild reaction after the first drug exposure, and halothane should not be administered within six months of a previous dose.

Phases of drug-induced liver injury

Symptoms of drug-induced hepatitis usually occur in three distinct phases: 1) an immediate, severe pre-icteric (before jaundice develops) condition causing moderate to severe neurological or gastrointestinal symptoms, 2) a period of improvement, and 3) a phase of severe liver injury with marked jaundice, elevated liver enzyme levels, increased gamma globulin levels, and liver tenderness that can be accompanied by kidney failure.

In those who recover, maximum serum bilirubin levels are seen after 2–3 weeks. People with severe toxicity experience liver atrophy and death from hepatic failure. If hepatic pre-coma or coma develops, mortality is as high as 70 percent. Liver damage is particularly extensive in persons who continue to use the offending drug after liver damage has started. For this reason, all medications that a person takes should be listed and considered suspect in persons with emerging liver disease.

Diagnosis

Liver enzyme tests and bilirubin levels are used to diagnose liver disease. Viral marker tests are used to determine if jaundice is due to viral infection. A careful medical and drug history can help diagnose liver injury due to toxins. The International Consensus Criteria for Drug-Induced Hepatoxicity have been developed to help determine if liver damage is drug-induced. These criteria include:

1. Time of drug intake compared to onset of symptoms is suggestive of drug injury if it occurs from 5–90 days and compatible with drug injury if less than 5 days or more than 90 days from initial drug intake.
2. Course of reaction after cessation of drug is very suggestive of drug injury when liver enzyme levels fall by 50 percent within 8 days after drug withdrawal; liver enzyme decreases of 50 percent within 30 days in hepatocellular disease and within 180 days in cholestatic illness.
3. Alternative causes of hepatitis have been excluded by other tests including liver biopsy
4. Positive response to re-challenge, with at least a doubling of liver enzymes, when the drug is re-administered, when available.

The reaction is considered "drug related" if all of the first 3 criteria are met, or if 2 of these criteria are met and the re-challenge test is positive.

Liver function tests

Hepatotoxins causing necrosis cause marked elevations of transaminase liver enzymes that reflect the extent of liver damage. Levels are typically higher than those seen in acute viral hepatitis. Alkaline phosphatase levels are slightly elevated, and bilirubin levels are moderately elevated.

In severe necrosis, plasma coagulation factors are depressed and the prothrombin time is elevated. In the early stages of necrosis, albumin levels are normal although they fall late in the clinical course and in chronic disease.

Blood levels of acetaminophen and alcohol are used to diagnose acetaminophen overdoses and alcohol abuse. In alcoholism, levels of the enzyme gamma glutamyl transferase (Gamma GT) are also elevated.

In microvesicular steatosis serum transaminase enzyme levels are modestly elevated to 5–20 times the normal range, and bilirubin levels are only moderately increased. The prothrombin time is usually prolonged, and low blood glucose levels may occur causing a condition of hypoglycemia.

Biopsy specimens cause characteristic symptoms of drug toxicity that are specific for the offending agent. Biopsy results are discussed further in chapter fifteen.

12

Metabolic Causes of Hepatitis

Hepatitis results from several metabolic disorders and inborn errors of metabolism that cause minerals, fat deposits, or amino acids to accumulate in the liver. These accumulations can directly destroy liver cells, interfere with liver function, and cause inflammation. Causes of metabolic hepatitis include: Wilson's disease, hemochromatosis, alpha-1-antitrypsin deficiency, galactosemia, fructose intolerance, tyrosinemia, non-alcoholic fatty liver disease (NAFLD), infantile giant cell hepatitis, obesity, and sarcoidosis. Fulminant hepatitis may also occur in conditions of shock. The metabolic causes of hepatitis and the effects on the liver caused by these abnormalities are described in chapter twelve.

Wilson's Disease

Wilson's disease is a rare inherited disease predominantly seen in young people characterized by increased deposits of copper in the body's tissues. Wilson's disease results in hepatic and neurological changes, deposits in the cornea known as Kayser-Fleischer rings, and lesions in the kidney and other organs. The Kayser-Fleischer ring is a greenish-brown ring near the margin of the cornea next to the sclerus (white of the eye) that results from deposits of copper.

Inheritance and prevalence

For disease to develop, both parents must contain the autosomal recessive gene on chromosome 13 responsible for Wilson's disease. The prevalence is about 1 in 30,000 and about 1 in 90 people are carriers [56] of this gene. Wilson's disease is seen worldwide but occurs most frequently in Jews of eastern European origin, Arabs, Italians, Japanese, Chinese, Indians and any community having a high rate of inter-marriage.

Copper

Copper is an essential trace element normally found in certain enzymes and proteins. Low levels of copper are normally found in the blood and tissues. Copper is required for the synthesis of hemoglobin and is found in the metabolic enzymes cytochrome oxidase, tyrosinase, monoamine oxidase, ascorbic acid oxidase, uricase, galactose oxidase and amino-levulinate dehydratase.

The major portion of copper (approximately 80 percent) found in red blood cells occurs as a constituent of the enzyme superoxide dismutase (erythrocuprein). This enzyme is also found in the liver and brain where it protects cells by scavenging the toxic free radical superoxide ions generated during aerobic metabolism. The remainder of copper found in red blood cells consists of complexes containing amino acids, which function to maintain normal dismutase enzyme activity.

Normal copper levels. Total levels of copper in red blood cells tend to remain stable at about 98 ug/dl or 15 umol/L even when there are deficiencies of dietary copper or increases in plasma or hepatic copper. In plasma, the liquid portion of blood, copper levels are higher than in red blood cells. The normal or reference range for copper in adults is 70–140 ug/dl (11–22 umolL) for males and 80–155 ug/dl (13–24 umol/L) for females.

The normal dietary intake of copper is 4 mg and about 2 mg of copper is absorbed and excreted daily after childhood. In Wilson's disease, only 0.2 to 0.4 mg can be excreted in bile, and about 1 mg is excreted in urine. Over time, copper accumulates causing a positive copper balance.

Ceruloplasmin. In plasma, copper is found in two forms: loosely bound and tightly bound to albumin and other plasma proteins. Only traces of free copper are found in plasma. Most copper, up to 95 percent, is tightly bound with globulin protein in a complex known as ceruloplasmin. The reference or normal range for ceruloplasmin is 25–43 mg/dl (250–430 mg/L). Copper linked or bound to albumin represents copper in transit (moving through the blood). In this form, levels increase after copper is ingested and fall after transport to the liver. Ceruloplasmin levels increase as levels of albumin-linked copper decrease.

Copper metabolism in Wilson's Disease

Wilson's disease is an autosomal recessive disease of copper metabolism first described in 1912 causing hepatitis, fibrosis, and cirrhosis. Onset of disease is usually in the second or third decade of life but occasionally it occurs as early as 4–5 years. Neonates normally have low ceruloplasmin levels and high levels of liver copper. This pattern normally changes during childhood and copper excretion becomes similar to that of adults. In Wilson's disease, this neonatal pattern of copper storage persists. Because the excretion of copper through bile is impaired, high levels of copper accumulate.

Disease Course in Wilson's Disease

The disease course resembles general copper poisoning and varies with age. In children, the liver is primarily involved. Later, neuropsychiatric changes become more common. After age 20, most patients have neurological symptoms.

SIGNS AND SYMPTOMS

The most common presenting signs and symptoms involve the nervous system and include rigidity, dysarthria, dysphagia (difficulty swallowing), tremor, incoordination, the Kayser-Fleischer ring described earlier in this section, and gait disturbances. Rarely, patients may have grayish-brown sunflower-shaped cataracts, similar to those caused by copper-containing foreign bodies.

Some patients, especially younger patients, may present with liver insufficiency ranging from loss of appetite to jaundice, portal hypertension and cirrhosis. Other patients have a combination of symptoms related to the liver and central nervous system.

At age 10–30 years, most patients show symptoms of chronic active hepatitis including jaundice, high transaminase enzyme values and elevated gamma globulin levels. Occasionally, patients present with fulminant hepatitis with progressive jaundice, hemolytic anemia (destruction of red blood cells), and renal failure. Patients may also present with cirrhosis and portal hypertension. Neurological changes usually occur 2–5 years after the onset of liver symptoms. Patients with chronic liver disease showing mental abnormalities such as slurring of the speech, hemolytic anemia, or early ascites should be screened for Wilson's disease.

NEUROPSYCHIATRIC SYMPTOMS

Although changes are usually chronic, the neurological changes seen in Wilson's disease may be acute and they can progressively worsen. Early changes include an extension tremor of the wrists, grimacing, difficulty writing, personality changes, limb rigidity, and slurred speech. The electroencephalogram (EEG) can show generalized non-specific changes that are sometimes seen in unaffected siblings.

LIVER TISSUE CHANGES

Wilson's disease causes a condition of liver cell destruction known as hepatolenticular degeneration. Copper deposits are distributed throughout the liver, and copper-rich fat granules are present. Normally the liver contains 55 ug/g of copper. In Wilson's disease, concentrations are usually greater than 250 ug/g. Liver changes include liver cell necrosis, fibrosis and cirrhosis. The liver cells show ballooning (swelling), multiple nuclei, clumps of glycogen, and fatty changes.

KIDNEY, BRAIN, AND OTHER ORGAN CHANGES

Wilson's disease can cause copper deposits to accumulate in the kidneys, musculoskeletal system, urinary tract, and brain. Signs and symptoms correspond to the primary site of damage. Increased renal copper can damage the renal tubules causing elevated amino acid levels, increased urine glucose and phosphorus levels, and kidney stones. Excess copper in the brain causes degenerative cell destruction in the basal ganglia.

Increased copper levels can cause the fingernails and toenails to have a bluish tinge. Skeletal changes reflect mineral loss and include premature osteoarthritis and joint pain caused by crystal deposits in joint fluid. Gallstones can be caused by increased red blood cell destruction. In addition, calcium metabolism can be altered causing a condition of parathyroid gland insufficiency (hypoparathyroidism).

Diagnosis

Wilson's disease is suspected in patients with hepatic or neurological symptoms or a family history of Wilson's disease. Blood tests for ceruloplasmin, copper and genetic tests for the Wilson's Disease gene (DNA test) are used for diagnosis. In Wilson's disease, plasma ceruloplasmin levels are greatly decreased, usually to less than 20 mg/dl. Plasma copper levels are decreased, and urine levels are markedly increased. Genetic tests for Wilson's disease show a homozygote mutation in the copper transporter gene (two alleles with the mutation, one from each parent) and should be treated even in the absence of symptoms. Liver biopsy showing an elevated liver copper level is used to confirm Wilson's disease.

IMAGING TESTS

Imaging tests are generally not required for diagnosis. Brain scans may show an enlargement of the ventricles, and MRI may show localized anatomical changes.

Treatment

The chelating compounds D-Penicillamine and trientine hydrochloride are used to bind and remove excess copper. Treatment used life-long is effective although at the onset improvement is slow, usually taking six months for noticeable effects. Failure to improve after two years of therapy suggests that irreparable tissue damage may have occurred. Elemental zinc is also used to reduce the absorption of dietary copper in patients who show a poor response to chelating agents.

Individuals with genetic test results indicating homozygous Wilson's disease respond well to treatment even in the absence of overt symptoms. Studies indicate that early treatment prevents copper accumulations and disease progression. Untreated, Wilson' disease is progressive and fatal. Fatality is also high in cases of fulminant hepatitis caused by Wilson's disease. Death is caused by liver failure and related bleeding abnormalities.

Pregnancy

Women with untreated Wilson's disease may have fertility problems and a higher rate of miscarriage. In women who become pregnant, both the mother and infant are considered at high risk. Women who are treated successfully and have nearly normal body copper levels regain fertility and are reported to have uneventful pregnancies and normal babies.

Iron Overload States and Hemochromatosis

Iron metabolism

Iron is derived from dietary sources and supplements. Iron is central to aerobic metabolism and is found in various enzymes and oxygen-binding components of protein. Depending on the body's stores, about 1–1.5 mg of iron is absorbed daily from the 10–20 mg of iron usually provided by diet. The iron is added to a nutrient pool and distributed as needed.

Some of the absorbed iron is stored in the form of ferritin, and some is linked to the carrier protein transferrin and transported to the body's cells. Degraded ferritin molecules are converted into a compound known as hemosiderin, which can be identified as blue granules in cells stained with special dyes.

Normally, the body contains about 4 grams of iron. About 3 grams of this iron are present in the protein components of blood (hemoglobin) and muscle (myoglobin) and in respiratory enzymes. About 0.3 grams of iron are stored in the liver and another 0.2 grams are stored in other tissues including the pancreas and adrenal glands.

Iron overload

In overdoses of iron supplements or in iron overload states resulting from multiple blood transfusions, hemochromatosis, and other iron overload states, excess iron directly damages liver cells and causes fibrosis. Iron causes cellular lipids to become rancid in a process of peroxidation, which, along with excess hemosiderin granules, damages cell membranes and interferes with cellular function. Iron increases collagen synthesis and excess iron leads to fibrosis. Biopsy specimens of the liver in iron overload show excess iron deposits in the form of hemosiderin granules.

Hemochromatosis

Hemochromatosis is a condition that causes the body to retain excessive amounts of iron. The normal controls that regulate iron uptake and release are disrupted in this condition, causing iron overload. Hemochromatosis is primarily caused by a genetic condition called hereditary hemochromatosis (HH). It may also occur secondary to conditions of disrupted red blood cell production (erythropoiesis) and in conditions of hemolytic anemia, including sideroblastic and sickle-cell anemias, and beta thallassemias. Hemochromatosis may also occur as a side effect of excessive iron therapy or from multiple blood transfusions.

HEREDITARY HEMOCHROMATOSIS (HH)

In hereditary hemochromatosis, men and women are affected equally although women do not usually show symptoms of disease until later in life due to the protection of blood loss in menstruation and childbirth. HH is rarely diagnosed before age 20, and the peak incidence is 20–40 years.

The classical picture in HH is of a lethargic, middle-aged man with bronze-tinged skin, enlarged liver, diminished sexual activity and loss of body hair, and joint pain. Many patients also have diabetes.

In HH, absorption of dietary iron is increased from the time of birth. When stored iron reaches toxic levels, absorption slows down. However, as the stored iron is distributed to the body, iron absorption increases again. Consequently, excess iron is stored in the liver, pancreas, endocrine glands, heart, skin and intestinal lining.

Disease course in HH and iron overload

Children rarely develop symptoms of hemochromatosis, but when they do they show a more acute disease course with increased skin pigmentation, endocrine changes and cardiac disease. Bronze pigmentation is due to increased melanin in the basal layer and an atrophied superficial epidermis, resulting in skin that is shiny, thin and dry with a gray-bronze cast. The liver may be enlarged and firm with fast progression to cirrhosis.

Typically, hereditary hemochromatosis is diagnosed in adults who present with symptoms of hepatitis, diabetes, heart disease or decreased pituitary function. About 70 percent of adults present with cirrhosis; 55 percent present with adult onset diabetes; 20 percent present with cardiac failure; 45 percent present with joint inflammation and pain; 80 percent present with skin pigmentation; and 50 percent present with sexual dysfunction. As liver damage increases, ferritin levels rise, and an increased ferritin level is one of the first signs of hemochromatosis. In other conditions of iron overload, iron levels, transferrin, ferritin, and total iron binding capacity (TIBC) tests aid with diagnosis.

Genetics

There are five major subtypes of hereditary hemochromatosis and a number of different subgroups. Most HH is caused by Type 1 HH. Hemochromatosis Type 1, which is considered classic HH, is an autosomal recessive disorder caused by a defect in the HFE gene on chromosome 6, which regulates iron absorption. There are at least 40 different alleles on this gene but most mutations occur on C282Y and H63D, which is the most common mutation. In Caucasians, about 0.5 percent of the population has a homozygote distribution (affected), and 8–10 percent of the population are heterozogyte carriers. In the United States about 1 million people are affected by HH. Carriers do not develop hemochromatosis but show disturbances of iron metabolism that lead to hemolytic anemia. The disease is most prevalent among individuals of Celtic descent, such as the Irish, Scottish, and Welsh.

Type 2 HH is also known as juvenile hemochromatosis. It is an autosomal recessive disorder that occurs in two distinct forms. Mutations on the HJV (hemojuvelin protein) gene are seen in HH Type 2A, and mutations on the HAMP (hepcidin protein) gene are seen in HH type 2B. These genes are both found on chromosome 2. Juvenile HH may occur in the teens but usually occurs in the second and third decades of life. Iron accumulates more rapidly than in adult-onset forms of HH. Congestive heart failure or arrhythmias caused by accumulations of iron in heart tissue may cause fatal heart failure before age 30.

HH Type 3 is caused by a mutation on the transferrin receptor gene (TFR2) on chromosome 7, and HH Type 4 is caused by a mutation on the SCL40A1 gene regulating ferroportin on chromosome 2. Type 4 HH is the only form that has an autosomal dominant pattern. Patients with HH Type 4 usually develop excessive iron stores in the Kupffer cells of the liver although their blood levels of iron may be low. Some Type 4 HH patients have high transferrin saturation with excessive iron stores in hepatocytes.

Diagnosis

Hemochromatosis is suspected in patients with signs of liver disease or diabetes with high levels of serum iron, percentage transferrin saturation and ferritin. Patients with HH usually have elevated ALT and AST enzyme levels, elevated serum iron transferrin saturation, increased serum ferritin, and biopsy specimens show high levels of iron in liver tissue. The combination of increased transferrin saturation (greater than 50 percent) with an increased ferritin (greater than 150 ug/l in women or greater than 300 ug/l in men) is more than 90 percent specific for hereditary hemochromatosis.

Hereditary hemochromatosis accounts for five percent of all cases of cirrhosis and is often confused with other forms of cirrhosis. Liver biopsy has been the traditional method of confirming diagnosis, with high levels of liver iron indicators of disease. In recent years, newer, genetic tests for the HE mutation are more often used to confirm diagnosis. In addition, MRI tests can also be used to measure liver iron levels.

OTHER IRON STORAGE DISEASES

Other conditions of iron storage can cause symptoms similar to those of hemochromatosis. These conditions include genetic mutations causing low transferrin levels; abnormal forms of ferritin related to bronchial cancer; porphyria cutanea tarda, erythropoietic siderosis, a condition of increased iron deposits in various body cells; and sideroblastic anemia.

Risk factors

Several factors contribute to increased iron stores. These include malnutrition resulting in protein deficiency, alcoholism, cirrhosis from other causes, chronic pancreatitis, hemodialysis procedures, medications containing iron, excess iron from blood transfusion especially in children, and abnormal transfer of iron through the placenta in the rare fatal condition of neonatal hemochromatosis.

Treatment

Iron can be removed in a process of venesection phlebotomy (removal of blood through a needle similar to withdrawing blood from blood donors) at rates as high as 130 mg/day. Large quantities of blood must be removed in the process. Phlebotomy of 500 ml removes about 250 mg of iron and tissues contain up to 200 times this amount. Phlebotomy is performed weekly or bi-weekly for about 2 years until the hemoglobin and iron levels fall into the normal range. Periodic monitoring of ferritin helps in determining when future phlebotomies are needed. The hormone erythropoietin, which increases red blood cell production, may be given to prevent anemia in patients with Type 4 HH.

Inborn Errors of Metabolism (IEM)

Inborn errors of metabolism (IEM) are rare disorders caused by genetic defects that result in the abnormal synthesis or metabolism of proteins, carbohydrates or fats. Although each IEM is a rare disorder, collectively IEMs are common disorders that can show up at birth or later in life. The incidence of IEMs is between 1 in 4000 and 1 in 5000 live births, and the prevalence of some IEMs is increased in certain ethnic groups. The effects or symptoms in IEMs are related to toxic accumulations of the compounds that would ordinarily be metabolized or by deficiencies of the compounds that are unable to be produced. IEMs are suspected when patients develop signs and symptoms consistent with metabolic disorders, especially if there is a family history of disease or early infant death. Blood and urine tests for amino acids and genetic profiles can be used to diagnose IEMs. The following IEMs can cause hepatitis.

Galactosemia

Galactosemia is a rare autosomal recessive disorder affecting one in 62,000 people characterized by low levels of blood glucose and reducing substances in the urine, and the inability to metabolize galactose, a constituent in milk. Affected infants lack the enzyme needed to metabolize galactose. Symptoms in galactosemia include vomiting, diarrhea, jaundice, liver damage, failure to thrive, cirrhosis, cataracts, kidney damage, and mental retardation, after ingesting milk. Many states now include galactosemia screening in their neonatal blood screening profiles.Treatment includes a diet free of milk and milk products.

Tyrosinemia

Tyrosinemia is a genetic disorder causing liver disease, low blood sugar, and kidney damage caused by the inability to metabolize the amino acid tyrosine. In severe liver disease, tyrosine crystals are found in urine.

Alpha-1-antitrypsin deficiency

Alpha-1-antitrypsin deficiency is an inherited condition occurring in approximately one in 5,000 live births. It is the most common genetic disease for which liver transplantation is done. In this condition, which is caused by a defective gene on chromosome 14, the liver's production of the amino acid alpha-1-antitrypsin is impaired. Without the normal protective properties of alpha-1-antitrypsin the lungs and liver are damaged.

The normal range for alpha-1-antitrypisin is 100–190 mg/dl. Alpha-1-antitrypsin deficiency is diagnosed by demonstrating very low blood levels of alpha-1-antitrypsin (less than 100 mg/dl) and with an alpha-1-antitrypisin genotype profile showing a ZZ or SS genotype causing a homozygous recessive disease. Carriers have a Z/non-Z or S/non-Z genotype. The genotype in unaffected people is non-Z/non-S. When results are inconsistent, a phenotype is performed.

Hereditary fructose intolerance (HFI)

Hereditary fructose intolerance (HFI) is an autosomal recessive disorder characterized by nausea, abdominal pain, liver inflammation, low blood sugar, and elevated urine fructose levels. Infants with this disorder appear normal at birth, only showing symptoms when fed formulas high in fructose or fruit juices. Fructose is a naturally-occurring fruit sugar, and it also occurs as a synthetic sweetener in foods and drinks. Patients with HFI also react to table sugar or sucrose, which is cane or beet sugar.

HFI is caused by a deficiency of the enzyme fructose-1-phosphate aldolase activity. This deficiency results in an accumulation of fructose-1-phosphate in the liver, kidney and small intestine. This accumulation, in turn, inhibits the normal breakdown of glycogen and the normal synthesis of glucose. The result is an extremely low blood sugar (hypoglycemia) following the ingestion of glucose or other sugars. Prolonged fructose ingestion in infants with this disorder ultimately leads to hepatic or renal failure and death. Treatment consists of a diet free of fructose and sucrose.

The incidence of HFI varies among different ethnic groups. Due to the difficulty in diagnosing HFI, the true incidence of this disorder is unknown but suspected to be about 1 in 10,000 persons. Diagnose is made by analyzing aldolase activity in liver biopsy specimens or by a fructose tolerance test in which fructose is administered intravenously under controlled conditions, and levels of glucose, fructose, and phosphate levels are tested. A DNA analysis is also available to test for hereditary mutations but a negative result does not rule out HFI because there may be other causes.

Lysosomal storage disorders

Lysosomal storage disorders are a group of hereditary disorders that interfere with the normal storage and processing of lipids. Several of these disorders, for instance cholesterol esterifcation defect secondary to a defect in cholesterol trafficking (formerly known as Neimann-Pick type C disease) can cause neonatal hepatitis.

Neonatal Hepatitis

Neonatal hepatitis is a condition of liver inflammation occurring from childbirth to the age of two months. Symptoms include jaundice, failure to thrive, enlarged liver and enlarged spleen. These symptoms are similar to those of biliary atresia, another liver disease seen in infancy caused by bile duct destruction. However, infants with biliary atresia have different biochemical abnormalities and show normal growth.

About 20 percent of all cases of neonatal hepatitis are caused by viral and bacterial infections contracted around the time of childbirth, including cytomegalovirus, rubella, congenital syphilis, toxoplasmosis, enteric infection, human immunodeficiency virus, viral hepatitis, and herpes. Most cases are not identified and referred to as idiopathic conditions. However, when family history indicates IEMs and the appropriate tests are used, diagnosis of neonatal hepatitis is often found to be caused by inborn errors of metabolism, cystic fibrosis, shock in congenital heart disease, conditions of giant cell hepatitis, and other infections in which the infectious agent cannot be identified.

Treatment depends on the type of virus isolated or inborn error of metabolism diagnosed. Neonatal giant cell hepatitis (idiopathic hepatitis) usually resolves on its own with no complications. Phenobarbital is sometimes used to increase bile secretion.

Non-Alcoholic Fatty Liver Disease (NAFLD)

Non-alcoholic fatty liver disease (NAFLD) is a condition of excess accumulations of fat in the liver caused by conditions other than alcohol abuse. NAFLD can occur in obesity, in diabetes, in rapid weight loss, as a complication of pregnancy, in tuberculosis, in malnutrition, as a consequence of intestinal bypass surgery for obesity, and as a side effect of certain medications, including corticosteroids, and excess vitamin A.

NAFLD is one of the most common liver disorders seen in the United States and may affect up to 24 percent of the population, including 90 percent of obese people and 50 percent of people with type II diabetes. People who carry excess weight around their abdomen or waist have a higher risk than people with lower body fat.

Fatty liver disease (steatosis)

Fatty liver disease or steatosis is caused by increased accumulations of fat in the liver. Fatty liver disease affects people of all ages, including children, although peak incidence occurs in people in their fifties. NAFLD is much more likely to occur in obese people and people with diabetes.

Patients with NAFLD usually are asymptomatic and are diagnosed incidentally during physical exams when an enlarged, smooth, firm liver is discovered. Liver function tests are often normal although transaminase enzyme and alkaline phosphatase levels may be slightly elevated. Patients with acute fatty liver are at risk of sudden death due to shock caused by pulmonary fat clots that block blood circulation.

DISEASE COURSE OF FATTY LIVER

Fatty liver by itself does not cause liver disease. However, it can lead to liver cell inflammation and steatohepatitis, and it can signify other metabolic problems. Steatosis in NAFLD is often accompanied by insulin resistance, liver cell inflammation, and fibrosis that can progress to cirrhosis, liver cancer, and liver failure.

Abnormalities of lipid metabolism, such as elevated cholesterol and triglycerides, in conjunction with NAFLD are seen in the condition called Metabolic syndrome or Syndrome X. About 56 percent of patients with NAFLD are reported to have Metabolic syndrome, and the prevalence is higher in patients with steatohepatitis.

Studies show that the fat accumulations in NAFLD are composed of fatty acids produced within the liver and also fats derived from diet. Excessive dietary fats and sugars contribute to NAFLD as the amount of dietary fat and sugar exceeds the liver's ability to process these substances. Insulin resistance also contributes to increased liver fat production.

Patients with NAFLD and hepatitis C usually have a more severe disease course than patients with hepatitis C alone. For this reason patients with hepatitis C who have fatty liver are treated with interferon even in the absence of other symptoms.

Non-alcoholic steatohepatitis (NASH)

Non-alcoholic steatohepatitis (NASH) is an advanced form of NAFLD in which steatosis is accompanied by inflammation and liver cell necrosis. Insulin resistance and lipid abnormalities are typically severe and about 88 percent of patients are reported to have Metabolic syndrome.

Patients with NASH may be asymptomatic or have mild symptoms of fatigue, malaise and abdominal discomfort. In about 20 percent of affected people, NASH progresses to cirrhosis. Because symptoms in NASH are often vague, liver disease may not be diagnosed until cirrhosis develops. This accounts for the high mortality rate in NASH. Patients with NASH also have a higher risk of progression to hepatocellular cancer than other patients with cirrhosis.

Diagnosis

NAFLD is suspected in patients with mild to moderate liver enzyme elevations, obesity, insulin resistance, or lipid abnormalities. Ultrasonography can be used to show large accumulations of fat in the liver. Computed tomography (CT) is a more sensitive technique that detects smaller fat accumulations. A definitive diagnosis requires a biopsy. Biopsy specimens show steatosis, inflammation, and, in advanced disease, fibrosis.

Treatment

If fatty liver is related to obesity, diabetes, or high lipid levels, treatment or better control of these conditions is the first step in treating fatty liver. Studies show that regular exercise and weight loss can slow disease progression. In NAFLD caused by intestinal bypass surgery, surgical reversal may be required. Drugs such as Actigall are being evaluated in clinical trials as treatments for NAFLD. Liver transplantation is rarely used as a treatment.

Miscellaneous Causes of Hepatitis

Sarcoidosis

Sarcoidosis is a chronic disease that causes the production of nodules containing nests of tissue cells. These nodules affect the function of the liver, lungs and lymph nodes. Sarcoidosis can cause an inflammatory process in the liver that progresses to hepatitis. Sarcoidosis is more common in African-Americans than other ethnic groups.

Shock (ischemic) liver

Shock caused by infection, trauma, or heart disease impairs blood circulation and interferes with cellular processes and organ functions. Shock can cause massive liver cell necrosis, causing a condition of hepatitis that can rapidly progress to fulminant liver failure.

13

Advanced Liver Disease

In most people, hepatitis resolves when infection clears, the offending drug or toxin is withdrawn, or medical intervention is successful in halting disease progression. Even when the liver is damaged, its tissue can regenerate. In acute hepatitis, treatment aims to reduce or ameliorate symptoms, stop the disease process, and prevent liver disease from progressing.

Acute infection that progresses to fulminant or chronic infection suggests disease that's resistant to treatment and on a course of its own. In fulminant infection, this course can rapidly progress, advancing toward liver failure and death. In chronic hepatitis, the disease course usually advances at a slower pace that can eventually lead to advanced conditions of fibrosis, cirrhosis, hepatocellular cancer, and liver failure. But even in chronic liver disease, occasionally the disease course can take a sudden turn and rapidly progress to fulminant liver failure. Chapter thirteen describes the various stages and types of advanced liver disease and the physiological changes that lead to liver failure.

Fulminant Liver Failure

Fulminant liver failure is defined as a potentially reversible condition resulting from severe liver injury or massive liver cell necrosis with onset of coma occurring within 8 weeks of the first symptoms of disease in the absence of preexisting severe liver disease. Subfulminant liver failure is a similar condition in which the mental changes and coma have a slower onset, taking 8 weeks to 6 months to appear. The term *acute liver failure* is used to describe either fulminant or subfulminant liver disease.

Acute liver failure represents a crisis situation in which massive liver cell necrosis or severe liver injury impair the liver's ability to function. This initiates a chain reaction affecting multiple organs, and death may occur even as the liver begins to recover. The inability to produce clotting proteins, process nutrients, and metabolize toxins leads to the characteristic features of: 1) hepatic encephalopathy and coma; 2) abnormal bleeding tendencies that predispose the patient to massive hemorrhaging; and 3) severe hypoglycemia, a condition of low blood sugar.

Causes of fulminant hepatitis

Fulminant hepatitis usually presents acutely in conditions of shock, viral infections, overdoses, idiosyncratic drug reactions, particularly reactions to antibiotics, and toxic exposures, including glue sniffing and ingestion of *Amanita* mushrooms (recent cases have been reported in France and California) [56]. Fulminant liver failure has also been reported in fatty liver of pregnancy and in hemodialysis patients exposed to contaminated water during dialysis. It can also emerge insidiously in patients with chronic disease. In cirrhosis, fulminant disease may develop rapidly when abnormal bleeding tendencies or infection precipitate liver failure.

Fulminant liver failure can be caused by all of the hepatitis viruses although it is very rarely seen in hepatitis C infection. Patients with hepatitis A typically have a more benign course although a higher mortality rate is seen in intravenous drug users and elderly patients.

Among the hepatitis viruses, hepatitis B is the most common cause of liver failure with a higher incidence in endemic areas. Patients with hepatitis B who are negative for hepatitis B surface antigen are presumed to have cleared the antigen quickly during massive cell necrosis. These patients have a higher survival rate than patients who are positive for surface antigen. Patients with hepatitis B who are co-infected with hepatitis D represent 50 percent of the fatalities in patients with HBV infection and liver failure.

Incidence and mortality

In the United States, about 2000 cases of fulminant liver failure occur each year. Of these, about 50 cases occur in children. In the absence of liver transplantation, which is the primary treatment for fulminant liver failure, the mortality rate in fulminant hepatic failure ranges from 60–80 percent.

Fulminant liver failure in children

In children, fulminant hepatitis can occur in accidental overdoses, viral and bacterial infections, as the initial presentation of Wilson's disease, and as a result of inborn errors of metabolism. Infants may present with vague symptoms of irritability, feeding problems, and sleep disturbances with a gradual progression to encephalopathy.

Hepatic encephalopathy

Hepatic encephalopathy is a characteristic feature of fulminant liver disease. Hepatic encephalopathy includes mental changes ranging from mild personality changes and drowsiness to profound coma. Onset is usually rapid, with rigidity and coma occurring within 24 hours. In patients with cirrhosis, episodes of encephalopathy can occur in intervals and appear to be triggered by certain factors such as gastrointestinal hemorrhage, sepsis, dehydration, constipation, or the use of sedatives.

Severity of encephalopathy can be graded using neurological tests and categorized into four distinct stages. Changes on encephalography (EEG) include: a bilateral slowing of normal alpha rhythm; appearance of delta waves; and in the later stages the appearance of triphasic waves. Cellular changes seen on biopsy are similar to those seen in Alzheimer's disease. Cerebral edema, a condition of increased fluid and swelling in the central nervous system, is commonly seen. Cerebral edema causes decreased blood flow within the brain, systemic hypertension and increased muscle tone leading to rigidity. Severe edema can raise blood pressure within the brain and injure the brain stem.

Brainstem injury is one of the most common causes of death in fulminant hepatic failure [10]. Other factors contributing to fatality include diminished levels of the actin scavenger, group-specific component (Gc) protein, which leads to abnormal actin deposits, massive hemorrhage, and metabolic hypoglycemia.

Circulatory changes

Acute liver failure results in a condition of vasodilation, which is a widening or stretching of blood vessels. Symptoms of vasodilation include flushed extremities, racing pulses, and pulsations in the small capillary blood vessels. In vasodilation, blood flow in the spleen is increased and blood flow in the kidneys is reduced. Cardiac output is increased, causing an abnormal heart rhythm or tachycardia, and a low blood pressure. Blood flow to the brain is reduced, contributing to the neurological changes in liver failure. Circulation in the lungs is also reduced, causing reduced levels of arterial oxygen saturation, which can lead to cyanosis and its associated symptoms of finger clubbing.

Coagulation defects

The liver's ability to produce clotting proteins is impaired in liver failure. This leads to decreased levels of factors II, V, VII, IX, and X, which causes prolonged prothrombin time (PT) and partial-thromboplastin time (PTT) levels. Blood PT and factor V levels are used to monitor the extent of liver damage. Gastrointestinal bleeding and ruptured esophageal varices are common manifestations of the clotting defects.

Infection

Infection is a common consequence of liver failure. Bacterial and fungal infections with progression to septicemia (blood infection) are related to indwelling catheters, a deficient immune response and corticosteroid or antibiotic treatment. Gram-positive organisms predominate in liver failure, suggesting that the skin may be the most important source of entry.

Fibrosis

The inflammatory process in hepatitis leads to microscopic changes in the liver consistent with scar tissue, causing a condition of fibrosis. Normally, the liver's stellate (star-shaped) cells store fat, vitamin A and protein molecules. In inflammation, stellate cells are activated by Kuppfer cells and immune system chemicals to produce collagen strands. These collagen strands are deposited in infected and injured cells to contain infection and injury. Normally, when infection or injury resolve, the collagen molecules dissolve and the affected stellate cells die, allowing the tissue to recover.

In chronic inflammation, ongoing collagen production increases and scar tissue forms. Fibrosis impairs the normal function of liver cells, reducing nutrient intake and decreasing the liver cell's ability to metabolize toxins. Blood flow also becomes impaired and contributes to cell death. In the early stages of fibrosis, damage is confined to the portal tracts of the liver. As fibrosis progresses, the damaged areas expand, causing a bridging fibrosis that extends between portal areas.

Diagnosis

Fibrosis is usually diagnosed by changes seen in liver biopsies. Several indexes, which are described in chapter fourteen, have been proposed for evaluating fibrosis based on laboratory results. In most protocols, the degree of fibrosis is predicted using liver enzyme levels, peptide levels, apolipoprotein levels, and platelet count. However, other causes of abnormal laboratory test results can affect results, interfering with the interpretation.

Contributing factors

Certain factors increase fibrosis. These include oxidative stress caused by antioxidant depletion related to alcohol abuse, drugs, and chronic liver disease; increased iron stores and deposits in iron storage disease; age, with advanced age causing increased vulnerability to oxidative stress; and fatty liver disease in conditions of obesity and diabetes. Fibrosis is also affected by nutrient status, severity of infection or injury, viral mutants, and immune system and collagen regulating genes.

Cirrhosis

Cirrhosis is the end stage of many types of liver disease that result in fibrosis. Factors influencing the progression of fibrosis to cirrhosis include severe liver injury, the length of ongoing inflammation, and the liver's response to damage. Cirrhosis is defined as diffuse liver fibrosis with nodular regeneration. The liver responds to injury by forming or regenerating new liver cells and producing collagen. When regeneration occurs with distorted changes in the form of nodules, and the collagen synthesis rate exceeds the degradation rate, cirrhosis develops.

While cirrhosis can occur as a consequence of any type of hepatitis, its two most common causes are alcoholic liver disease and chronic hepatitis C infection. Common symptoms include fatigue, loss of appetite, weakness, weight loss, abdominal pain and jaundice. About 20–30 percent of patients with chronic viral hepatitis develop cirrhosis. Of these about 3–5 percent develop hepatocellular carcinoma annually [28].

Compensated cirrhosis

In compensated cirrhosis, liver function remains adequate, and biochemical tests such as liver enzymes only show mild elevations. Patients may have characteristic symptoms such as firm liver enlargement, vascular spiders, reddened palms, and ankle swelling. Some patients may remain compensated until they die from other causes, and others progress into decompensated disease and liver failure or they develop severe complications such as gastrointestinal bleeding.

Decompensated cirrhosis

In decompensated cirrhosis, liver function and general health fail. Symptoms of jaundice, muscle wasting, weight loss, ascites, and fever are common. Jaundice indicates that liver damage has exceeded the capacity for regeneration. As disease progresses symptoms of hepatic encephalopathy, clotting abnormalities and circulatory problems develop. Urine urobilinogen levels are high, serum albumin levels are low, and alkaline phosphatase levels are moderately elevated. About 25,000 people die from cirrhosis annually in the United States.

Causes of cirrhosis

Cirrhosis is a serious condition resulting from progressive liver disease related to alcohol excess, chronic viral hepatitis, autoimmune hepatitis, a small number of drug toxicities, the autoimmune disorder primary biliary cirrhosis described later in this section, and in several metabolic and inherited liver disorders. Untreated, only 30 percent of patients with cirrhosis survive 5 years after their initial diagnosis.

Diagnosis

Diagnosis is made through liver biopsy. Tissue changes include fibrosis and liver nodules. Nodules less than 3 mm in diameter are seen in micronodular cirrhosis, and nodules from 3 to 5 mm in diameter along with thick bands of fibrous tissue are seen in macronodular cirrhosis. In mixed cirrhosis both types of lesions are seen. Micronodular cirrhosis is seen in the early stages, with conversion to the macronodular stages taking about two years. While these descriptions are helpful, it's more important in terms of prognosis and treatment to describe the etiology or cause of cirrhosis as determined by cellular changes or medical history.

Treatment

Liver damage cannot be reversed but treatment can stop or delay further progression, including progression to hepatocellular cancer. Primary treatment includes medications to ameliorate symptoms and specific therapies related to the cause of cirrhosis, such as interferon and anti-viral compounds for cirrhosis related to viral hepatitis. When complications cannot be controlled, liver transplantation is necessary. Survival after liver transplant for cirrhosis is 80–90 percent.

Primary biliary cirrhosis (PBC)

Primary biliary cirrhosis is a slowly progressive autoimmune liver disease that primarily affects women, with a peak incidence in the fifth decade of life. PBC is only rarely seen in people younger than 25 years. PBC is characterized by liver inflammation and destruction of the bile ducts. As a consequence, bile secretion is decreased and toxic substances are retained within the liver. These eventually cause further liver damage, fibrosis, cirrhosis and liver failure. Antimitochondrial antibodies are present in 90 to 95 percent of patients with PBC and they are often present before clinical signs appear.

Hepatocellular Carcinoma (HCC)

Hepatocellular cancer (HCC), a cancer that originates in liver cells (hepatocytes), is also known as primary liver cancer. It is the fourth most common cause of cancer worldwide and its incidence is steadily increasing because of the increased number of individuals with chronic viral hepatitis.

Risk factors

Certain factors influence the development of HCC. For instance, males are twice as likely to develop HCC as females, and individuals with iron overload have a high risk. Individuals who have used oral contraceptives for 8 years or longer or who have used anabolic steroids are also at high risk.

In hepatitis B infection, patients with high viral titers (greater than 10^5 virions/ml) are 7 times more likely to develop HCC as patients with low viral titers. In addition, Taiwanese patients with subtype C are 5 times more likely to develop HCC as patients with other subtypes.

Other risk factors for HCC include hepatitis C, moderate alcohol intake (more than 30 grams ethanol per day), severe fibrosis, cirrhosis, family history of liver cancer, and advanced age. Patients with both hepatitis B and hepatitis C are at a particularly high risk for HCC. Alcohol itself does not cause HCC but it promotes disease progression in individuals who develop hepatitis from other causes.

The hepatitis B virus is reported to inactivate an enzyme that normally protects the liver from cancer. HCC is more prevalent in countries in which hepatitis B infection is endemic, such as Nigeria, Benin, Singapore, Taiwan and Hawaii. In the United States and Europe, the prevalence of liver cancer is low. Environmental risk factors for HCC include chronic alcohol abuse, the mold aflatoxin B, plant alkaloids in certain teas, nitrosamines in charbroiled meats, vinyl chloride exposure and carbon tetrachloride exposure.

Disease course

Liver cancer develops slowly, usually over 30–40 years. It begins in the liver with the sporadic appearance of new cell populations. These new cell populations show clonal expansion by cell proliferation. The expanded clones or nodules serve as models for new clones with subtle changes. Over time, a malignant cell (neoplasm) line occurs and its growth is unrestricted leading to the development of liver cancer.

Viral genotypes

Clinical evidence indicates that certain viral genotypes found in specific populations are associated with a higher risk for HCC. For instance, subtype C of HBV is associated with risk for HCC in Taiwanese patients. In Alaska, where HCC is common, serologic evidence of HCV infection is low, whereas in Spain, 75 percent of patients with HCC show evidence of HCV infection.

Diagnosis

Abnormal laboratory results in HCC include increasingly high levels of the liver tumor marker alpha-fetoprotein (AFP), increasing ALT, AST, and alkaline phosphatase levels, hypoglycemia (low blood sugar), polycythemia (increase in red blood cells), hypercalcemia (elevated serum calcium), and increased fibrinogen (a clotting protein).

CT scan and MRI can be used to detect the presence of tumors and masses, and angiogram can be used to detect abnormal blood flow through tumors. Liver biopsy shows the presence of cancerous growths.

Sclerosing Hepatitis

A sclerosing form of hepatitis with rapid progression to fibrosis has been reported to occur in patients following liver transplants.

End-Stage Liver Disease

End-stage liver disease refers to acute liver failure that is resistant to treatment and conditions of decompensated cirrhosis. End stage liver disease is diagnosed in patients with abnormal liver function tests with symptoms of jaundice, ascites, edema, encephalopathy, coagulation defects, and malnutrition.

Priority for liver transplantation is based on a mathematical score known as the Model for End stage Liver Disease (MELD). The MELD score is based on blood levels of bilirubin, creatinine (indicator of kidney function) and prothrombin time, an indicator of coagulation defects.

14

Diagnosing Hepatitis

A diagnosis of hepatitis is a two-step process: 1) assessment of liver function — liver function tests, including enzyme and protein levels, are used to evaluate liver cell damage and also the liver's ability to carry out its normal functions; 2) determining specific causes of liver disease — specific diagnostic tests such as viral markers or copper levels. This chapter describes the various blood and imaging tests used to help diagnose hepatitis, determine its underlying cause, and monitor its response to treatment.

Blood Tests

Liver function tests include a number of different blood tests that assess liver damage as well as liver function. Included are liver enzyme levels, protein levels, and bilirubin tests. When abnormal liver profile or liver function test results suggest a diagnosis of hepatitis, other blood tests are used to see if the liver's function is impaired. For instance, the prothrombin time (PT) is commonly used to assess the liver's ability to synthesize clotting proteins. Other specialized tests such as ferritin levels and viral marker tests are used to determine the specific cause of liver disease.

Initial blood test results, which are known as baseline levels, help in establishing a timeframe that indicates if hepatitis is in its early infective stages or winding down. For instance, in viral hepatitis enzyme levels rise early and often fall within a week of disease onset. People with fulminant disease may show falling enzyme levels even while their condition is deteriorating. Serial tests are performed over time to help assess the disease course, response to treatment, and determine if complications are developing.

Liver enzyme level

Enzymes are proteins that enhance chemical reactions. For instance, the enzyme bromelain aids digestion, and enzyme-based detergents degrade the chemical bonds of stains. In the body, enzymes are constantly facilitating chemical reactions. In the liver, enzymes help convert food into energy, regenerate new cells, produce hormones and other proteins, detoxify chemicals, and eliminate wastes. The most important liver enzymes are the transaminase enzymes and the cholestatic enzymes.

When liver cells are damaged, transaminase enzymes spill from the cells and pour out into the blood circulation. When the bile ducts are inflamed, injured or blocked, cholestatic enzymes spill into the blood circulation. Enzyme levels, therefore, help determine the causes of liver disease. In evaluating the laboratory results, enzyme levels must be compared to specific reference or normal ranges. A slightly elevated transaminase enzyme level along with a markedly elevated cholestatic enzyme level suggests cholestatic liver disease rather than liver cell damage.

The extent of the enzyme elevation, while helpful in gauging improvement, doesn't necessarily correlate with disease severity. Certain conditions, described at the end of the enzyme section, are associated with specific enzyme changes.

TRANSAMINASE ENZYMES

Transaminase or aminotransferase enzymes include:

1. aspartate aminotrasferase (AST, formerly called SGOT)
2. alanine aminotransferase (ALT, formerly called SGPT)

ALT is primarily found in the liver, making it a more specific indicator of liver damage. Smaller amounts of ALT are found in skeletal muscle, kidneys, heart, muscle, and pancreas. In most cases, an elevated ALT suggests liver disease, whereas an elevated AST can have other causes. Besides residing in the liver, AST is also found in significant amounts in the heart, kidneys, and muscles. In liver cell injury, levels of both AST and ALT are elevated. An elevated AST level in a patient who has a normal ALT level suggests the elevated AST is a result of damage to other organs besides the liver.

Transaminase enzymes are usually normal in people with stable cirrhosis and metastatic liver disease. Slight to modest elevations of transaminase enzymes are seen in obesity, diabetes mellitus, alcohol abuse, drug reactions, and circulatory failure. Levels 2–10 times the normal range are seen in infectious mononucleosis, Wilson's disease, autoimmune hepatitis, protease inhibitor deficiencies, drug-related hepatitis, and immediately after passing gallstones. Marked elevations, more than 10 times the reference range, are seen in massive hepatic necrosis (for instance, acetaminophen overdoses), viral hepatitis, severe alcoholic hepatitis and severe ischemia.

Table 14.1 Enzyme reference values

Note: these are the most commonly used ranges;
values may vary depending on the testing method used.

ALT: The reference range for ALT is 2–45 IU/l

AST: The reference range for AST is 2–40 IU/l

ALP: The reference range for Alkaline phosphatase is 35–130 IU/l

Gamma GT: The reference range for Gamma glutamyl transferase (GGT) is 3–60 IU/l

Aldolase: The reference range for aldolase is <6 U/L

Cholinesterase: The reference range for cholinesterase is 8–18 UU/L

Lactic dehydrogenase (LDH): The reference range for LDH is 100–190 U/L

CHOLESTATIC ENZYMES

The cholestatic enzymes alkaline phosphatase (ALP) and gamma glutamyl transferase (GGT or Gamma GT) are increased in conditions in which bile flow is impaired, including bile duct defects and liver cell injuries that impair bile release. GGT is primarily produced in the bile ducts, whereas ALP is also found in bone, and smaller amounts are found in the placenta, bile ducts, intestines, and kidneys. When both GGT and ALP are increased, the liver is presumed to be responsible. If only ALP is elevated, and the cause is uncertain, an alkaline phosphatase fractionation test can be used to help determine if the elevation is from bone or liver.

Levels of alkaline phosphatase rise in cholestasis and to a lesser extent in liver cell damage. Levels of GGT rise in cholestasis and in hepatocellular disease. Levels are also increased by certain drugs and in alcoholism, even in the absence of liver disease, and occasionally in metastatic liver cancer. A high elevation of ALP in the presence of normal or only modestly elevated AST and ALT levels suggests disease of the bile ducts. An isolated elevated GGT with no other liver test abnormalities does not need to be further evaluated unless there are other risk factors and clinical signs of liver disease.

Other liver enzyme levels

Certain liver enzyme tests, such as lactic dehydrogenase (LDH), were once widely used to help diagnose liver disease. Because these enzymes are primarily elevated in other conditions, they are no longer routinely used to diagnose hepatitis except in the case of diagnostic challenges and special circumstances.

ALDOLASE

Aldolase is an enzyme found in various tissues and muscles that facilitates the breakdown and conversion of energy of the sugars glucose, fructose and galactose. Aldolase levels are increased in conditions of muscle damage, including the rhabdomyolysis caused by certain drugs, and in acute hepatitis.

CHOLINESTERASE

Cholinesterase is an enzyme produced by the liver necessary for metabolism of the neurotransmitter acetylcholine. Decreased levels are seen in hepatocellular disease, especially cirrhosis, and reflect diminished synthesis and malnutrition. Decreased levels of cholinesterase cause increased susceptibility to chemicals.

LACTIC DEHYDROGENASE (LDH)

Lactic dehydrogenase is an enzyme found in cardiac muscle and, in lower concentrations, in the liver. Marked increases in LDH are seen in patients with cancers that affect the liver.

Enzyme elevations in hepatitis

The transaminase enzymes and the alkaline phosphatase level are the primary tests used to diagnose and monitor hepatitis. The predominant enzyme to rise and the pattern of enzyme elevation can help differentiate the various types of hepatitis. The degree of enzyme elevation and the ratio of ALT relative to AST also vary in different types of hepatitis. Before the discovery of hepatitis C and blood tests to identify HCV infection, blood donors in the United States were tested for ALT, and donors with high levels were excluded.

ACUTE HEPATITIS

In the early stages of acute hepatitis AST levels are typically higher than ALT levels. Liver cells contain one and a half to two times as much AST as ALT. However, AST has a shorter half-life of 18 hours (time in the circulation before breaking down) than ALT, which has a half-life of 48 hours. Therefore, after one or two days of illness, ALT is typically higher than AST. Later in the disease course, if fibrosis or cirrhosis develop, the AST: ALT ratio can rise as liver damage exceeds liver cell regeneration.

In acute hepatitis caused directly by toxins or shock, AST and ALT levels increase rapidly, often to extremely high values, accompanied by a marked increase in prothrombin time. Peak abnormalities usually occur 24–48 hours after onset of injury and then rapidly fall to normal (according to their half-life). In acute hepatitis caused by viral infections, cell damage occurs over time and inflammation persists. Consequently, AST and ALT levels rise slowly, reach a plateau and then fall gradually over the course of several weeks. Prothrombin time are usually only elevated in severe cases.

ALCOHOLIC HEPATITIS

Alcohol injures liver cells directly, and it causes an immune response capable of cellular injury. Alcohol increases AST release and inhibits ALT production, causing a higher AST than ALT value. AST and ALT levels are only minimally increased compared to levels seen in other forms of hepatitis. In alcoholic hepatitis, AST rarely rises higher than 300 IU/l, and the ratio of AST to ALT is often greater than 2:1.

Transaminase enzyme levels are elevated in all types of liver disease. Usually, the highest levels are seen in severe cases of acute viral hepatitis, toxin or drug-induced hepatic necrosis, and ischemic hepatitis related to circulatory shock. Moderate transaminase elevations, usually 3–20 times the normal range are seen in acute or chronic hepatitis and alcoholic hepatitis.

CHRONIC HEPATITIS

Chronic hepatitis is almost always a clinically apparent disease. Symptoms are vague and mild and typically, diagnosis is made when elevated enzyme levels are detected. Usually, AST and ALT levels are elevated less than four times the upper limit of the reference range. In many cases, levels only show slight elevations and sometimes levels are only sporadically abnormal. Occasionally, 5–10 normal levels may separate elevated levels [28]. In some cases ALT levels are continually normal although mild signs of liver damage are seen on biopsy. Other laboratory tests in chronic hepatitis usually remain normal unless complications from chronic hepatitis develop.

Bilirubin and urobilinogen levels

Bilirubin is the end product resulting from the normal destruction of red blood cells and muscle. In the liver, bilirubin is metabolized and excreted. When liver cells are damaged or the production of bilirubin is increased, bilirubin spills out into the blood and levels of total bilirubin, primarily indirect bilirubin, are elevated. When total bilirubin rises to 3 mg/dl or higher, jaundice develops.

Increased amounts of bilirubin are seen in hemolytic conditions characterized by excessive red blood cell destruction and in conditions in which the liver cannot conjugate bilirubin or transport it through bile ducts. In the benign condition known as Gilbert's syndrome, bilirubin cannot be properly metabolized in the liver. This causes an elevation of indirect bilirubin although there are no related symptoms or signs of liver disease.

BILIRUBIN

In the blood, the bile pigment bilirubin is found in both its unconjugated or indirect form and in its conjugated or direct (polar) form. Levels of indirect bilirubin reflect bilirubin that has not yet been conjugated in the liver, for instance, bilirubin caused by the breakdown of red blood cells in neonatal jaundice. Direct bilirubin reflects bilirubin that has been conjugated in the liver. When liver cells are damaged, direct bilirubin is released into the blood circulation. Levels of total bilirubin measure both indirect and indirect bilirubin. Total bilirubin levels are used to measure the severity and progression of jaundice.

Levels of direct bilirubin more than 50 percent of the total suggest post-hepatic rather than hepatic jaundice, for instance cholestatic liver disease. Levels of direct bilirubin between 20 and 40 percent of the total value suggest hepatic liver disease.

Table 14.2 Bilirubin reference ranges

Total bilirubin reference range: 0.1–1.2 mg/dl
Indirect bilirubin reference range: 0.1–1.0 mg/dl
Direct bilirubin reference range: 0.2–0.4 mg/dl

Increased levels of indirect bilirubin are seen in: hemolytic states, extensive liver cancer, Gilbert's syndrome, toxins causing hemolysis (excessive breakdown of red blood cells), and neonatal jaundice.

Increased levels of direct bilirubin are seen in: viral or toxic hepatitis, alcoholic hepatitis, drug related hepatitis, cirrhosis, bile duct disorders, and cancer of the pancreas or common bile duct.

Blood glucose and hypoglycemia tests

Patients with hepatitis may have hypoglycemia, a condition of low fasting blood sugar. They may also show evidence of reduced liver glycogen stores. The severity of the hypoglycemia increases with increased liver cell damage, with severe hypoglycemia a characteristic finding in fulminant liver disease.

Reference rate for fasting glucose: 60–100 mg/dl

UROBILINOGEN

Urobilinogen is an intermediate product formed during the conjugation of bilirubin. Urine urobilinogen levels are increased in hemolytic jaundice and in viral hepatitis. In viral hepatitis increased urine urobilinogen may be the first change seen. Urine urobilinogen is measured as a semi-quantitative test with positive results graded from 1–4, with 4 indicating highest concentrations.

Protein levels

One of the liver's major functions is protein synthesis. Synthesis may be impaired in liver disease, and proteins may be released from injured cells. Some proteins, such as fibrinogen, haptoglobin, C3 complement, and alpha-1-antitrypsin are also released during inflammation. The proteins commonly measured to assess liver function include albumin, clotting proteins, and immunoglobulins.

ALBUMIN

The two major constituents of protein include albumin and globulin. Albumin is the major protein that circulates in the blood. Here, it carries or transports other substances including drugs and hormones. Albumin is produced in the liver and secreted into the blood, where it helps maintain fluid levels within tissues. Low levels of albumin lead to a release of fluid from tissues, causing a condition of edema. Individuals with chronic liver disease, especially those with cirrhosis, frequently have low albumin levels. Low albumin levels are seen in liver disease, malnutrition, and in some kidney disorders.

Reference range for albumin: 4.0–5.0 mg/dl

PROTHROMBIN TIME (PT)

The liver produces several different clotting proteins. When levels are deficient the blood's ability to clot is impaired. The time it takes blood to clot can be measured in a blood test called the prothrombin time (PT). During the testing process the amount of time that it takes for a specimen to clot is compared to a normal control, and a ratio known as the INR is calculated. Vitamin K can usually return the PT level to normal unless liver disease is particularly severe.

Reference range for prothrombin time= 9–11 seconds
Reference range for INR= 0.8–1.2

IMMUNOGLOBULINS

Immunoglobulins (Ig) are a class of proteins with several subtypes, including gamma globulin (IgG). Immunoglobulin proteins are produced in the liver and by white blood cells. Increases in specific immunoglobulins are seen in various liver diseases. For instance, levels of immunoglobulin G are increased in hepatitis C and autoimmune hepatitis, and levels of immunoglobulin A are increased in alcoholic liver disease.

Blood ammonia tests

Ammonia is a nitrogen-rich compound primarily produced in the colon during the metabolism of protein. As it passes through the liver ammonia is further metabolized to urea by hepatocytes. Certain factors, such as genetic mutations, can interfere with the metabolic process causing elevated blood ammonia levels (hyperammonia).

Severe or chronic liver failure, particularly in fulminant liver disease and advanced cirrhosis, can impair normal ammonia metabolism and cause hyperammonia. Ammonia levels are also elevated in most conditions of hepatic encephalopathy and in Reye's syndrome which is primarily a central nervous system disorder with only minor changes in liver function. The fasting ammonia level is helpful in diagnosing Reye's syndrome and in helping to determine if conditions of encephalopathy are related to liver dysfunction. The reference range for ammonia is 15–45 ug/dl or 11–32 umol/L.

Blood lipids tests

The liver plays a major role in producing, transporting, and metabolizing fatty lipid substances, primarily cholesterol, phospholipids, and triglycerides. The liver produces most of the body's cholesterol and a smaller amount, about 15 percent of the total cholesterol stores, is derived from diet. The liver metabolizes lipids into bile acids that are used to form cell membranes, hormones, and lipoproteins. Impaired lipoprotein synthesis, in turn, contributes to fatty liver.

About one-third of the fatty acids consumed daily are processed by the liver where they are either transformed into triglycerides or oxidized. Oxidation usually occurs in the fasting state, and transformation into triglycerides occurs in the non-fasting state. Excess triglyceride production results in a condition of fatty liver. In fatty liver, triglycerides lodge into liver cells displacing other cellular components. Triglyceride levels are usually increased in hepatitis and fatty liver disease.

Elevations of cholesterol are commonly seen in cholestatic liver disease although the reasons for this increase are uncertain. Fasting and states of malnutrition reduce cholesterol production. Consequently, in patients with advanced cholestatic tumors cholesterol levels may be normal [56].

Hematology tests

The complete blood count (CBC) is used to evaluate the red blood cell count, white blood cell count, platelet count, and red blood cell morphology. If anemia is present, the red blood cell count and its protein content, hemoglobin, are decreased. In hemochromatosis, the red blood cell count and hemoglobin are usually increased. The parameter most likely to be affected in hepatitis, however, is the platelet count.

Platelets are small blood components necessary for blood clotting. In hepatitis, the spleen often becomes enlarged and traps platelets intended for the blood circulation. Consequently, a low platelet count, which causes a condition called thrombocytopenia, may be seen in hepatitis. Thrombocytopenia causes an increased bleeding tendency, characterized by bruises. The reference range for platelets is 150–375K/ml. Patients with platelet counts less than 50K/ml are considered at risk for abnormal bleeding.

Renal (Kidney) Function Tests

Kidney function may be impaired by immune complex deposits as an extrahepatic manifestation or complication of alcoholic cirrhosis or viral hepatitis. More often, decreased renal function and renal failure occur as a complication of fulminant or end-stage liver disease. In end-stage liver disease, the kidneys show no abnormalities. Their inability to function is due to alterations in renal blood flow, causing a condition of hepatorenal syndrome. Kidneys removed from dying patients with hepatorenal syndrome assume normal function when transplanted into transplant recipients [54].

The tests most often used to evaluate kidney function are the blood urea nitrogen (BUN) and creatinine tests, which measure the kidney's ability to clear protein. Both of these tests are elevated in kidney disease.

Reference range for BUN= 8–23 mg/dl

Reference range for creatinine= 0.1–0.6 mg/dl

Fibrosis Indexes and Tests

Several protocols for evaluating fibrosis or liver function based on laboratory test results have been proposed, and several blood tests have been developed for evaluating fibrosis. The most commonly used protocols are the Child-Turcotte Class modified by Pugh, which is often called the Child class, and the APRI index. The FibroTest and FibroSpect tests are new experimental procedures used to evaluate the degree of fibrosis in patients with hepatitis C who prefer to not have liver biopsies.

Child-Turcotte Class

In the Child-Turcotte class, liver function is graded from A through D, with patients in class A having a higher predicted survival rate. This index is particularly important in assessing a patient's suitability for liver transplantation. The index is based on measures of albumin, bilirubin, prothrombin time, and the demonstration of ascites or encephalopathy.

APRI Index

The APRI index is a calculated index derived from laboratory test results used to assess the severity of liver damage. The calculation is based on the laboratory's reference range for AST and the patient's AST result and platelet count.

FibroSpect

The FibroSpect test developed by Prometheus Laboratories is used to evaluate degrees of cirrhosis in patients with hepatitis C. Results are reported in a range from 0–4, indicating no liver scarring to severe liver scarring. Its use in evaluating fibrosis in other types of liver disease is under evaluation.

FibroTest

Manufactured in France, the FibroTest is a commercial test that is also able to determine staging in fibrosis in hepatitis C.

Other tests for fibrosis and cirrhosis

The liver biopsy remains the gold standard for detecting and evaluating fibrosis and cirrhosis. However, certain blood test abnormalities are typically seen in cirrhosis, and these results offer insight into the progression of liver disease. Abnormalities seen in liver disease that has progressed to fibrosis or cirrhosis include: elevated iron, ferritin, transferrin, and alpha-fetoprotein, and a low platelet count.

Tests for Metabolic Disorders

Metabolic causes of hepatitis are diagnosed by using specific tests, such as iron and transferrin levels in suspected hemochromatosis or fructose tolerance tests for hereditary fructose intolerance. Certain genetic tests for amino acid and other mutations can also be used. For instance, the HFE gene test for the C282Y homozygote is used to diagnose hereditary hemochromatosis. Other tests used to diagnose metabolic causes of hepatitis are described in chapter twelve.

Tests for iron overload disorders

Although iron and ferritin levels are typically increased in hemochromatosis, elevations of these levels are also seen in any condition of hepatocyte injury as the liver cell contents are spilled into the blood circulation. Conditions of acute inflammation occurring in other organs can also falsely elevate these results. In patients with viral hepatitis or other conditions of liver cell necrosis, the results of liver function tests may be identical to that seen in iron overload disorders.

Also, in sudden presentations of acute iron overload, iron levels may not show significant elevations. When diagnosis is in doubt, genetic tests, liver biopsy, and imaging tests capable of detecting iron stores may be necessary. There are five distinct types of hereditary hemochromatosis: Type 1, Type 2A, Type 2B, Type 3, and Type 4.

The gene mutations characteristic of hereditary hemochromatosis can be identified with blood tests. For hereditary hemochromatosis Type 1, one of two different mutations of the HFE gene known as C282Y and H63D mutations, are seen. Genetic mutations at gene JHV (hemojuvelin) are seen in hemochromatosis Type 2A, and mutations in the transferrin receptor 2 (TFR2) are seen in hemochromatosis type 2. A mutation of the SLC 40A1 gene that regulates the protein ferroportin is seen in hemochromatosis type 4.

Biopsy has the advantage of being able to measure iron content corrected for age and to predict the degree of fibrosis or cirrhosis. Bone marrow aspirations are not recommended as the iron content in marrow is not adequate for a proper determination of iron stores.

Liver Autoantibody Tests

In autoimmune disease, the immune system produces antibodies that react with the body's cells and tissue. Autoantibodies to liver cells are seen in autoimmune liver diseases, such as autoimmune hepatitis, although occasionally low titers of liver antibodies are seen in viral hepatitis and other autoimmune conditions. For instance, anti-mitochondrial antibodies, which are always seen in primary biliary cirrhosis, are sometimes seen in low titers in patients with the autoimmune thyroid disorder Graves' disease. The liver autoantibody tests used to diagnose autoimmune liver disorders are described in chapter ten.

Viral Markers

Most patients with elevated transaminase enzymes, jaundice or other signs and symptoms of liver disease will be tested for hepatitis viruses.

The basic screening tests for viral hepatitis detect viral antigens and antibodies, and the more specific confirmatory tests measure viral DNA or RNA.

Viral antigens and antibodies

Viruses are made up of various specific protein components known as viral antigens. These viral antigens can be identified in blood tests to diagnose viral infection. Viral antigens, however, may not show up for several weeks to several months after the onset of infection, and in most cases viral antigens only persist for short periods.

As the disease resolves, the immune system attempts to clear the virus by producing specific antibodies that can sometimes neutralize or destroy the viral antigens. Tests for viral antibodies can be used to diagnose current and past infections. The earliest antibodies produced by the immune system are IgM antibodies. The presence of IgM HAV antibodies, for instance, indicates active HAV infection. Over time, the immune system produces longer acting IgG antibodies. Tests for IgG antibodies are used to detect past infection or immunity from vaccinations.

HEPATITIS VIRAL PANELS

Viral panels include several different tests that measure either antigens or antibodies to HAV, HBV and HDV using enzyme immunoassay, chemiluminescence or recombinant immunoblot assays. In patients who show evidence of hepatitis B infection, tests for hepatitis D may also be performed. Equivocal results for HAV IgM and HBcIgM suggest that the patient is forming antibodies that haven't yet reached the detection limit or that acute infection is resolving and the titer is dropped. Equivocal reports are reported as such with a recommendation that the test be repeated in 1–2 weeks.

Tests for hepatitis E are used in patients from or who have recently traveled to endemic regions. Nucleic acid tests for viral particles are used to confirm infection, determine the level of infectious particles, and monitor treatment response. Genotype profiles are used to determine the type and subgroup of HBV and HCV.

Hepatitis testing is important in four periods of patient care: 1) time of diagnosis, using genotype testing to identify types of hepatitis that are more aggressive or more difficult to treat; 2) during therapy to see if viral load is falling in response to therapy; 3) at the completion of therapy to determine if there is an end therapy response; and 4) 6 months after the completion of therapy using nucleic acid tests to see if there is a sustained response to therapy [1].

Table 14.3. Viral hepatitis markers

Hepatitis A: HAV IgM antibody; anti-HAV IgM

Positive test indicates acute hepatitis A (HAV) infection; HAV IgM shows up early in infection and persists for 2–6 months.

Hepatitis A: HAV IgG antibody; anti-HAV IgG

Positive test indicates past infection; HAV IgG appears toward the end of acute illness and persists for several years, causing life-long immunity.

Hepatitis A: HAV Ab; total anti-HAV, measuring IgG and IgM antibodies

Positive test indicates past infection or immunity; if HAV IgM is negative; a positive total HAVAb test indicates past infection.

Hepatitis B: HBsAg; hepatitis B surface antigen

HBsAg appears from 6 days to several months after infection, and it also appears transiently within 8 days of HBV and combined HBV/HAV vaccines; seen with HBcIgM in acute infection; with HBeAg indicates active, replicating virus; persists with HBcAb in HBV carriers; normally clears within a few weeks to a few months in infection as the clinical course subsides; if HBsAg clears before HBsAb appear in the circulation (window period), infection may be missed.

Hepatitis B: HBsAb; hepatitis B surface antibody

HBsAb forms as HBsAg clears from the blood in infection; occurs and persists after HBV vaccinations indicating protective immunity; may occur in patients with active HBV infection who are actively infected with escape mutants

Hepatitis B: HBc IgM, hepatitis B core IgM antibody

HBcIgM appears early in infection before HBsAb; indicates early or acute HBV infection within the preceding 4–6 weeks

Hepatitis B: HBcAb, hepatitis B core total antibody, includes IgG and IgM

HBcAb in the absence of HBcIgM indicates exposure to HBV with recovery/immunity; persistent HBcAb and HBsAg indicates chronic infection

Hepatitis B: HBcAg; hepatitis B core antigen

Primarily used to detect core antigen in liver biopsy specimens; indicates acute active infection

Hepatitis B: HBeAg, hepatitis Be antigen

HBeAg has traditionally been associated with HBV infectivity; however escape mutants can prevent HBeAg production and expression, masking infectivity; Patients with negative HBeAg who have detectable HBV DNA are considered to be

Table 14.3.(cont.)

Hepatitis B: HBeAb; hepatitis Be antibody

Hepatitis C: HCVAb, hepatitis C antibody, measurement of both IgG and IgM HCV antibodies.

Hepatitis C: HCVAb by RIBA; recombinant immunoblot assay

Hepatitis D: HDV Ag; hepatitis D antigen

Hepatitis D: HDV IgM; hepatitis D IgM antibodies

Hepatitis D: HDV Ab; hepatitis D antibody

Hepatitis E: HEV IgG; hepatitis E IgG antibody

Hepatitis G: HGV Ab; hepatitis G antibody

more resistant to conventional therapy than patients who are positive for HBeAg.

HBeAb appears as HBeAg clears from the blood; associated with lower-level or recovering acute infection or response to therapy with lower levels of HBV DNA and lowered transaminase enzyme levels; also seen in chronic HBV infection in which HBeAg has cleared or infectivity persists due to escape mutants.

Positive results are seen in both active and past infection; positive results are reported as a signal/cutoff ratio s/c that compares the strength of the test reaction to a normal control. Results with S/C values <8.0 are not predictive of a true HCV result and require repeat or additional testing; S/C values >8.0 indicate highly predictive, >95 percent confidence, of a true anti-HCV status; in acute HCV infection the appearance of HCV antibodies may be delayed for several months, making tests for HCV RNA better indicators of acute disease. False positive antibody screen results may occur and S/C values <8.0 require additional or repeat testing.

Alternate procedure used to confirm positive HCVAb test results, although, with determination of HCVAb and the introduction of tests for HCV RNA, this test is no longer widely used.

HDV Ag in the presence of HBsAg occurs in acute HDV infection

HDV IgM antibodies are seen in acute HDV infection

HDV antibodies are seen in HDV infection; titers higher than 1:1000 indicate active viral replication.

HEV IgG antibodies are seen in approximately 93 percent of acute HEV infections; negative results may occur in early HEV infection before antibodies emerge and in past, resolved HEV infections.

Total HGV antibodies indicate acute or past infection

H=hepatitis; A,B,C,D, E, G=type of virus; V=virus; Ag=antigen; Ab=antibody; IgM=immunoglobulin M antibody; IgG=immunoglobulin G antibody; HBc= hepatitis B core protein; HBs= hepatitis B surface protein; HBe= hepatitis Be protein;

Nucleic acid testing (NAT)

Molecular biology techniques are used to identify specific viral particles. Small amounts of viral material in body fluids can be tested directly or amplified for better recovery. With these analyses, the level of viral RNA or DNA (viral load) in a certain amount of blood, usually one ml, can be determined. Because viral particles are present in the blood before the immune system is able to produce detectable antibodies, infections can be diagnosed days or weeks earlier than with antibody tests. Consequently, positive NAT results can be used to confirm a positive viral antibody screening test. However, a negative NAT test result doesn't clarify whether an antibody screening test result is a true positive. In the case of specimens with low positive (<8.0 S/C ratio) HCV antibody results that test negative for HCV RNA, the CDC recommends repeating the antibody test with a RIBA method [13].

Various methods are used for direct NAT testing, such as the polymerase chain reaction (PCR) technique, reverse transcriptase (RT) PCR, target-amplified direct nucleic amplification (TMA) tests and the branched chain DNA (bDNA) HBV tests. These tests are designed to detect unique nucleic acid sequences. Because bDNA assays are less sensitive than other methods they are no longer used as much today, and they are not recommended for diagnosing HCV infection or determining treatment endpoints [13].

Table 14.4. Viral hepatitis nucleic acid tests (viral load) and indications

HBV DNA (PCR), Qualitative	Measures HBV DNA polymerase enzyme; to help determine if treatment is indicated; indicator of chronic infection when present 6 months after the onset of acute HBV infection; monitor treatment response; demonstrates viral replication
HBV DNA, Quantitative	To help determine if treatment is indicated; indicator of chronic infection when present 6 months after the onset of acute HBV infection; monitor treatment response; demonstrates viral replication; indicates emergence of resistant variant mutants;
HBV DNA (bDNA)	Limited dynamic range with sensitivity of 500 IU/ml; no longer recommended

Table 14.4 (cont.)

HCV RNA, Qualitative (PCR)	Measures level of HCV RNA polymerase enzyme; detects acute infection prior to seroconversion (antibody production); confirm positive antibody test results; differentiate between resolved and active infection; demonstrate resolution of infection; Limit of detection (LOD) for Roche Diagnostics Cobas Amplicor HCV test = 50 IU or approximately 100 copies/ml; LOD for Bayer Versant TMA test= 5.1 IU/ml or approximately 10–20 copies/ml; HCV PCR by TaqMan real time technology with a dynamic range as high as 28,800,000 IU/ml.
HCV RNA, Quantitative	Predict and monitor response to antiviral therapy; differentiate active asymptomatic infection from disease resolution; not a strong prognostic indicator as patient samples contain a broad concentration range of HCV virions although they offer benefits for therapy stopping strategies. The Heptimax viral load test is one of the most sensitive tests with a reportable range of 5 IUs/ml to 8.3 million IUs/ml; the Roche Diagnostics Cobas Amplicor HCV Monitor Test has a detection range of 600–500,000 IUs
HCV branched DNA (bDNA) test	Less sensitive than qualitative and quantitative assays for HCV RNA; Bayer Versant HCV vDNA test reference range= 615–8 million IUs.

Viral load interpretation

Qualitative measurements are more sensitive but results for these tests are only reported as positive or negative. Using a qualitative test with a detection limit of 100 eq/ml, test results greater than 100 are considered positive, and results below 100 are considered negative. The virus may be present, but if its value is lower than that of the detection level, it is considered negative.

Quantitative measurements of HBV DNA or HCV RNA detect viral load, which is a measure of the amount of viral material present in a specific volume of blood. Viral load levels range from not detectable to several hundred million international units (IUs). Each different testing method has a different sensitivity limit or low level of detection. In general, the lower the pre-treatment viral load, the more likely it is that a person will respond to treatment.

Branched DNA tests

Branched DNA tests for hepatitis B and C, while less expensive than tests for DNA or RNA, are seldom used because they lack the sensitivity of the other tests.

DNA or RNA polymerase (PCR tests)

Tests for DNA or RNA polymerase report levels of viral enzymes and may be used as qualitative tests to indicate negative or positive results, based on a cut-off range. They generally have a greater sensitivity than quantitative tests. Factors affecting viral enzyme production could also influence the results, including different rates of replication in mutant species.

Units of measurement

Viral load may be measured in copies/ml, eq/ml, or IUs/ml. The World Health Organization recommends using IUs for measuring viral load. Tests that report viral load in other units of measurement include a conversion formula for converting results into IUs. Most of these formulas are based on 2–5 viruses for each international unit. If conversion formulas aren't available, results in eq/ml are divided by 3 to determine IUs. For instance, the average viral load of hepatitis C is 3.2 million eq/ml or 1 million IU/ml.

Log changes

When evaluating a response to treatment, changes in log are more important than the actual viral count. A one log change is a 10-fold increase or decrease. For instance a viral load of 1,000 indicates a 2-log decrease from a previous count of 100,000.

Treatment evaluation

A decrease in viral load during treatment indicates a good treatment response. Treatment causes a complete virological response if it reduces viral load to an undetectable level. After 12 weeks of treatment, a 2-log decrease in viral load or non-detectable viral levels indicates a good treatment response.

Viral Genotype Tests

Shortly after diagnosis of HBV or HCV infection, viral genotype tests are used to determine the specific viral subtype. Several different methods, such as line probe assay and the recently introduced HCV DupliType assay with increased sensitivity, are available using molecular genetic techniques.

Specific treatment protocols are used depending on the particular viral genotype a patient has. For instance, patients with type 2 or type 3 HCV receive combination treatment for 24 weeks compared to 48 weeks or longer in patients with type 1 HCV. Genotypes in HBV infection are helpful in determining mutant strains with resistance to specific treatments.

Tests for other infectious causes of hepatitis

In instances of suspected hepatitis virus not caused by the common hepatitis viruses, other tests may be used to help with diagnosis. For instance, blood tests that show antibodies to cytomegalovirus, Epstein-Barr virus, and bacterial antigens can be used to help diagnose other infectious causes of hepatitis.

Tumor Markers

Many cancer cells produce specific proteins, hormones and enzymes at a much higher rate than what is normally seen. Elevated levels of these compounds can be used as tumor markers to help diagnose various cancers. However, many of these proteins are only elevated in certain stages of cancer. In addition, elevations may be seen in more than one type of cancer, and levels may also be elevated in other benign conditions. Thus, elevated tumor marker levels can suggest specific diseases but not provide a definitive diagnostic tool.

Alpha-fetoprotein (AFP)

Alpha-fetoprotein (AFP) is a protein produced during fetal development by the fetal yolk sac and by the liver. Levels in maternal blood are elevated during pregnancy, with peak concentrations seen early in the second trimester of pregnancy. In adults, increased levels indicate tumor elements or increased liver cell regeneration. Increased AFP levels are seen in patients with liver cancer, hepatitis, and liver cirrhosis. In patients with fulminant hepatitis, a low AFP is an ominous sign and indicates that the liver is not producing new cells and repairing itself.

The reference range for AFP is 0–20 ng/ml. Moderate elevations, usually less than 100 ng/ml, are seen in acute and chronic hepatitis, cirrhosis, liver tumors, pregnancy, cystic fibrosis, stomach cancer, and pancreatic cancer. In liver cancer, the AFP is usually markedly elevated with levels generally higher than 400 ng/ml. With successful treatment for HCC, the AFP will usually fall to normal levels and rise in the event of recurrences. However, not all types and stages of HCC cause an increased AFP, and a normal AFP is not reassurance that there is no evidence of HCC.

Imaging Tests

In patients suspected of having hepatitis, imaging tests are not usually included in the diagnostic workup. However, certain imaging tests may be used to see if the liver is enlarged or shrunken, and to check for anatomical abnormalities, masses, cysts, abscesses, and gallstones. Routine X-rays can be used to detect gallstones that are not calcified when they are suspected, but the following imaging tests are more commonly used today: ultrasonography (ultrasound, sonograms); radionuclide imaging; computerized axial tomography (CT, CAT) scans; and magnetic resonance imaging (MRI) techniques.

Ultrasonography

Ultrasonography is a procedure in which sound waves are used to produce images. It is the least expensive technique for creating images of the gallbladder and biliary tract. In distinguishing causes of jaundice, ultrasound can tell if the cause is bile duct obstruction or blood flow obstruction caused by cysts.

Liver sonograms, which are performed on patients after fasting to ensure an empty stomach, can show abnormal masses and changes in size. Overall, sonography is better for detecting structural changes than diffuse tissue changes. Ultrasound is often used in conjunction with liver biopsy to guide the surgeon to the area of the liver in which abnormalities are present.

ELASTOGRAPHY

Elastography, using a FibroScan technique, is an ultrasonography procedure used to measure the stiffness of liver tissue. Used in conjunction with chemistry tests for the evaluation of fibrosis, elastography offers a non-invasive method of grading fibrosis in patients with liver disease.

Radionuclide imaging

In radionuclide imaging, a radioisotope such as technetium is injected intravenously. The isotope travels through the circulation and ultimately is taken up by the liver. The liver is then scanned using gamma rays. This technique is particularly helpful for detecting blockages in the cystic duct and gallbladder inflammation.

CT scans

Computerized axial tomography scans, which use gamma radiation, show the liver in relation to its surrounding organs. Changes in mass caused by tumors or fatty deposits can be seen on CT scans. CT scans are usually used to further study masses seen on sonograms. Various CT techniques in which multiple images are taken are sometimes used to evaluate the liver's function over a period of time.

MRI

Magnetic resonance imaging (MRI) is similar to CT scanning although it does not use radiation. MRI can detect changes in density occurring in tissue caused by tumors, cysts, calcifications, and fat deposits. MRIs are particularly helpful for evaluating fatty liver, conditions of iron overload and related conditions.

15

Liver Biopsy

In liver biopsies, one or more small samples of liver tissue are removed with a needle aspiration or surgically. Theses tissue specimens are then sent to the laboratory where they are examined under a microscope. During this examination, pathologists check for cellular changes and tissue abnormalities indicative of specific liver diseases.

Biopsy results reveal the nature of liver cell injury and damage and they can be used to classify the cellular injury according to its severity and progression. Chapter fifteen describes the procedures used in liver biopsy. In addition this chapter explains how biopsy results are used to diagnose liver disease and evaluate disease severity.

Needle Biopsy of the Liver

In 1833, the physician Paul Ehrlich performed the first liver biopsy in an effort to study the impaired glucose metabolism of a diabetic patient. Although several other physicians followed his lead, the liver biopsy remained in the back shadow of medicine until the 1930's at which time it became a popular procedure in both France and the United States. In the following decade, liver biopsy was embraced as the primary diagnostic tool for investigating the high incidence of viral hepatitis among armed forces returning from World War II.

Before the discovery of hepatitis C in 1989, biopsies were still widely used to diagnose patients with suspected hepatitis who tested negative for hepatitis A and hepatitis B. Today, with sensitive tests for diagnosing hepatitis C and autoimmune hepatitis, biopsies are performed less often. Biopsies aren't as sensitive as viral marker tests for diagnosing viral hepatitis. However, biopsies are still considered necessary for assessing the extent of liver scarring, fatty infiltration, and liver damage in patients with certain forms of liver disease including chronic hepatitis and alcoholic liver disease.

Liver biopsy is also helpful for identifying drug-related acute liver disease when the medical history is unclear and for establishing the cause of elevated liver enzymes in patients with fatty liver disease. Certain infections, such as syphilis or herpes, can be identified by biopsies when the cause of liver disease in uncertain. Biopsies are often performed after liver transplants to help determine the source of new liver problems.

What to expect

Most biopsies are performed in radiology or gastroenterology departments of hospitals or surgical clinics and are scheduled for the early morning. Occasionally, liver biopsies are performed during surgical procedures.

How to Prepare

Patients must avoid taking any medications that interfere with the blood's ability to clot for at least ten days before a scheduled biopsy. These include blood thinners such as Coumadin; analgesics, including aspirin, nonsteroidal anti-inflammatory medications such as ibuprofen and naproxen, cyclooxygenase inhibitors such as Celebrex and Vioxx, and supplements containing vitamin E, ginkgo biloba, ginseng, and garlic.

Within one week of the procedure, the patient's liver function status, blood count, platelet count, and clotting ability are evaluated with laboratory tests. Patients with abnormal bleeding times, anemia, low platelet counts, or poor platelet function may require treatment or blood product transfusion before a biopsy can be performed. The blood group and type are also tested and a specimen is retained so that blood can be crossmatched quickly in the event blood transfusions are needed.

Indications

Liver biopsies are performed on patients with suspected liver diseases, liver masses, or an enlarged liver. In some liver diseases, a biopsy helps determine the best course of treatment. For instance, before treatment for viral hepatitis, a biopsy may be needed to assess the progress of the disease and its course. In patients with small atrophied livers or ascites, an adequate biopsy specimen may be difficult to obtain and the risk of inadvertently puncturing other organs is increased.

Biopsy procedures

In some cases, a mild sedative or analgesic is administered intravenously to help relax the patient. Patients are asked to lie on their right side or on their back with their right arm beneath their head.

The doctor is usually able to locate the liver by tapping on it. The surface skin is then cleaned and covered with sterile towels. Into the clean dry surgical area, the doctor injects a local anesthetic agent, usually lidocaine, to numb the surface area. Once the anesthetic takes hold, the doctor inserts a needle into the liver for a fraction of a second and a sample of liver tissue is removed. The biopsy sample typically contains one or two small slivers of liver tissue. In the event that the sample is insufficient, the doctor may have to repeat the needle stick.

Once the procedure is complete, the area is bandaged and the patient is instructed to lie on his right side or back for a period of two to six hours. During this time, the patient's vital signs will be taken regularly.

MENGHINI AND OTHER TECHNIQUES

The Menghini needle removes liver tissue through aspiration and is particularly helpful for patients with cirrhosis. Tissue samples may be fragmented during removal but the procedure is quick, safe, and effective. Tru-Cut needles and Biopty guns with attached needle may also be used depending on the preference of the physician.

A short needle is available for pediatric patients. Pediatric patients are often treated with pentobarbital and a local anesthetic.

BLIND AND GUIDED TECHNIQUES

In the blind technique, the doctor aims for an area of the liver after inspecting the surface. In fine-needle guided biopsy, a specific direct location is targeted, making it particularly helpful for diagnosing tumors.

ULTRASOUND-GUIDED BIOPSY

An ultrasound procedure is often performed simultaneously with the biopsy to help guide the needle insertion.

COMPUTERIZED TOMOGRAPHY (CT)-GUIDED BIOPSY

Where a precise area of the liver needs to be biopsied or there are other imposing organs or interfering fat layers, a CT scan can be used to guide the needle insertion.

LAPAROSCOPY

In laparoscopy, a thin lighted tube or laparoscope is inserted through an incision made in the abdominal wall, and other internal organs are moved away by introducing gas into the abdomen. Instruments may be passed through the laparoscope or through separate puncture sites to obtain biopsy specimens.

TRANSVENOUS OR TRANSJUGULAR LIVER BIOPSY

In patients with abnormal bleeding tendencies or ascites, a radiologist may perform a transvenous or transjugular liver biopsy. In this procedure a needle is inserted through a catheter into a vein that connects to the portal vein, and a biopsy sample can be obtained. This type of biopsy is indicated in patients with bleeding tendencies, coagulations disorders, failed percutaneous biopsies, small livers, and in uncooperative patients.

SURGICAL LIVER BIOPSY

Liver biopsy samples may be obtained during open abdominal operations such as exploratory laparotomies. In patients with abnormal bleeding tendencies or other risk factors, patients are often transfused with fresh frozen plasma containing clotting factors before surgery.

Difficulties

Failure to obtain a good biopsy sample is most likely to occur in patients with cirrhosis who have ascites. The tough cirrhotic liver can be difficult to pierce and only a few cells may be obtained. Difficulties also occur in pulmonary emphysema because the liver is pushed downward by the low diaphragm.

After the procedure

After the procedure is complete, the patient is required to remain for several hours for observation and monitoring of vital signs. Studies show that most complications that arise from biopsy emerge within the first few hours after the biopsy although complications can occur within the first fifteen days after the procedure. After patients are discharged they are advised to stay within an hour's drive of the surgical facility.

Complications

Possible complications include excessive bleeding from the puncture site and damage to adjacent organs particularly the kidney, colon, and gallbladder. Excessive bleeding occurs in less than 1 percent of patients and is most likely to occur in patients with abnormal bleeding tendencies. In cases where the gallbladder is accidentally punctured, bile can leak into the abdominal cavity causing a condition of peritonitis. Bleeding is the most common complication and peritonitis is the second most frequent complication of liver biopsy. Mortality from liver biopsy is extremely low, ranging from 0.01 to 0.1 percent. Deaths from hemorrhage usually occur in patients with a poor prognosis.

A small number of patients, about 2 percent, may develop hematomas, which are characterized by blood clots or fibrosis, or bruising at the puncture site. Hematomas may be accompanied by fever and rarely delayed hemorrhage [56]. In about five percent of patients vascular fistulas may occur and cause abnormal bleeding. In most cases fistulas spontaneously heal.

A transient infection can also occur, especially in patients with cholangitis. Septicemia, which is a systemic blood infection, is rarely seen and usually caused by infection with *Escherichia coli*.

Biopsy Specimens

A satisfactory biopsy specimen is 1–4 cm long, weighs 10–50 mg, and contains tissue from four portal zones. Often, three consecutive samples are taken by redirecting the biopsy needle through a single puncture. Specimens from livers with cirrhosis tend to crumble and have an irregular contour due to nodules, whereas in fatty liver, specimens have a pale greasy texture. Cholestasis causes the liver to be green, and metastatic tumors often cause the tissue to appear white.

Specimens are immediately fixed or preserved in formaldehyde solutions and fixed into thin tissue layers that can be stained and studied. A variety of different stains can be used to study copper and iron stores, the age of the cells, active collagen synthesis, viral antigens, and fatty deposits.

Biopsy Results

Because most types of liver disease are diffuse, affecting liver tissue consistently, a small amount of tissue can reveal a great deal of information. When tumors are suspected, a specific area of tissue is removed. Biopsy results indicate if the cells are healthy or if there are signs of necrosis, cancer, cholestasis, viral infection, cirrhosis, steatosis or inflammation. Certain signs of necrosis, such as balloon-like swelling, are characteristic of viral hepatitis. The most important finding in liver biopsy is the stage of liver disease, characterized by the degree of fibrosis or cirrhosis.

Sections of tissue are routinely stained for iron content. Copper deposits are also seen in stained preparations, appearing as black-brown granules in patients with cholestasis and occasionally in patients with advanced Wilson's disease. Special stains can also be used to identify alpha-1-antitrypsin globules in patients with alpha-1-antitrypsin deficiency.

Tissue specimens are also examined with electron microscopy. Electron microscopy is particularly valuable for identifying tumors, and storage disorders such as Wilson's disease.

Necrosis

Liver cell destruction is known as liver necrosis. When necrosis involves individual hepatocytes or small groups of cells, it's called focal necrosis. When several regions of focal necrosis are seen, the term spotty necrosis is used. This is a characteristic finding in acute hepatitis. Confluent necrosis refers to substantial areas of liver-cell death and, accompanied by signs of inflammation, it is most often seen in viral or drug-induced hepatitis. Confluent necrosis without inflammation is seen in shock, heart failure, and acetaminophen overdoses.

Piecemeal necrosis is a process of erosion of liver tissue at its junction with portal tracts accompanied by inflammation. Necrosis is described as bridging when it extends from portal venules to portal tracts. Bridging necrosis is seen in acute hepatitis and in acute phases of chronic hepatitis.

Cholestasis

Cholestasis refers to the presence of visible bile in tissue sections. Bile may occur in the form of acute patches near the cell canaliculi or as intrahepatic (between cells) bile plugs or deposits forming duct-like structures. Canalicular cholestasis is mostly seen in acute hepatitis, cholestatic drug jaundice and large bile-duct obstructions. Intrahepatic cholestasis is seen as a result of certain drugs, such as oral contraceptives, in sepsis, pregnancy and in lymphomas.

Viral hepatitis

Unlike bacterial infection, which causes acute inflammatory changes on liver biopsy, viral hepatitis is characterized by an infiltration of liver tissue with white blood cells, primarily lymphocytes and macrophages, and cellular changes consistent with liver cell damage. Kuppfer cells may also be swollen and most or all tracts are affected.

The normal liver plate or cellular architecture is lost in viral hepatitis, and this feature distinguishes viral hepatitis from liver cell damage caused by cholestasis. In viral hepatitis, liver damage is most severe in zones 3 near the terminal hepatic venules. Certain areas of tissue in zone 3 may show increased cellular damage, which is called spotty necrosis. Acute hepatitis A is also associated with necrosis in zone 1.

The damaged cells usually appear swollen with balloon degeneration, characterized by granular, pale-staining cytoplasm. Abundant acidophil bodies, which are cell inclusions associated with increased cell destruction, may also be seen in the cell cytoplasm. Acidophil bodies are seen in other liver diseases but in viral hepatitis they are markedly increased.

Samples of liver tissue can also be stained and investigated for viral components. Orcein staining shows hepatitis B surface antigen in the hepatocyte as a uniform, finely granular, brown material known as a ground-glass appearance in patients with chronic hepatitis B. With immunofluorescent stains, the distribution of hepatitis B, C and Delta viral antigens may be demonstrated. In viral hepatitis the cells appear swollen and the cell nuclei are irregular in shape. Increased chromatin and multiple nuclei may be seen in some infected cells.

Drug-induced and alcoholic hepatitis

The changes in drug-induced hepatitis are similar to those of viral hepatitis although drug-induced hepatitis is more likely to show sharply-defined necrosis near the hepatic venules, granulomas, steatosis, damage to small bile ducts and a poorly developed inflammatory reaction. Some toxins, such as vinyl chloride, copper sulphate, and vitamin A can also cause portal hypertension in the absence of cirrhosis. And although necrosis in drug-induced hepatitis is usually not as severe as that of viral hepatitis, some drugs, such as phenytoin (dilantin) and paraminosalicylic acid can cause prominent necrosis.

Chronic occupational exposure to heavy metals such as beryllium and copper can cause sarcoid-like granulomas in the liver, lungs, and other organs. More than 60 different drugs cause hepatic granulomas, including allopurinol used for gout, aspirin, chlorpromazine, quinine and tolbutamide.

In alcoholic hepatitis, cell ballooning is more prominent and acidophil bodies are rarely seen. However, other inclusions known as Mallory bodies are commonly seen in damaged hepatocytes, and fibrosis may be seen. The Mallory body is a dramatic form of hyaline protein degeneration that occurs in damaged hepatocytes.

Mallory bodies are seen in alcoholic liver disease, Indian childhood cirrhosis, Wilson's disease, chronic cholestatic disease such as primary biliary cirrhosis, liver damage after intestinal bypass for obesity, liver toxicity caused by perhexilene maleate, chlorphentramine, thioridazine, nifedipine, stiboesterol, glucocorticoid steroids, and amiodarone, and hepatocellular carcinoma. In Western societies, the Mallory body is most commonly found in alcoholic hepatitis.

Autoimmune hepatitis

Biopsy is a valuable tool in autoimmune hepatitis, but it may be impossible to perform if coagulation defects are present. When biopsy is performed, tissue changes are similar to those seen in viral hepatitis. However, autoimmune disease is a chronic condition frequently causing a piecemeal necrosis, characterized by an erosion of liver cells at the interface of connective and liver cell tissue. This causes a cell clustering known as a liver-cell rosette formation. Signs of inflammation, liver cell swelling, regeneration, and collapse of the liver plate may also be seen. In some cases biopsy in autoimmune hepatitis may be necessary to determine if cirrhosis is also present.

Classification of Disease

The classification of disease severity is based on the type of liver injury, degree of inflammation and necrosis, and the stage, which is determined by the degree of fibrosis. Stage in the METAVIR scoring system, which is commonly used to classify fibrosis in biopsy specimens, ranges from F0, which is no fibrosis, to F4, which indicates cirrhosis. In the METAVIR system disease activity is graded from A0 to A3, with A0 indicating no activity and A3 indicating severe activity.

A single score of liver disease can also be determined by using the Histologic Activity Index, which correlates fibrosis with necrosis and inflammation.

Cirrhosis

In cirrhosis, the normal structure of the liver is replaced by nodules separated by fibrous tissue. The size of nodules is measured and used to tell if cirrhosis is micronodular, with nodules 3 mm or smaller, or macrondular with nodules greater than 3 mm. A macronodular, shrunken, extensively fibrotic liver is seen in advanced cirrhosis. The nodules in macronodular cirrhosis may also be disorganized and difficult to differentiate because of their poor resemblance to normal tissue. When there is tissue regeneration, cirrhosis can be difficult to diagnose.

16

Conventional Treatment

Although hepatitis is an ancient disease, the realization that chronic disease can cause serious symptoms up to 30–40 years later has made it apparent that more effective treatments are needed. Consequently, clinical researchers are investigating new therapies, and current therapies are constantly changing. Chapter sixteen describes the primary treatment options available for patients with hepatitis. However, because many potential treatments are undergoing clinical trials, specific therapies and drug combinations can be expected to change as newer specific treatments are discovered.

Overall, treatment for hepatitis depends on its cause. For instance, antiviral therapies such as interferon and nucleoside analogues are used to reduce viral replication in viral hepatitis, and immunosuppressant treatments that slow down or suppress the immune system are used to slow disease progression in autoimmune hepatitis. Chapter sixteen describes the conventional treatments available for hepatitis, including liver transplants, and it explains how clinical trials are used to evaluate new therapies.

Liver Care

For the success of any treatment protocol, general liver health must be taken into consideration. Alcohol use is one of the biggest deterrents to successful treatment. Certain drugs and chemicals can also damage the liver and interfere with treatment. For example, marijuana and corticosteroids are both reported to interfere with interferon therapy. Prevention is also an important part of liver health. Vaccines against other hepatitis viruses, for instance hepatitis A vaccines for persons with hepatitis B or hepatitis C, are recommended to prevent further injury to the liver.

A nutrient-rich diet is essential for liver health, and patients who maintain a normal body weight show a better response to various anti-viral therapies. A diet low in saturated fats is also an important factor in recovery from non-alcoholic fatty liver disease. Because their importance to treatment is so important, the lifestyle changes that influence liver disease and treatment are described in a separate chapter, chapter eighteen.

New Therapies and Clinical Trials

Before new therapies are released to the general public, they are tested on a small segment of the population in clinical trials conducted in four different phases. If adverse effects are seen in early phases, the study may be discontinued. And although not all patients in a study are given the studied drug, if results of the studied drug are particularly promising in early phases, more study participants may be given early access to the drug. Some clinical trials also evaluate complementary therapies that are used in conjunction with or in place of conventional medicines.

Patients with viral hepatitis who do not show a good response to current available therapies are generally good candidates for clinical trials. However, patients considering entering clinical trials must check certain details. Some clinical trials can interfere with medical insurance coverage since many HMOs and PPOs will not cover clinical trials, and if patients become ill during trials, their medical expenses may not be covered. It's important for patients to check with their insurance companies and also the clinical trial coordinator to clarify what costs are covered.

It's also important to find out what investigators are participating in the study and to see if there is a financial incentive that might bias results, particularly if the marketing branch of pharmaceutical companies are involved. Phase 4 studies are usually post drug (FDA) approval studies, which may be funded by the marketing arms of the pharmaceutical company rather than the research arms. Patients may want to be leery of phase 4 studies. Phase 2 & 3 are usually pre-approval studies funded by the research divisions of pharmaceutical companies designed to find out if the drug works in the way it is intended. Available clinical trials for both conventional and alternative therapies can be found with Clinical Trial Information in the resources section.

Treatment for Hepatitis A

The hepatitis A virus (HAV) causes an acute illness that is often not diagnosed until the late stage of infection when the virus is already clearing. Most HAV infections completely resolve within 1–2 months. The incubation period is typically 15–60 days after exposure with a mean of 30 days. Individuals who have been exposed to HAV, for instance during institutional epidemics, are usually treated with gamma globulin as a form of passive immunization to help prevent infection. When acute HAV infection occurs, treatment is typically geared toward relieving symptoms. Analgesics such as acetaminophen, using less than 2 grams daily, are used for fever and pain.

No specific management is necessary for most patients with uncomplicated infection. Most patients feel better when they avoid fatty foods, which may cause digestive discomfort. HAV infection that progresses to fulminant hepatitis requires hospitalization and supportive therapies.

Treatment for Hepatitis B and Hepatitis C

Interferon Therapies

Interferon is the primary therapy for hepatitis B and hepatitis C. Interferon is a naturally occurring immune system protein known as a cytokine. Interferon was first discovered in the late 1950s by researchers Isaacs and Lindermann at the National Institute for Medical Research in London [52]. These researchers observed that cells colonized by viruses could not be infected by other viruses. The researchers demonstrated that infected cells produced a protective protein, which they named interferon.

Cytokines are normally produced by the body's white blood cells to help us fight infection and destroy cancerous cells. In infection, interferons bind to specific cell surface receptors and induce profound antiviral, antiproliferative (interfere with viral replication), and immunomodulatory (regulate the immune response) effects.

Interferons inhibit the viral life cycle at several phases, including cell entry, RNA synthesis and protein synthesis. Interferons also induce immune system markers known as HLA class I antigens to appear on the liver cell membrane. These markers promote lysis or destruction of infected hepatocytes by inducing the production of T suppressor lymphocytes with cytotoxic (capable of destroying cells) potential and they increase the activity of another cytokine known as interleukin-2. Interferon also induces the production of T helper cells that help kill off the hepatitis C viruses. Through these steps in the immune response, interferons help reduce the viral load and they help eradicate viruses. In addition, interferon is reported to repair the scarring or fibrosis caused by infection with hepatitis B or C.

NATURAL VS SYNTHETIC INTERFERONS

The body normally produces interferons in response to infection. Recombinant and synthetic interferons have been manufactured for use in hepatitis B and C that are identical to the naturally occurring interferons. Both natural and manufactured forms of interferon-alpha (IFN-α which is produced by lymphocytes and monocytes), interferon-beta (IFN-β which is produced by fibroblast cells), and interferon-gamma (IFN-γ which is produced by helper CD4 T lymphocytes) have been found to bind to the same cell receptor causing similar efficacy and treatment effectiveness.

Alpha, beta, kappa, and omega interferons are class I interferons, and gamma interferons are class II interferons. Class III interferons include three different types of interferon lambda. Most of the manufactured interferon products are alpha interferons. Interferons are administered by intramuscular (IM) or subcutaneous injection. Pegylated compounds are formed by combining interferon with pegylated glycols. Pegylated interferons are longer-lasting, reducing the number of injections to once weekly and providing a better treatment response than regular interferon compounds.

INTERFERON ANTIBODIES

Unfortunately, the immune system recognizes the manufactured or recombinant interferons as foreign substances. Consequently, immune system cells can produce antibodies that neutralize or inactivate recombinant interferon products during the course of therapy, making the interferon therapy ineffective. Patients with hepatitis C who relapse during therapy are usually found to have IFN-_ binding antibodies. In some but not all studies, switching these individuals to natural interferon usually restores effectiveness.

INTERFERON PRODUCTS

Recombinant interferon is genetically engineered or produced synthetically. Several products are currently FDA approved, and a number of other interferons that specifically target the liver are under investigation. Interferon treatment alone (monotherapy) is effective for about 50 percent of patients with hepatitis B and 30 percent of patients with hepatitis C [52]. Approved products for hepatitis include:

1. interferon alpha-2b, recombinant (Intron A manufactured by Schering-Plough, Kenilworth, NJ, which was approved for hepatitis C in 1991 and hepatitis B in 1992 and for extended use in chronic HCV in 2003; PEG-Intron (peginterferon alpha-2b) is the first pegylated interferon approved for hepatitis C in 2001; the combination of Intron A with ribavirin (Rebetol) is known as Rebetron. Intron is also approved for Roferon A and is also used for malignant melanoma, hairy cell leukemia, condlyoma acuminata (venereal warts), and AIDS-related Kaposi's sarcoma

2. interferon alpha-2a recombinant (Roferon A manufactured by Hoffman-LaRoche, Inc., Nutley, NJ), which is also identical to natural alpha-2a interferon and approved in 1996 for the treatment of hepatitis C infection. Roferon A is also used for chronic myelogenous leukemia (CML), hairy cell leukemia, and AIDS-related Kaposi's sarcoma.

3. consensus interferon, the first bio-engineered product, which is also called alfacon-1 (Infergen, first manufactured by Amgen with rights sold to Intermune in 2001); approved for the treatment of hepatitis C in 1997.

4. pegylated interferons: pegylated interferon alpha-2a (Pegasys), a longer-acting interferon was introduced by Hoffman LaRoche in 2002 and it was approved for hepatitis C in 2002 and for hepatitis B in 2005; pegylated alpha-2b (PEG-Intron) manufactured by Schering-Plough was approved for hepatitis C in 2001.

Other products used in controlled and uncontrolled trials include:

interferon alpha-n3 (Alferon manufactured by Interferon Sciences) and interferon alpha-n1 (Welferon manufactured by Glaxo Wellcome Inc., Research Triangle Park, NC)

SIDE EFFECTS OF INTERFERON

Interferon has certain unpleasant side effects that cause about 10 percent of patients to stop treatment, and another 10–40 percent of patients need to reduce their dosage. Initial flu-like side effects may occur during the first 3–4 weeks of treatment. These typically persist up to 12 hours after injections and include persistent nausea, loss of energy, joint aches, chills, headache, muscle aches, dizziness, stuffed nose, and loss of appetite. These side effects are usually treated with 1–2 tablets of 325 mg acetaminophen taken one hour before and four to six hours after injections. Dehydration should be prevented by drinking 32–64 ounces of water daily. Administering the injection at bedtime can reduce side effects unless this causes insomnia. Ginger capsules, using 2–3 500 mg capsules can be used to reduce nausea and inflammation.

Long-term side effects include fatigue, bone marrow suppression, thrombocytopenia (low platelet count), neutropenia (decreased count of neutrophil white blood cells), increased susceptibility to bacterial infection, diarrhea, abdominal pain, pancreatitis, alopecia (hair loss), rash, itching, menstrual irregularities, anemia, depression, tinnitus, insomnia, psychosis, seizures, suicidal ideation, cognitive changes, irritability, eye dryness, visual changes, dry mouth, mouth ulcers, vaginal dryness, decreased libido, nail changes (brittleness and splitting), and depression.

In addition, about one percent of patients develop autoimmune thyroid disease, which can be detected by routine thyroid function tests. A nutrient-rich diet and preventing dehydration can help with fatigue. If significant psychiatric symptoms persist, treatment may need to be stopped. Patients on interferon should have routine blood counts at 1, 2, and 4 weeks after starting interferon, and therapy should be discontinued if platelet counts fall below 30K/ml or white blood cell counts fall below 750/ml [38].

Nucleoside Analogs

Nucleoside analogs include a class of antiviral compounds, such as lamivudine, which reduces levels of viral DNA polymerase in hepatitis B, and ribavirin, which reduces levels of RNA polymerase in hepatitis C. These compounds interfere with viral replication by interfering with production of the enzymes necessary for viral replication. Nucleoside analogs are primarily used in conjunction with interferon as mainstay treatments for hepatitis B and C.

Common side effects of nucleoside analogs include headache, diarrhea, fatigue, abdominal pain, muscle aches, increased lipid levels, cough, and skin rashes. Severe side effects include lactic acidosis, a condition of increased lactic acid, enlarged liver, and steatosis. These symptoms may occur after therapy has been stopped.

Treatment for Hepatitis B

Some researchers report that interferon deficiency causes the body to launch an incomplete immune response resulting in the chronic carrier state in patients infected with HBV [56]. This explains why most infants become chronic carriers. The immune system does not become fully mature until about age 2 years.

Interferon alpha 2a (Intron) was approved by the FDA for the treatment of chronic hepatitis B in 1992, and Peginterferon alpha-2a (Pegasys) was approved in 2005. The nucleoside analogue lamivudine (Epivrir) was approved in 1998, followed by adefovir (Hepsera) in 2002 and entecavir (Baraclude) in 2005. Prior treatments such as prednisone, adenine arabinoside, and acyclovir were limited by their ineffectiveness and their potential toxicity and are no longer used. Several other nucleoside analogues, including valtorcitabine are being studied for their use in chronic HBV.

Treatment with either interferon, Nucleoside analogs, or a combination of both may decrease the incidence of disease progression in patients with chronic HBV infection. In some cases, treatment totally eradicates HBV and in others it slows the disease course. Patients with chronic HBV infection with transaminase levels more than double the normal range or who show evidence of significant inflammation on liver biopsies are good candidates for therapy.

Interferon therapy in HBV

The usual dose of interferon alpha-2a is 5 million units administered daily or 10 million units administered three times each week injected subcutaneously or intramuscularly (IM) for twelve–sixteen weeks. Pegasys is usually administered once weekly. HBV DNA levels usually decrease within days of initiating interferon treatment and remain detectable through 8–12 weeks of treatment. At about week 8, a rise in ALT and AST levels occurs, which is referred to as a flare.

This expected flare, which is also seen in nucleoside analog therapy, occurs as infected hepatocytes are lysed or destroyed. This flare can result in a tenfold increase in ALT and AST levels and possibly cause hepatic failure. For this reason, caution must be used in treating patients who have progressed to cirrhosis. After the flare, levels of HBV DNA are usually negative. Ultimately, liver biopsy specimens show reduced inflammation and hepatocellular necrosis. Replicative forms of HBV disappear from the liver.

About three-six months after starting interferon, HBeAg disappears and HBeAb appears, and ALT levels return to normal. HBsAg clears in about 25 percent of patients within 12 months after the appearance of HBeAb, usually patients treated with interferon soon after acquiring HBV infection. In some cases, HBsAg disappears years after interferon therapy.

Patients who do not respond to interferon therapy (non-responders) do not usually respond to re-treatment at higher doses. Treatment options include the addition of Nucleoside analogs if they aren't part of the initial treatment plan or entry into a clinical trial evaluating a new therapy.

COST OF TREATMENT

Interferon is an expensive treatment and frequently needs a letter of authorization showing medical necessity from the physician before it is covered by medical insurance. Medicare covers the cost of interferon therapy but requires that injections be administered in the doctor's office or by a Medicare-approved nurse in the patient's home. Patients not on Medicare are able to self-administer their injections. For people who do not have insurance or who have insurance that does not cover interferon therapy, there are several programs listed in the resources under the section Drug Treatment Financial Assistance that provide financial assistance.

Predictors of response

Certain groups are more likely to respond well to interferon. These include: ALT greater than 100 IU/L; HBV DNA less than 100 pg/ml; female gender; age younger than 40 years; short duration of disease; active hepatic inflammation; heterosexuality; HIV negative, and non–Asian origin [52]. When Nucleoside analogs are added, the response in Asians is dramatically improved. Overall, studies show indicate that the best response is seen when pegylated interferon is used [50].

The primary criteria for a successful response are a loss of HBV DNA and HBeAg from the serum. Although loss of HBsAg is desired, it is not necessarily observed at the end of therapy. Clinical trials of interferon therapy from 1976 on show that interferon therapy for chronic HBV causes long-term effects in most patients treated with either 5 or 10 million units of interferon three times weekly for four months.

People most likely to develop lamivudine resistance include those who initially have high HBV DNA levels and high ALT levels and people who show signs of advanced disease in liver biopsy procedures.

Nucleoside analogs in HBV

Nucleoside analogs are oral medications given alone as a form of monotherapy or, more commonly, they're administered in conjunction with interferon. Available compounds include lamivudine, adefovir, and entecavir. Lamividudine, the first drug of this class used for HBV, is used most often although many patients develop resistance to lamivudine within 1–3 years. Flares are also likely to occur if the medication is stopped before HBeAg conversion to HBeAb.

Studies have shown that adefovir is a potent inhibitor of both wild-type and lamivudine-resistant HBV and can be effectively used in patients showing resistance to lamivudine. However, adefovir needs to be administered indefinitely because withdrawal of therapy is generally associated with viral reactivation. Mutants with resistance to adefovir can also occur. Studies in which 10 mg of adefovir was used daily showed a 43 percent HBeAg to HBeAb conversion rate at 144 weeks and a 56 percent rate of HBV DNA suppression to less than 1,000 copies at 144 weeks [50].

Entecavir is a potent antiviral reported to clear HBV DNA within hepatocytes. Entacavir resistance has been seen in patients resistant to lamivudine. The choice of what antiviral medications to use is based on the patient's genotype, HBV DNA count, and the physician's experience.

Antiviral medications

Most patients with acute hepatitis B are able to clear the virus and are not treated with antiviral medications. These treatments are used for patients with chronic hepatitis B infection. Patients eligible for interferon therapy must usually demonstrate positive HBsAg, HBeAg or HBV DNA for at least 6 months, indicating that they have chronic infection. In addition they must have an elevated ALT during this time period and a liver biopsy showing evidence of chronic hepatitis.

Other criteria may include age over 18 years and compensated liver disease (most liver function is intact). Exclusions for interferon therapy include pregnancy, other serious medical illnesses, positive human immunodeficiency virus (HIV), renal insufficiency, and active drug or alcohol abuse.

Studies of interferon use in children show a similar response as that seen in untreated children. Studies of Italian children show that 70 percent convert HBeAg to HBeAb, and become HBV DNA negative before adulthood, and 29 percent clear HBsAg before adulthood [52].

Thymosin

Thymosin is a polypeptide hormone normally produced by the thymus gland. In adults, the function of the thymus gland gradually declines and levels of thymosin are low. Used therapeutically in clinical trials, thymosin alpha-1 (Zadazin, manufactured by SciClone Pharmaceuticals) is reported to stimulate the immune system and help eradicate HBV. Thymosin used in combination with interferon is reported to be particularly effective in persons with HBV who have pre-core mutants and are negative for HBeAg. Thymosin is still under investigation in clinical trials.

Special circumstances in Treatment of HBV

In certain circumstances, the usual therapies used for HBV infection are not recommended. These are described in the following sections.

PATIENTS WHO ARE HBEAG AND HBV DNA NEGATIVE

Patients with HBsAg who are negative for HBeAg and HBV DNA tend to be older and may have more advanced liver disease. There is no well defined treatment for individuals in this group other than general supportive measures. Ursodeoxycholic acid is a safe non-toxic bile acid that can be helped to reduce symptoms such as itching. Patients with HBV DNA who test negative for HBeAg (15 percent of patients with HBV in the U.S.) may have pre-core mutations and would be recommended for treatment.

PATIENTS WITH CIRRHOSIS

Patients with HBV-related cirrhosis are usually only treated with interferon if they have a positive HBsAg and HBV DNA and normal prothrombin time, albumin, and bilirubin levels. A corticosteroid may be used in conjunction with the interferon in cirrhotic patients. Most patients with cirrhosis show an exacerbation or worsening of HBV infection. This flare is usually caused by immune destruction of HBV-infected liver cells. Patients with cirrhosis should only be treated with interferon under the guidance of an experienced hepatologist, a physician specializing in liver diseases.

PATIENTS WHO ARE ASIAN

Most patients with chronic HBV infection are infected at birth or during childhood and have been infected for a long time. Many of these patients have normal ALT levels and biopsy results consistent with chronic hepatitis B, indicating that they have developed HBV tolerance. In clinical trials, only 15 percent of Asian patients treated with interferon demonstrated subsequent loss of HBeAg, and 29 percent showed evidence of interferon antibodies [52]. However, a greater response was seen in patients using pegylated interferon with lamivudine. Asians also show a better response to lamivudine monotherapy than non–Asians. Among Asian patients receiving liver transplants, HBV recurrence is reported to be high.

PATIENTS WITH HBV AND DELTA VIRUS INFECTION

Individuals with concurrent HBV and delta virus (HDV) infection are candidates for interferon therapy. However, the response rates are poorer than in patients with HBV alone, and in patients who respond, relapse is common. HDV tends to inhibit HBV replication and most patients with HDV have lower HBV DNA levels. As HDV infection improves, viral replication of HBV can increase. This results in eventual relapse after a seemingly successful treatment in the majority of treated patients.

INFANTS OF POSITIVE MOTHERS

Infants born to mothers with HBsAg are vaccinated shortly after birth with the recombinant HBV vaccine (followed by two consecutive doses at intervals of several months) and also administered HBIG. In full-term babies of normal weight, this treatment results in a 95 percent rate of protection. In premature low-weight infants, the response rate is poor. It's recommended that vaccination be postponed until these babies' possessive weight reaches 2 kg or two months of age. Babies who are vaccinated will show transient positive tests for HBsAg for up to 8 days. This could be misinterpreted as a true positive HBsAg result. Tests for HBsAg that are positive in newborns shortly after vaccination should be repeated after several weeks.

Children who become HBsAg carriers should be counseled on their increased risk for developing liver diseases including hepatocellular carcinoma (HCC) and advised to avoid alcohol. Among patients infected at birth the lifetime risk for HCC is 50 percent in males and 20 percent in females [15].

Treatment for Hepatitis C

Patients with chronic hepatitis C are treated with a combination of interferon and a nucleoside analog, usually ribavirin (Copegus), which is a guanosine analog. The goals of treatment are to suppress viral replication, reduce inflammation, and prevent further disease progression. Patients with acute HCV are sometimes treated with a short course (1–3 months) of interferon to help prevent chronic infection. This protocol is based on studies showing that treatment administered within 12 weeks of disease onset can totally eradicate HCV. However, HCV rarely causes acute symptoms, and most patients do not realize that they are infected until they develop symptoms of chronic HCV disease.

The National Institutes of Health 2002 Consensus Statement recommends that all persons with chronic HCV receive antiviral therapy. However, ALT levels frequently fluctuate in patients with HCV. The decision to treat chronic HCV depends on a number of factors, such as genotype, viral load, symptoms, biopsy results, and side effects associated with treatment. Patients with chronic hepatitis C should discuss treatment options with their physicians. Regardless of whether treatment is started or postponed, patients with chronic hepatitis C should have frequent blood tests to assess their aminotransferase enzyme levels and liver function tests.

Treatment based on HCV genotype

The HCV genotype is an important consideration for the type of treatment used and the duration of treatment. Pegylated interferon and ribavirin are used in all three genotypes. Genotype 1: a sustained virologic response is seen in approximately 45 percent of people using interferon and ribavirin for 48 weeks; Genotype 2 and 3: a sustained virologic response is seen in up to 80 percent of people treated for 24 weeks or 48 weeks if fibrosis or cirrhosis are present; Genotype 4, 5, and 6: a sustained virologic response is seen in about 45 percent of people. Patients typically receive weekly injections of pegylated interferon. Usually, genotypes 1, 4, 5, and 6 receive 1,000–1,200 mg ribavirin daily, and genotypes 2 and 3 receive 800 mg ribavirin daily.

A sustained virologic response is based on HCV RNA levels of less than 5 IU/ml six months after discontinuing therapy. Some patients relapse within the first few months after discontinuing therapy and some patients relapse after many years. Therefore, it's important to have regular ALT and HCV RNA levels after stopping treatment.

TREATMENT DURATION

Most protocols, depending on genotype, recommend using therapy for 24–72 weeks, although in some cases treatment may be stopped after 12 weeks if an appropriate response isn't noted. In the Tera-VIC-4 study, an improved response was seen when therapy was extended to 72 weeks rather than 48 weeks [50]. Because the treatment of HCV is in its pioneer stages, changes to the usual dosing protocols can be expected.

TREATMENT FAILURE

A common reason for treatment failure is the production of new mutant HCV strains that have resistance to therapy. Other reasons cited for drug failure include older age, obesity, genotype 1, higher viral loads, conditions of fatty liver or cirrhosis, African-American or Hispanic patients, male gender. Studies also show that insulin resistance can also contribute to drug resistance, presumably due to fatty liver disease and changes in levels of the protein leptin. High levels of insulin may also reduce the body's natural production of interferon and its ability to launch an effective immune response.

In patients with genotypes 2 who are receiving treatment, risk factors for treatment failure include male gender, history of alcohol abuse, standard rather than weight-based treatment doses, and presence of liver biopsy changes indicating advanced disease.

FACTORS INFLUENCING REMISSION

Certain factors are known to influence permanent remission from HCV. These include: female gender, low body weight, low viral load, typically less than 2,000,000 IU/ml, ethnicity other than African-American, age less than 40 years at the time of infection, and the absence of cirrhosis.

People who show a 2 log drop, for example from 20,000 to 200, after three months of anti-viral therapy are most likely to have a sustained virologic remission. Most people who have relapsed after treatment with interferon and ribavirin attain sustained remission when they are re-treated with pegylated interferon and ribavirin. The introduction of pegylated interferon is the treatment of choice for HCV.

Types of interferon

Studies show improved results when pegylated interferon is used. However, when response is poor, other forms of interferon may be used, including consensus interferon or interferon alfacon-1 (Infergen) or gamma interferon-1b (Actimmune).

Side effects of Ribavirin

The side effects of interferon were described earlier in this chapter. Ribavirin has some specific side effects that must also be considered in HCV therapy. The most serious side effect of ribavirin is its propensity to cause anemia, a condition also associated with hepatitis C. Patients on interferon and ribavirin must have regular blood counts and changes in hemoglobin level may require a change in dosage of antiviral medications. In most cases, lowering the dose helps correct the anemia. Other side effects include rash, itching, shortness of breath, and nausea.

RIBAVIRIN IN PREGNANCY

Ribavirin is known to cause birth defects and should not be used during pregnancy. Two forms of birth control are recommended while on ribavirin and for six months after discontinuing therapy. In December, 2004 the FDA changed the labeling of peginterferon alpha-1 (Pegasys) to indicate that its use with ribavirin (Copegus) is contraindicated in women who are pregnant and in men whose female partners are pregnant. Ribavirin has been classified as FDA Pregnancy Category X. A registry of pregnancy exposures is being compiled. Contact information can be obtained at 800–593–2214 or at www.ribavirinpregnancyregistry.com. Questions regarding the safety of ribavirin can be addressed to Roche's Drug Safety Department at (800) 526–6337.

Weight-based therapies

The prevalence of HCV in African-Americans is about 2–3 times that seen in the white population in the United States. African-Americans have traditionally been under-represented in clinical trials and evidence-based studies show that they have a poorer response to antiviral drug therapies. Studies of African-Americans with genotype 1 HCV in which the ribavirin dose was based on weight rather than a fixed dose show a 21 percent sustained response compared to a 10 percent response in patients receiving a fixed dose [50]. Based on these studies, weight-based therapies are considered superior.

Treatment of HCV in co-infection with HIV

Results of the PRESCO trial, the largest study conducted of patients co-infected with HIV/HCV, which began in 2002, show a similar response to interferon and ribavirin than that seen in patients infected with only HCV. Co-infected patients in the study were required to have CD4 T-cell counts of at least 300 cells/ml; in addition, they could not be on the antiviral drug didanosine. All patients in the trial agreed to abstain from alcohol and drugs and they could not have severe neuropsychiatric symptoms. Patients with HCV genotype 1 or 4 were treated for 12–18 months, and those with genotype 2 or 3 were treated randomly for either 6 or 12 months. All patients received peg-interferon along with 1000–1200 mg ribavirin daily [49].

Early studies, before current drug therapies were introduced, showed faster HIV progression in patients coinfected with HCV. More recent studies do not show this finding. In studies of co-infected pregnant women, the CD4+ count stayed stable or improved and there were no increases of HIV RNA or progression to death.

HCV in pediatric patients

HCV is rarely seen in infants, occurring in approximately 3 percent of HCV positive mothers. Risk of perinatal infection has not been linked to breastfeeding, but because HCV infection is known to occur in breast-fed infants of these mothers, breastfeeding is not recommended, especially in mothers with high levels of HCV RNA. Even though vertical transmission of HCV is inefficient, it appears to be the main cause of pediatric HCV transmission. HCV in children causes mild symptoms and a low rate of spontaneous recovery with a higher incidence of severe liver disease in adulthood. Inteferon alpha 2a is used for the treatment of HCV in the pediatric population.

Other therapies

Thymosin-alpha 1 (Zadaxin), which is described in the section on hepatitis B, has not yet been FDA approved for HCV infection. However, clinical trials show that its use with pegylated interferon for chronic HCV is promising. Because thymosin is frequently included in alternative medicine protocols, its use is described in the following chapter.

Ursodeoxycholic acid, which is the primary treatment for primary biliary cirrhosis, is used to reduce the effects of toxic bile salts in patients with HCV. Although it helps to reduce symptoms, this compound has no effect on viral load.

Future HCV therapies

Many therapies are undergoing clinical trials or being investigated for their use as a treatment in HCV infection. Two of the most promising treatments include the compound isatoribine (Anadys Pharmaceuticals), a toll-like receptor 7 inhibitor, shown to significantly reduce viral load in phase Ib of clinical trials; and Zadaxin (thymalfasin) used in conjunction with Pegasys and ribavirin in people who failed treatment with combinations of interferon and ribavirin. Zadaxin showed significant improvement with few side effects.

Other investigational treatments include: Actimmune, albuferon, BILN-2061, colchine, the caspase inhibitor IDN 6556, interferon beta, interleukin 10, interleukin-11, perfenidone (PFD), the HCV protease inhibitor SCH 6, rituximab for treating hepatitis C-associated cryoglobulinemic vasculitis; merimepodib (MMPD) used in addition to Pegasys and Copegus; internal ribosome entry site (IRES) inhibitors that inhibit the virus from binding the ribosome of hepatocytes; inhibitors of RNA-dependent RNA polymerase to halt viral replication; inhibitors of the enzyme NS3/4A serine protease to halt viral replication; and inhibitors of nucleoside triphosphatase (NTPase)/RNA helicase to halt viral replication. Anti-sense oligonucleotides are also under investigation. Although these compounds interfere with the assembly of viral proteins, they are large molecules that cannot be absorbed by the body in their present form.

Treatment for Alcoholic Hepatitis

Discontinuing alcohol use can stop disease progression in most cases of alcoholic hepatitis. Corticosteroids are used to reduce inflammation in patients with alcoholic liver disease. Corticosteroids are reported to improve short-term survival in patients with severe alcoholic hepatitis.

Treatment for Non-Alcoholic Fatty Liver Disease (NAFLD)

Gradual, moderate weight loss is reported to improve liver enzyme levels and liver tissue changes in patients with non-alcoholic fatty liver disease (NAFLD). In one study in which this is described, nutritional intervention consisted of a low-fat, low-sugar diet and the medication Orlistat (xenical), a fat blocker. Patients experienced an average weight loss of 6.7 kg and experienced improved liver function (39).

Treatment for Autoimmune Hepatitis (AIH)

Patients with autoimmune hepatitis are usually treated with immuno-suppressant medications that slow their immune system down, reducing the production of autoantibodies. Other therapies in use are described in chapter ten. In patients who are resistant to medical therapy, liver transplants are used. Approximately 20–30 percent of patients who have liver transplants for AIH may experience a recurrence of disease after several years. Immunosuppressant medications are used to prevent recurrence.

Some patients do not show a good response to medical treatment. Patients who do not show a 50 percent reduction in transaminase enzyme levels after six months of treatment with immunosuppressant may need to consider liver transplantation.

Patients with cirrhosis

Treatment for cirrhosis is primarily supportive and used to control symptoms. Treatment may also include nutritional supplements, and drugs known as prostaglandin analogs that can reduce collagen production.

Liver Transplants

In patients with fulminant liver failure or end-stage liver disease, liver transplantation may be the only treatment for survival. Liver transplantation is the surgical replacement of a diseased liver by all or part of a donated liver. Approximately, 5,000 liver transplants are performed in the U.S. annually.

However, finding a replacement donor can be difficult. In March of 2003, 80,719 individuals in the United States were on lists awaiting an organ transplant, and in 2002, transplant surgeries were performed on 24,791 individuals who received organs from 12,739 donors [24]. Each day about 17 people on the waiting lists die before they are able to receive an organ.

In addition to limited organ supplies, for an organ transplant to be successful, the host's immune system must accept and respond appropriately to the donated organ. Otherwise, the immune system rejects the organ and reacts to its presence, causing an inflammatory process that ultimately destroys the organ over a period of days to months. Symptoms of rejection include fever, flu-like symptoms, hypertension, edema, changes in heart rate, and shortness of breath. Although rare, a severe acute rejection necessitates the immediate removal of the organ.

The three-year survival rate for liver transplants is about 75 percent. Traditionally, immunosuppressant drugs have been used to slow down the immune system and keep it from rejecting the grafted organ. These medications, unfortunately, can have serious side effects including increased risk of infection. A newer approach called mixed chimerism is under investigation. This procedure involves transplanting a small amount of bone marrow from the donor at the same time as the liver transplant. This helps the recipient recognize the grafted organ as if it were his own, reducing the risk of rejection.

In hepatitis B

Patients with chronic HBV infection are considered poor candidates for orthotopic liver transplant primarily because re-infection affecting the grafted liver is common. These patients often progress to liver failure within 6 months to 2 years after transplantation. Fibrosing cholestatic hepatitis occurs in about 25 percent of transplanted HBV patients, and it has a high mortality rate. Patients with a lower risk of HBV recurrence and a better survival rate include those with HDV infection and those who are HBeAg and HBV DNA negative.

The use of long-term intravenous HBIG passive vaccination following transplant in European studies showed a lower recurrence of re-infection. However, HBIG is very expensive and not approved for intravenous use in the United States [52]. Prostglandin E and lamivudine used following transplant are also associated with a lower recurrence of HBV infection and of fibrosing cholestatic hepatitis.

In hepatitis C

Chronic hepatitis C that doesn't respond to treatment may necessitate liver transplant. Recurrence is likely in most patients in whom the virus has not been eradicated. Recurrent HCV following transplant appears to follow three patterns: one third of patients progress to cirrhosis rapidly after 2–4 years; one third progress to cirrhosis slowly over a period of 10–15 years; and one third will experience good health for many years before developing any problems related to HCV. Liver biopsy results one year after transplant give an indication of the future course. If no scarring has developed in one year, slow progression is likely. If signs of fibrosis are seen, progression may be more rapid, and antiviral treatment is recommended.

Artificial livers

A bio-artificial liver using pig cells has been developed by researchers at Cedars-Sinai Medical Center in Los Angeles and is currently being investigated. The initial trial showed that this device improved the survival rate by more than 20 percent. However, the company that conducted the trial is no longer in business, and a second trial is required before the device can be approved by the FDA.

Treatment for Hepatic Encephalopathy

Treatment for hepatic encephalopathy has traditionally involved a low protein diet based on the idea that with less protein to metabolize, ammonia levels would be reduced. Studies show that although ammonia is increased in most cases of hepatic encephalopathy and may contribute to symptoms, diet has little effect on outcome. Newer therapies include liver detoxification, reduction in hypertension within the brain, and the use of L-ornithine and L-aspartate amino acids to reduce brain edema.

Treatment for Coagulation Defects

Recombinant factor VIIa, a genetically engineered clotting factor is used in cases of impaired clotting related to liver failure that does not respond to vitamin K or fresh frozen plasma blood products. Recombinant factor VIIa quickly normalizes the prothrombin time (PT) level and improves blood clotting and fluid balance.

Treatment for Liver Cancer

Surgery and radiation are the primary treatments for liver cancer. Traditional surgery may be performed to remove the tumor or cryosurgery can be used. In cryosurgery a probe capable of freezing and destroying cancerous cells is inserted into the tumor. When tumors have grown too large or have invaded major blood vessels or other organs, chemoembolization or percutaneous ethanol injections can be used.

Chemoembolization involves the injection of chemotherapeutic agents such as doxorubicin and cisplatin directly into the artery that feeds the tumor. Chemoembolization is a non-surgical option that preserves healthy tissue while destroying the blood vessels that supply the tumor. The procedure can be repeated as needed to arrest tumor growth or progression. In percutaneous ethanol injection, ethanol is injected directly into the liver tumor to destroy cancer cells.

17

Complementary Medicine

Interferon production in the body depends on adequate levels of vitamin C. Onions and carrots strengthen the immune system, increasing its ability to fight infection and prevent the development of autoimmune disease. These and similar facts form the basis for including complementary medicine in hepatitis treatment plans.

Complementary medicine refers to therapies, such as herbs, dietary supplements, and energy healing therapies such as acupuncture that are generally outside the realm of conventional medicine. The goals of complementary medicine for patients with hepatitis include: 1) to strengthen the liver in an effort to help it clear infectious microorganisms and regenerate healthy tissue; 2) to modulate and strengthen the immune system so that it responds appropriately to infection and liver cell damage and 3) to promote general health so that all of the body's organs and systems contribute to the process of healing and recovery. Chapter seventeen describes complementary therapies used for hepatitis.

Integrative Medicine

The use of complementary medicine in conjunction with conventional treatment is known as integrative medicine. This approach is used by hepatologists, internists, gastroenterologists, integrationist physicians, and other practitioners of conventional medicine. Complementary medicine may also be prescribed by naturopaths or herbalists. Complementary medicine can includes therapies that can interact with or interfere with conventional medicines and they can have side effects that make them a poor choice for hepatitis despite being effective at reducing symptoms. For this reason, complementary medicine in hepatitis should always be used under the direction of a licensed practitioner.

Prescription medicine and side effects

One of the advantages of appropriately used complementary medicine is its ability to reduce the need for or the dose of some prescription medications. Annually, more than 100,000 people die as a result of severe reactions to prescription medications, making prescription drug side effects the fourth leading cause of death in America [72]. The 2006 safety goals for hospitals include greater awareness of prescription drug side effects and family involvement, which is intended to facilitate a faster recognition of adverse effects. Key problems with prescription medications include individual variation in dose requirements and the inability of drugs to target only specific organs.

Individual response to a specific drug can vary from 4 to 40 fold depending on the person's size, general health, and their ability to absorb, metabolize, and eliminate drugs.

Nutraceuticals

Nutraceuticals refer to the active medicinal ingredients found in natural substances, such as plants and herbs. For instance, the herb milk thistle contains several active compounds, notably silymarin and silibinin. Both of these compounds help prevent toxic liver damage and help the liver regenerate faster by increasing protein synthesis if liver cells are damaged.

Plant-based healing remedies

Plant-based healing refers to the use of herbs as well as fresh fruits and vegetables that are rich in antioxidant vitamins. The allicin in garlic and the polyphenols in green tea are examples of plant-based healing remedies.

Nutritional supplements

The nutritional supplements recommended by the Life Extension Foundation (see Resource section) for the treatment of liver disease include: choline, 1500 mg daily, to reduce fat deposits in the liver; acetyl-L-carnitine, 1000 mg taken twice daily, to help maintain liver cell mitochondria and increase energy; and the following antioxidants: vitamin C, using 2500 mg daily; vitamin E, 400 IU daily, CoQ10: 100-300 mg daily; N-acetylcysteine (NAC), 600 mg daily; alpha lipoic acid, 250 mg 2-3 times daily; selenium, 200 mcg daily, and zinc, 30 mg daily. Because vitamin B3 (niacin) disrupts healthy methylation, it should be avoided by people with liver disorders, and the following B vitamins should be taken individually: B1 (thiamine, using 500 mg daily; B2 (riboflavin, 75 mg daily; B5 (panthothenic acid), 1500 mg daily; B6 (pyridoxine) 200 mg daily; B12 (cobalmin), using one 5 mg sublingual lozenge 1-5 times daily, and folic acid, using 800 mcg daily. Also, vitamin K2, in a dose of 45 mg daily, has been reported to decrease the risk of progression to hepatocellular cancer in patients with chronic viral hepatitis.

In addition, S-adenosylmethionine (SAMe) is needed to synthesize glutathione and has been found to restore liver function related to damage caused by hepatitis C. The suggested dose is 400 mg used 3 times daily. SAMe should not be taken on an empty stomach. The compound polyenylphosphatidylcholine (PPC), has also been shown to prevent the development of fibrosis, cirrhosis, and lipid peroxidation caused by alcohol consumption. The product HepatoPro, available in the United States, contains pharmaceutical-grade PPC and is recommended at doses of 900 mg 2-3 times daily.

Herbal Medicine

A number of traditional Chinese herbal tonics and formulas such as HepatoPlex One have been developed by Misha Cohen and her colleagues. These preparations are designed to help alleviate symptoms of chronic hepatitis C and reduce elevated liver enzyme levels. Contact information for Misha Cohen and her Chicken Soup Clinic can be found in the resource section.

Herbs

Herbs used for hepatitis include herbs such as ginger that are known to reduce inflammation, herbs such as neem that have anti-viral properties, and herbs such as milk thistle that help regenerate liver tissue and repair the effects of toxins. Herbs should not be used in patients with obstructive liver disease and they should only be used under the direction of one's physician. The following list includes herbs designated as safe by the FDA when used in recommended doses.

Table 17.1 Herbs used for hepatitis

Baical skullcap (*Scutellaria baicalensis*): anti-inflammatory properties, reduces jaundice and symptoms of fever and chills in viral hepatitis, improves sleep and stimulates bile production; contraindicated in patients with obstructive bile disease; used in tonics or as tea containing 3-9 grams of the powdered root three times daily.

Boldo (*Peumus boldus*): Leaves of the boldo plant, which are found in South America and China, are used to reduce pain and inflammation in hepatitis and reduce toxic damage; reduces pain, fatigue, and sleep disturbances in hepatitis; used as a tea, tincture or as capsules, using up to 3 grams daily.

Ginger (*Zingiber officinale*): extracts of the ginger root are used to reduce inflammation and nausea in patients with hepatitis; the fresh root is used and capsules containing 500 mg ginger root extract are used 2-3 times daily.

Green tea (*Camellia sinensis*): catechins present in green tea are rich in antioxidants and are reported to offer liver protection similar to that of milk thistle; recommended dose is 1-2 capsules containing 725 mg each or 5-10 cups of green tea daily.

Kamalahar: Ayurvedic herb used for the treatment of viral hepatitis; in clinical trials kamalahar reduced liver enzyme levels and bilirubin levels without causing adverse side effects.

Milk thistle (*Silybum marianum*): the seeds, roots and leaves are used to regenerate damaged liver tissue, tone, restore and normalize liver tissue, reduce inflammation and stimulate bile production and flow; shown in clinical trials to reduce liver enzyme levels and relieve bloating, abdominal pressure and sleep disturbances in patients with hepatitis, cirrhosis, and drug toxicity; the most effective remedy for poisoning with Amanita phalloides mushrooms; available in tinctures, capsules, teas, powders and whole seeds, using 250-500 mg daily. Several clinical trials have been conducted using milk thistle extracts alone or in combination with conventional therapy. Results are available at http://nccam.nih.gov/clinicaltrials/hepatitis. htm.

Neem (*Azadirachta indica*): plant extracts from the bark, seeds, and leaves of the tree, which is native to India; used as a pesticide and in Ayurvedic medicine; proven to be effective in studies for the treatment of viral hepatitis and acetaminophen induced liver damage; should not be used in autoimmune hepatitis or in pregnancy; available in capsules or as a tea used five times daily; information on clinical trials of neem available at http://www.neemtreefarms.com/immune.html, and at http://www. neemamerica.org.

Reishi (*Ganoderma lucidum*): used in hepatitis to reduce pain, improve liver enzyme levels, strengthen the immune system, improve sleep and help regenerate the liver; not to be used in persons with bile duct obstruction; used as a powder, tincture or tablets, using up to 3 grams daily.

Turmeric (*Curcuma longa*): used in hepatitis for its anti-viral effects against hepatitis B and for its protective activity in patients with drug induced hepatitis; reduces the lipid peroxidation that occurs in liver damage and reduces inflammation; protects against tumor formation, including hepatocellular carcinoma; not to be used in patients with bile obstruction; used as a powder, paste, capsule, or tonic; used as a powder one teaspoon is used from 1-3 times daily.

Precautions

Dandelion root and licorice root should be avoided because of their potential side effects. Dandelion is rich in vitamin A, which can be toxic to the liver. Licorice root is known to elevate blood pressure, promote sodium retention, causing electrolyte imbalances and increase stores of iron within the liver. Extracts of glycrrhizin, the active ingredient of licorice root, have been studied in clinical trials and shown to offer no significant benefits.

COLLOIDAL SILVER

Colloidal silver is sometimes used in programs for treating hepatitis. However, it can cause serious side effects and is not recommended by the FDA.

Glandular Extracts

Glandular extracts are preparations containing tissue proteins and peptides. Extracts from the thymus gland and liver are used for hepatitis.

Thymus extracts

The thymus gland is an immune system organ that produces and stores immune system T lymphocyte cells and also hormones, peptides, and cytokines that aid in the immune response. The thymus gland is efficient in childhood, but over time loses its functional abilities. Crude extracts of glandular thymus derivatives include the oral preparations Thymic Fractions 1402 A, Complete Thymic Formula, Immunoplex 402, NatCell thymus extract, and Thymosin fraction 5, and injectable thymosin, Thymosin-alpha-1 (Zadaxin).

Liver extracts

Liver glandular extracts have been used for treating liver disease since at least 1896 [26]. In clinical trials using liver extracts for three months, patients had reduced liver enzyme levels compared to patients receiving placebos [26]. Capsules and tablets containing liver extracts are available. Pre-digested formulations are easier to absorb.

Liver formulas

The tonic Liv.52/Liver Care manufactured by the Himalayan Drug Company and Himalaya USA has been available for the treatment of liver disorders, including hepatitis and alcoholic liver disease, for more than 50 years. Its effectiveness has been confirmed in clinical trials dating back from the 1960s. Liv.52/Liver Care contains a number of carefully selected herbal components and minerals that help heal the liver as well as herbs that reduce the side effects that may be caused by the therapeutic herbs. Studies of patients with viral hepatitis showed a faster reduction in liver enzymes than that seen in patients treated with conventional medications and B vitamins [26].

Another product, Hep-Forte, manufactured by Marilyn Neutraceuticals contains glandular extracts, vitamins and minerals that support liver health.

Oral digestive enzymes

Digestive enzymes aid in digestion and assist with the removal of toxic substances from the blood. Clinical trials involving the German compound Phlogenzym showed results similar to those of interferon but without the side effects associated with interferon. The product Wobenzym, which is available in the United States, is comparable and its recommended dose is 5 tablets taken on an empty stomach used three times daily [26]. Because this product is a natural blood thinner it is not recommended for patients with bleeding tendencies, and it should only be used with approval from one's physician.

Cleansing Diets

Cleansing diets are used to help detoxify the liver and reduce its workload. Cleansing diets include enzyme therapies, vegetable extracts to restore the alkaline balance, fluid replacement, and herbs to provide energy. Cleansing diets should only be undertaken with approval from one's physician. More information on cleansing diets can be found at the Alternative Medicine Clinic of San Francisco at http://www.biotherapy-clinic.com.

Energy Healing

Energy healing dates back to 500 B.C. when the Pythagoreans recorded observing a halo of light energy surrounding the body. In Eastern medical traditions, the body's energy force is known as ch'i or qi, and blockages or disruptions of the body's energy are responsible for disease. The goal of energy healing is to correct blockages in the flow of chi energy along their paths through the body, which are known as meridians.

In hepatitis, energy healing is used to help restore liver function and reduce inflammation. Energy healing should only be performed by a certified practitioner with experience in treating hepatitis.

Acupuncture and acupressure

Acupuncture points or acupoints are found on various locations on the body where meridians emerge at the surface. Acupoints correspond and control energy flow in various organs. In acupuncture, needles are used to manipulate acupoints and correct energy imbalances. Moxibustion is a form of acupuncture employing heat from burning substances, usually herbs, to facilitate the manipulation.

In acupressure, acupoints are stimulated by pressure rather than needles. Acupressure isn't as intensive a therapy as acupuncture, but it is effective for reducing symptoms and improving energy.

18

Lifestyle Influences and Prevention

Diet, exercise, chemical exposures, substance abuse, exercise routines, stress reduction techniques, and general lifestyle all influence healing. In hepatitis, these factors are particularly important. Chapter eighteen describes some of the major lifestyle influences in hepatitis.

Diet and the Immune System

An efficient immune system is essential for good health. A healthy immune system fights and eradicates infectious agents, protects us from autoimmune disease, and helps the body's tissues repair after injury. Certain foods promote immune system health and reduce inflammation, whereas other foods, particularly processed and fast foods, compromise and weaken the immune system, interfering with its function and promoting inflammation.

Table 18.1 Anti-inflammatory chemicals found in food

Polyphenols: phytochemicals such as acanthocyanins that protect against free radicals are found in colorful fruits, including blueberries, blackberries, strawberries and raspberries.

Quercetin: anti-inflammatory antioxidant compound with natural antihistamine properties found in red grapes, apples (especially red delicious varieties), red and yellow onions, garlic, and broccoli.

Antioxidants: nutrients that protect against the free radicals that cause inflammation found in carrots, winter squash, tomatoes, leafy green vegetables, arugula greens, endive, bell peppers, sweet potatoes, beets, kiwi, artichokes, yams, cantaloupe, spinach, and kale.

Omega-3-fatty acids: nutrients essential for tissue repair that reduce inflammation found in seafood, particularly wild salmon, light tuna, mackerel, sardines, anchovies, dark greens, walnuts, and flaxseed oil.

Oleic acid: works with omega-3-fatty acids to reduce inflammation; found in macadamia nuts and almonds.

Green tea: catechins in green tea reduce inflammation because of their high levels of antioxidants.

Fiber: helps with digestion and detoxification found in whole grains, fruits and vegetables.

Coffee: chemicals in coffee have been found to reduce progression to liver cancer in patients with hepatitis.

Digestive enzymes: chemicals such as bromelain and papain that promote liver function and reduce inflammation are found in pineapples and papayas.

Table 18.2 Foods/Substances that promote inflammation to be avoided in hepatitis

Arachidonic acid: pro-inflammatory compound found in beef, lamb and pork with smaller amounts in chicken, dairy products and eggs.

Omega–6 oils and Saturated fats: pro-inflammatory compounds found in vegetable oils, trans fats in crackers, fried foods, fast foods, processed foods.

Alcohol: promotes inflammation; poor prognosis when used in patients with hepatitis; abstinence may reverse liver damage and improve the response to treatment; it is recommended that patients with viral hepatitis abstain from alcohol to help prevent progression to cirrhosis.

Food additives: promote inflammation and add to the liver's chemical load; found in processed and pre-packaged foods.

Pesticides: promote inflammation, damaging to the liver; found in unwashed fruits and vegetables.

Recreational drugs: increase workload of the liver, reducing its function; ecstasy and cocaine injure liver cells, increasing liver damage in patients with hepatitis.

Prescription and over-the-counter drugs, herbal medicines: all drugs and chemicals are metabolized by the liver and many substances can injure the liver; all drugs should be used only with approval of one's physician to avoid further liver injury and dangerous drug interactions. Whenever new medications are added, transaminase enzyme, alkaline phosphatase, and bilirubin levels should be routinely performed at baseline, every two weeks for the first month, and monthly for the next three months to assess patients for possible drug-related hepatotoxicity.

Dietary supplements: certain dietary supplements, such as vitamin A, beta carotene, mixed carotenoids, iron, and niacin can injure the liver and should be avoided or only used in multi-vitamins under the direction of a physician. Note: multivitamins free of iron are available.

Exercise

Moderate exercise, such as walking or yoga, is important for immune system health as well as liver health. Exercise helps stimulate the circulation, improves digestion, and helps transport oxygen to the liver and other tissues. Strenuous exercise, such as long-distance running, should be avoided because it can stress the immune system and weaken its function.

Experts report that the side effects of anti-viral therapy are tolerated better in people who continue to work and remain active even if they need to reduce their working hours. Exercise offers a number of benefits for patients with hepatitis. In addition to helping maintain muscle mass and strength, exercise helps reduce stress and depression, strengthens the cardiovascular system, and helps maintain intestinal function.

Psychoneuroimmunology (PNI)

Psychoneuroimmunology (PNI) is the scientific study of the interrelationship between the immune system, nervous system, and endocrine system. Also known as the mind-body connection, PNI explains how nervous system effects such as stress can injure immune and endocrine function.

PNI is an important concept for patients with hepatitis because immune system health is the key to healing. The harmful effects of stress can be reduced by various stress reduction techniques, including meditation, deep breathing exercises, the Chinese discipline of Qi Gong, which focuses on breathing and movement, and certain exercises such as yoga and tai chi. Treating endocrine disorders, such as thyroid disorders that may develop during interferon therapy, is essential for improving both immune and nervous system function. For optimal healing in hepatitis, immune system, endocrine system, and nervous system health must all be taken into consideration.

Glossary

Abdomen. Area below the rib cage and above the legs that contains the stomach, liver, spleen and bowels.

Abscess. Localized lesion containing pus resulting from infection.

Acetaminophen. Analgesic; ingredient in many over-the-counter painkillers, such as Tylenol.

Acinus. Functional anatomic unit of the liver, adjacent to the portal triad, consisting of a diamond-shaped mass of liver tissue that's supplied by a terminal branch of the portal vein and of the hepatic artery and drained by a terminal branch of the bile duct.

Acute. Short-term self-limiting condition of sudden onset.

Acute hepatitis. The first stage of hepatitis; acute hepatitis has a sudden onset with symptoms ranging from mild to severe and typically resolving within six months.

Acute liver failure. Rapid onset of liver failure associated with clotting disturbances.

Acquired immune deficiency syndrome (AIDS). Blood borne disease caused by infection with the human immunodeficiency virus (HIV).

Adefovir dipivoxil (Hepsera). An oral nucleoside analogue drug that interferes with the replication of the hepatitis B virus approved for the treatment of chronic hepatitis B infection September 2002.

Adipose tissue. Fatty body tissue occurring anywhere in the body including other organs.

Alanine aminotransferase (ALT). Liver enzyme formerly known as serum glutamic pyruvate transaminase or SGPT. When liver cells are damaged high amounts of ALT are released and spilled into the blood circulation, causing elevated blood levels.

Albumin. A protein synthesized exclusively by the liver that assists in maintaining blood volume in blood vessels. Low levels of albumin or hypoalbuminemia are seen in several liver disorders and in conditions of poor health and nutrition. In severe liver disease, albumin production is impaired. If albumin levels in the blood fall too low, fluid seeps from blood vessels causing edema or ascites.

Alkaline phosphatase (ALP). Enzyme found primarily in the liver and bones although smaller amounts may be found in the intestines, kidneys and placenta. In liver disease, alkaline phosphatase is released from damaged liver cells, and high levels spill out into the blood circulation. An elevation of ALP in patients with normal or only slightly elevated ALT and AST levels suggests diseases of the bile ducts.

Alpha-1-antitrypsin deficiency. Genetic disease that can affect multiple organs including the liver. This condition causes the liver to produce defective alpha-1-antitrypsin and these molecules can lead to a metabolic form of hepatitis.

Alpha fetoprotein (AFP). AFP is a protein increased in pregnancy and in patients with certain forms of cancer, including liver cancer. The blood level of AFP is used as a tumor marker to help diagnose liver cancer. AFP levels are routinely performed in patients with chronic hepatitis B infection.

ALP. *See* Alkaline phosphatase.

ALT. *See* Alanine aminotransferase.

Alternative medicine. Therapies used to treat illness that are not included in the scope of conventional medicine.

Amino acids. Nitrogen-containing molecules that are the building blocks of protein; all protein consists of many different amino acids, and the particular arrangement of these molecules determines the protein's properties.

Ammonia. A nitrogen-rich breakdown product of amino acids; levels of ammonia are elevated in hepatic encephalopathy, hepatic coma and other conditions.

Ampulla of vater. Small opening in the duodenum that leads to the common bile ducts.

ANA. *See* Antinuclear antibody.

Analgesic. Medication used to reduce symptoms of pain.

Anemia. A condition characterized by low levels of red blood cells or hemoglobin.

Angiogenesis. The development of new blood vessels, of special concern in tumors.

Anicteric. Without jaundice, normal bilirubin level

Antibiotic. Drug used to destroy bacteria; antibiotics have no effect on viruses.

Antibody. Immunoglobulin protein produced by the immune system in response to foreign antigens, such as viruses; antibodies provide immunity or protection from another encounter with the antigen, they help fight infection, and they serve as markers or evidence of prior exposure to the foreign particle or passive immunity from vaccination.

Antigens. Protein particles usually foreign to the body, such as bacteria or viruses, capable of eliciting an immune response and production of specific antibodies.

Anti-HAV IgG antibodies. Antibodies formed in response to exposure to the hepatitis A virus or to HAV vaccination, which generally persist for life.

Anti-HAV IgM antibodies. Antibodies formed in response to exposure to the hepatitis A virus that persist during active HAV infection and diminish within a few months after disease onset.

Anti-HB core antibodies (Anti-HBcAb). Antibodies formed in response to hepatitis B infection.

Anti-HB e antibodies (anti-HBeAb). Antibodies that are formed in hepatitis B infection as the disease begins to resolve and the virus clears.

Anti-HB surface antibodies (Anti-HBsAb). Antibodies formed in response to exposure to the hepatitis B virus or to hepatitis B vaccination. This antibody provides protective immunity against hepatitis B.

Anti-HB surface antigen (HBsAg). Protein found on the surface of the hepatitis B virus (HBV) that may be detected in blood during active infection and in hepatitis B carriers.

Anti-HCV antibodies. Antibodies formed in response to exposure to the hepatitis C virus.

Anti-HDV antibodies. Antibodies formed after exposure to the hepatitis D virus.

Anti-inflammatory. Substances capable of reducing inflammation.

Antinuclear antibody (ANA). Broad class of autoantibodies directed at cell nuclei that are seen in numerous autoimmune disorders, including lupus and autoimmune hepatitis; further tests must be done to determine the specific type of ANA present.

Antioxidants. Nutrients and other substances that are able to quench or neutralize the free radicals that contribute to aging and disease; many vitamins and minerals have antioxidant properties and are used in alternative medicine healing protocols.

Antiviral. Substances with the ability to halt viral replication often used as a treatment for hepatitis.

Apoptosis. Programmed cell death of all the body's cells; for instance, red blood cells undergo apoptosis 150 days after they're formed. Diseases such as hepatitis increase apoptosis.

Arrhythmia. Condition of irregular heartbeat.

Aspartate aminotransferase (AST). Enzyme formerly known as serum glutamic oxalacetic transaminase (SGOT) found in the liver, heart and kidneys; high levels of AST are seen in liver inflammation and liver cell injury.

Ascites. Fluid accumulation in the peritoneal cavity that occurs in portal hypertension, cirrhosis and other advanced liver diseases.

AST. *See* Aspartate aminotransferase.

Asterixis. An uncontrollable type of hand tremor typically seen in early hepatic encephalopathy; liver flap.

Asymptomatic. Without apparent disease symptoms.

Autoantibodies. Group of antibodies produced during the autoimmune response that target the body's proteins, generally associated with specific autoimmune diseases.

Autoimmune. An immune system reaction in which immune system cells react with the body's own self components, such as the proteins in various body cells.

Autoimmune hemolytic anemia (AIHA). Autoimmune disorder associated with destruction of red blood cells, resulting in anemia.

Autoimmune hepatitis. Condition of hepatitis caused by immune system changes that damage and destroy liver cells.

Ballooning degeneration. Hydrophic swelling of a hepatocyte characteristically seen in hepatitis.

Benign. Harmless, not associated with disease development.

Bile. Bitter, dark green or gold substance consisting of salts, pigments, cholesterols, proteins and other chemicals needed for digestion and detoxification that is produced and secreted by liver cells; bile is also stored in the gallbladder where it's released as needed.

Bile acids (bile salts). Sterols manufactured by the liver that help solubilize bile and aid in the production and elimination of cholesterol.

Bile duct. One of several openings in the liver that transport bile into the intestines and the gallbladder.

Bile ductile. Small bile ducts found at the edges of the portal triads, which feed into the interlobular bile duct.

Biliary tract. Gallbladder and bile ducts, which collectively help transport bile; also known as the biliary system or biliary tree.

Bilirubin. Yellow pigment produced by the liver during the breakdown of red blood cells and other bodily proteins, which is found in bile; small amounts are released into the blood circulation daily, and these amounts increase in conditions of increased red blood cell destruction, in liver disease and in obstructive biliary disease. In liver disease, bilirubin levels rise, causing a condition of jaundice.

Biopsy. Procedure in which a small amount of tissue is removed during surgery or by local aspiration and studied for evidence of cellular change. *See also* Liver biopsy.

Bloodborne infection. Infection contracted by exposure to blood that is contaminated with infectious bloodborne organisms, such as hepatitis or immune deficiency viruses that can be transmitted through blood.

Body mass index (BMI). A calculation based on height and weight used to determine body mass and define obesity.

Branched DNA (bDNA) test. Blood test used to reveal the presence of minute quantities of DNA and RNA from specific organisms, such as HCV.

Bridging necrosis. Necrosis linking two portal areas or a portal area and a central area commonly seen in chronic hepatitis.

Bruit. Increased blood flow through a bodily organ, which can be heard during a physical examination with a stethoscope.

Budd-Chiari syndrome. Rare liver disease in which the veins that drain blood from the liver are blocked or narrowed.

Candidiasis. Infection caused by the *Candida* fungus, which normally is present in the gastrointestinal tract. Infection occurs when a change, such as the introduction of antibiotics or immunosuppressant medications, causes *Candida* overgrowth.

Carbohydrates. One of the three main classes of food that serve as a source of energy for the body, including the sugars and starches found in breads, cereals, and fruits; in the liver carbohydrate stores are converted into glycogen.

Carbohydrate-deficient transferrin (CDT). Chemical substance found in the blood that is increased in patients with alcohol abuse.

Carcinoma. A new growth, cancer, or malignant tumor.

Cardiac disease. Any of several different disorders affecting the heart and its function.

Carrier. A person, usually in apparently good health, who has been infected with an organism, such as HBV or HCV that is never cleared from the body. Carriers are capable of infecting and causing disease in others.

CAT scan. *See* Computerized axial tomography.

CBC. *See* Complete blood count.

Centers for Disease Control and Prevention (CDC). Federal organization dedicated to the prevention and control of communicable diseases. The CDC monitors and conducts extensive research into infectious diseases and makes this information available to the general public.

Chemiluminometric immunoassay (CIA). Laboratory procedure with greater sensitivity and specificity than enzyme immunoassays that is used for the detection of viral markers.

Cholangitis. Infection or inflammation in the bile ducts sometimes seen in patients with gallstones or primary sclerosing cholangitis.

Cholestasis. Condition of impaired bile flow caused by liver cell defects or bile duct obstruction.

Cholestatic jaundice. Jaundice caused by failure of conjugated bilirubin to be sent to the gut. (Characterized by an elevated direct bilirubin.)

Cholestatic liver enzymes. Liver enzymes primarily increased in obstructive liver disease such as gamma-glutamyl transpeptidase (gamma GT) and alkaline phosphatase (ALP).

Cholesterol. Lipid or fatty substance produced in the liver and normally found in the blood, brain, liver and bile. Cholesterol is both produced and metabolized in the liver.

Chromosomes. Thread-like structures in the nucleus of an animal or plant cell that contain deoxyribonucleic acid (DNA).

Chronic. Condition that persists long-term or that appears to resolve but remains in a latent stage and causes recurring disease symptoms at a later time.

Chronic hepatitis. Condition of hepatitis showing continued persistence of viral markers or viral DNA or characteristic cellular changes on biopsy that persist for more than 6 months after disease onset.

CIA. *See* Chemiluminometric immunoassay.

Cirrhosis. Liver disease characterized by fibrosis and scaring of the entire liver to a degree that is sufficient to interfere with normal liver function. Cirrhosis can ultimately lead to hepatocellular cancer, liver failure and death.

Clinical trials. Carefully controlled trials usually conducted by universities in affiliation with pharmaceutical companies for the purpose of studying the efficacy and safety of potentially new medical treatments.

Clotting factors. Proteins produced in the liver that allow blood to clot at the site of an injury. In advanced liver disease, a deficiency of clotting factors is a poor prognostic sign.

Coagulopathy. Disorder of blood clotting that causes a bleeding tendency and abnormal blood clotting tests, particularly an elevated prothrombin time.

Co-infection. Simultaneous infection with two infectious agents, such as HBV and HDV.

Common bile duct. Duct or tube that carries bile from the liver to the small intestine.

Complete blood count (CBC). A blood test which measures levels of blood cells, including the white blood cell count; the proportions of the different types of white blood cells; the red blood cell count; the red blood cell parameters, such as hemoglobin count; and the platelet count.

Complications. New medical problems that arise as a result of treatment or as consequence of disease; side effects.

Computerized axial tomography (CAT). Diagnostic imaging procedure that produces cross-sectional horizontal and vertical detailed images of bones, muscles, fat and organs.

Conjugated bilirubin. Bilirubin that has been conjugated to glucuronic acid, making it water soluble; direct bilirubin.

Confluent-lytic necrosis. Death of clusters of hepatocytes attributed to humoral immunity or the immune system's response to liver injury.

Councilman (acidophil) body. Single-cell necrosis (apoptosis) of a hepatocyte, typically in hepatitis, occurring as a result of attack by a T-killer cell.

Course of infection (disease course). Stages an infection goes through from initial exposure to the onset of symptoms and resolution.

Cryptogenic cirrhosis. Condition of cirrhosis in which the cause is not evident. Cryptogenic cirrhosis accounts for 5–15 percent of patients with chronic liver diseases in the United States.

Cytokines. Hormone-like proteins that are secreted by immune system cells that regulate the intensity and duration of the immune response.

Cytotoxic substances. Substances capable of destroying cells.

Decompensated cirrhosis. Advanced form of cirrhosis in which liver function is impaired. Symptoms include ascites and/or jaundice, weakness, muscle wasting, weight loss, bruising, finger clubbing, low blood pressure, vascular spiders, enlarged liver, enlarged spleen, mental changes, and fever. Jaundice in decompensated cirrhosis implies that liver cell destruction exceeds the liver's capacity for regeneration.

Deoxyribonucleic acid (DNA). Component found in the cell of living matter that carries hereditary identifying genetic information.

Dialysis. *See* Hemodialysis.

DNA. *See* Deoxyribonucleic acid.

DNA polymerase. An enzyme essential to the replication of DNA viruses. DNA polymerase can be measured to indicate levels of viral replication.

Dubin-Johnson syndrome. Inherited form of chronic jaundice with no apparent cause.

Dysphagia. Difficulty swallowing usually caused by blockage or injury to the esophagus.

Edema. Accumulation of fluid in the soft tissues outsides of blood vessels, particularly in the ankles although in severe edema fluid can also accumulate in the abdomen.

EIA. *See* Enzyme immunoassay.

ELISA. *See* Enzyme-linked immunosorbent assay.

Encephalopathy. Brain function abnormality causing confusion, disorientation and symptoms of dementia. *See* Hepatic encephalopathy.

Endoscope. Small, flexible tube with a light and a lens on the end used in medical procedures for the study of the stomach, duodenum, colon or rectum.

Endoscopy. Procedure in which an endoscope is used to study and treat damaged organs, for instance in the repair of varices.

Entecavir. An oral nucleoside analogue drug that interferes with the replication of hepatitis B. In April, 2005, Entecavir became the third oral drug approved for the treatment of hepatitis B.

Enteral nutrition. Procedure in which food is passed through tubes places in the nose, stomach and intestines; tube feeding.

Enzymes. Naturally occurring chemical substances that assist or catalyze chemical reactions.

Enzyme immunoassay. Laboratory method that detects the presence of antibodies to specific viruses used as an initial screening test for infectious diseases.

Enzyme-linked immunosorbent assay (ELISA). Diagnostic blood test used to detect antibodies, including viral antibodies.

Epidemiology. Field of medicine that studies the incidence, distribution, and control of disease in a population that helps determine ways disease can be prevented.

Epithelium. Inner and outer tissue covering of organs including those of the digestive tract.

Esophageal varices. Stretched or ruptured veins in the esophagus commonly seen in advanced liver diseases.

Fatty liver. Condition characterized by increased amounts of fat in liver cells; occurs in obesity, alcoholism, as a complication of pregnancy, and in hepatitis; also called steatosis.

Fecal fat test. Test that measures the amount of fat present in stool specimens.

Feces. Stool.

Fibrosis. Scar formation resulting from the repair of tissue damage; in the liver extensive fibrosis is called cirrhosis.

Fistula. Abnormal passage between two organs or between an organ and the outside caused when damaged tissues come into contact with one another and join.

Flavivirus. Group of related viruses including the viruses that cause yellow fever, St. Louis encephalitis and hepatitis C.

Focal necrosis. Death of individual cells, evidenced either by Councilman bodies or lytic necrosis. Inside the lobule, liver cell destruction is viewed as focal lobular necrosis and is seen in smoldering hepatitis from any cause.

Fulminant hepatitis. Acute potentially-life threatening condition of hepatitis occurring within eight weeks from the onset of symptoms characterized by encephalopathy.

Gastroenterology. Branch of medicine that studies the function and diseases associated with the esophagus, stomach, pancreas, intestines and liver.

Gastrointestinal tract. Large, muscular tube that extends from the mouth to the anus through which food passes, is absorbed, digested, and excreted.

Genotype. Pattern of genetic information that is unique to a group of organisms or viruses including the subtle minor differences in composition that may affect the way a particular viral genotype responds to treatment. Genotypes are helpful in determining optimal treatment protocols.

Giant cell hepatitis. Relatively common pattern of liver injury occurring primarily in children associated with autoimmune hepatitis; in adults this condition can have features suggesting a viral origin that occasionally occurs after liver transplants and has a rapidly progressive course.

Gilbert's syndrome. Fairly common mild disorder causing increased bilirubin levels in the absence of liver damage.

Glomerulonephritis. Kidney disorder associated with inflammation of the small convoluted mass of capillaries necessary for blood circulation in the kidneys often associated with immune complex deposits.

Glomerulus. One of the blood filtering structures that comprise the nephron, the functional unit of the kidney.

Glycogen. Carbohydrate formed from glucose metabolism that serves as a source of energy; glycogen is primarily stored in the liver and, to a lesser extent, muscle cells.

Granuloma. Mass of red, irritated tissue that emerges on various tissues, including the liver.

Ground glass hepatocytes. Distinctive hepatocytes seen in chronic hepatitis B infection. The ground glass cytoplasm is caused by an unusual accumulation of a cytokeratin material.

Guillain-Barré syndrome. Autoimmune disorder affecting the central nervous system, damaging the protective myelin sheaths that cover nerves; also called acute idiopathic polyneuritis.

HAV. *See* Hepatitis A virus.

HBc. *See* Hepatitis B core antigen.

HBe. *See* Hepatitis Be antigen.

HBIG. *See* Hepatitis B immune globulin.

HBsAg. *See* Hepatitis B surface antigen.

HBsAb. *See* Hepatitis B surface antibody.

HBV. *See* Hepatitis B virus.

HBV DNA. Nucleic acid particles of HBV that can be measured as a marker of active viral replication and infectivity. Tests for HBV DNA are used to confirm diagnosis of active infection, determine the need for treatment, and monitor treatment response.

HCV. *See* Hepatitis C virus.

HCV RNA. Nucleic acid particles of HCV that can be measured as a marker of active viral replication and infectivity. Tests for HCV RNA are used to confirm diagnosis, determine a need for treatment, and monitor the treatment response.

HDV. *See* Hepatitis D virus.

HELLP syndrome. Serious condition of hemolysis, elevated liver enzymes and low platelets occurring in pregnancy that often resolves after delivery.

Hemochromatosis. Disease of iron metabolism leading to increased storage of iron within the liver, which can lead to conditions of hepatitis and cirrhosis.

Hemodialysis. Procedure used for patients with kidney disease in which toxins and waste products are removed from the blood.

Hemoglobin. Main protein component of the red blood cell consisting of a protein-iron complex that serves as the vehicle for the transportation of oxygen from the lungs and carbon dioxide from blood cells back to the lungs.

Hemolytic anemia. *See* Autoimmune hemolytic anemia.

Hemolytic jaundice. Jaundice due to excessive destruction of red blood cells.

Hemophilia. Condition caused by an absence or deficiency of Factor VIII, a clotting factor necessary for proper blood clotting.

Hepatic artery. Artery that transports oxygenated blood from the heart to the liver.

Hepatic encephalopathy. A condition seen in advanced liver disease that usually precedes hepatic coma related to increased levels of ammonia, glutamates, and other chemicals released during the liver's metabolic processes; symptoms range from altered mood to stupor.

Hepatic failure. End stage liver disease in which the liver fails to function.

Hepatic vein. The vein that carries blood away from the liver.

Hepatitis A virus (HAV). Organism responsible for infectious hepatitis or hepatitis A.

Hepatitis B core antigen (HBcAg). Protein component of the hepatitis B virus that occurs early in the course of hepatitis B before antibody production begins.

Hepatitis B core antibody (HBcAb). Immunoglobulin protein that develops after exposure to the hepatitis B virus early in infection before hepatitis B surface antibodies are produced; indicator of active hepatitis B infection.

Hepatitis B e antigen (HBeAg). Protein component of HBV that occurs early in the course of HBV infection.

Hepatitis B immune globulin (HBIG). A passive vaccine containing antibodies to hepatitis B used as a post-exposure treatment for people exposed to hepatitis B, including newborns born to mothers with hepatitis B.

Hepatitis B surface antigen (HBsAg). Protein component found on the surface of HBV; its presence can be used as an indicator of active infection or a persistent carrier state.

Hepatitis B surface antibody (HBsAb). Immunoglobulin protein that develops after exposure to HBV or after HBV vaccination that indicates immunity to HBV.

Hepatitis B virus (HBV). Organism responsible for serum hepatitis or hepatitis B infection.

Hepatitis C virus (HCV). Organism responsible for HCV infection.

Hepatitis D virus (HDV). Delta agent; a type of hepatitis virus found only in patients with HBV infection that causes superinfection or co-infection with HBV. HDV is primarily seen in recipients of multiple blood transfusions, including patients with hemophilia or those undergoing renal dialysis, and among people who share contaminated needles.

Hepatitis E virus (HEV). Organism responsible hepatitis E infection.

Hepatitis F virus (HFV). Organism responsible for hepatitis F, which has not yet been proven to be clinically significant.

Hepatitis G/GB virus (HGV). Organism responsible for hepatitis G/GB infection.

Hepatocellular carcinoma (HCC). Primary liver cancer; a malignant liver tumor (hepatoma) that can occur as a consequence of cirrhosis that can develop as a consequence of chronic HBV or HCV infection.

Hepatocellular jaundice. Jaundice due primarily to failure of hepatocytes to properly take up or conjugate bilirubin.

Hepatocyte. Parenchymal (tissue) cells of the liver containing a well-developed substructure of organelles, including mitochondria, endoplasmic reticulum peroxisomes, lysosomes and Golgi apparatus.

Hepatologist. Physician, usually a gasteroenterologist, who specializes in the treatment of individuals with diseases of the liver and its functions.

Hepsera. *See* Adefovir

HEV. *See* Hepatitis E virus.

HFV. *See* Hepatitis F virus.

HGV. *See* Hepatitis G/GB virus.

HIV. *See* Human immunodeficiency virus.

Human immunodeficiency virus (HIV). Retrovirus that causes HIV infection and AIDS.

Humoral immunity. Type of immune response in which B lymphocytes produce antibodies directed against infectious agents and elicit the production of toxic immune system chemicals capable of destroying infected cells.

Icteric. Yellow tinged skin, eyes or tissues; jaundiced.

Icterus. *See* jaundice.

Immune complex. Combination of linked antigen, usually an infectious particle, with its specific antibody; immune complex can be small and soluble or large and capable of interfering with the function of tissue cells.

Immune system. System of organs and cells working together to protect the body from infection and malignancy.

Immunity. Condition of resistance to specific infectious agents conferred by active or passive antibody production, including prior infection and vaccines.

Immunoglobulin (Ig). Protein normally found in the body that's used in antibody production; thus, immunoglobulins and antibodies are often used interchangeably. There are several different classes of immunoglobulins including IgA, IgM, IgG, and IgD. The earliest antibodies produced in response to viral infection are IgM antibodies. These persist for several months and are followed by the production of IgG antibodies. IgG antibodies usually persist for life and confer immunity.

Infection. Condition caused by the body's direct contact with harmful microorganisms.

Incidence. The number of new infections occurring in a given period of time within a specific community.

Injecting drug use. The use or abuse of drugs administered directly into the bloodstream by intravenous injection.

Interferon. Naturally occurring defensive cytokine produced by the immune system in response to infection; interferons can also be produced synthetically and used as a form of treatment for viral infections.

Inteferon Alpha-2b (IntronA). A drug that mimics naturally occurring interferon. It is administered three times weekly for hepatitis B and is the first drug used for the treatment of hepatitis B.

Intravenous. Administration of medications through the veins

Jaundice. Yellowing of the eyes, skin and tissues resulting from excess bilirubin in the bloodstream; also known as icterus.

Laparoscope. Narrow tube with a tiny video camera attached that is used to observe the inner surface of organs and bodily structures.

Laparotomy. Surgical procedure in which the abdomen is opened and the abdominal structures investigated or treated.

Lesion. Abnormal tissue caused by injury or malignancy.

Liver biopsy. The removal and study of small pieces of liver tissue obtained through needle aspiration for the purpose of determining liver damage, inflammation or infection.

Liver enzymes. Several different enzyme proteins, including ALT and AST, that are used in the liver's metabolic processes; when liver cells are damaged, liver enzymes spill out into the blood circulation, causing elevated blood levels.

Liver function tests (LFTs). Liver function tests are blood tests that help assess the functioning of the liver and determine liver cell damage; LFTs include tests for liver enzymes, albumin and bilirubin.

Lobular disarray. Loss of the normal radial arrangement of liver plates within the lobule, typically with severe distortion of the sinusoids. The hallmark biopsy finding in acute hepatitis.

Lupoid hepatitis. Former term used to describe autoimmune hepatitis. *See* Autoimmune hepatitis.

Lupus. Referring to the characteristic rash seen in patients with lupus disorders; lupus stems from the word wolf and early reports described this butterfly-shaped facial rash as wolf-like; referring to any of the lupus disorders, including discoid lupus, system lupus erythematosus, and neonatal transient lupus.

Lymph node. Accumulation of lymphoid tissue organized as definite lymphoid organs situated along the course of the lymphatic vessels.

Lymphocyte. Type of white blood cell primarily involved in the immune system's response to infection. Lymphocytes can be further divided into subtypes such as natural killer cells, T helper cells (CD4 cells), and T suppressor cells (CD8 cells).

Lysosomes. Dense organelles containing deposits of iron, lipofuscin, bile pigments, and copper found in liver cells that contain hydrolytic enzymes that act as scavengers.

Macrophage. Large mononuclear phagocytic (capable of engulfing other cells, bacteria and viruses) cell of the tissues that exists as either a wandering type or a fixed type that lines the capillaries and sinuses of organs such as the bone marrow, spleen, liver, and lymph nodes; macrophages phagocytize, process and present infectious particles to T lymphocytes and they engulf, thereby removing, damaged and infected tissue cells.

Massive necrosis. Complete or near-complete cell destruction, with most of the hepatocytes on a biopsy slide appearing dead due to poisoning, viruses, medication reactions, or ischemia.

Metabolism. The breaking down of compounds, such as drugs and food, into simple molecules that can be absorbed by the body's cells.

Monocyte. Type of white blood cell resembling tissue macrophages found in the peripheral blood and tissues with phagocytic properties.

Mucosal lining. Lining of the gastrointestinal tract organs that produces mucus.

Myoglobin. Major protein component of muscle tissue, which is released from damaged muscle cells. Myoglobin blood levels are used as indicators of muscle injury.

NAT tests. *See* Nucleic acid amplification tests.

Natural killer (NK) cell. Specific type of lymphocyte programmed to attack and destroy cells damaged and infected by viruses and other microorganisms.

Needle-stick. Accidental puncture of the skin during procedures in which needles or other sharp instruments are used to gain entry into blood or bodily organs.

Non-A, non-B hepatitis. Term used until the late 1980s to describe conditions of apparent viral hepatitis not caused by hepatitis A or B;

Nucleic acid amplification tests (NAT). Laboratory procedure used to detect nucleic acid, either RNA or DNA, to aid in the diagnosis of specific substances, such as viruses. In NAT methods, the specimen is treated in a matter that amplifies the amount of nucleic acid present in the sample. NAT tests are superior for diagnosing viral hepatitis since they detect specific viral particles.

Paracentesis. Procedure requiring local anesthesia used to drain excess fluid or ascites by inserting a needle into the abdomen and withdrawing fluid.

Parenteral. Administered through injection rather than orally.

PCR. *See* Polymerase chain reaction.

PEG. *See* Polyethylene glycol.

PEG-interferon. Pegylated interferon; compound containing both polyethylene glycol and interferon used in the treatment of hepatitis that is longer-acting than regular interferon products and typically used weekly.

Peliosis hepatitis. Hepatitis characterized by a random distribution of large blood-filled cavities or nodules that may be lined with sinusoidal cells.

Percutaneous transmission. Mode of transmitted substances, including infectious microorganisms, into the body through the skin, for instance by injection.

Pericarditis. Inflammation of the serous membrane lining the pericardial sac surrounding the heart and the organs of the great vessels; in pericarditis pericardial swelling can cause symptoms resembling those of a heart attack with pain appearing in the middle or left front of the chest and radiating back to the shoulders; untreated pericarditis can cause scar tissue to form in the pericardial sac, restricting the heart's movement.

Perinatal transmission. Mode of transmission occurring during childbirth.

Phenobarbital. Long-acting barbiturate used as a sedative or anticonvulsant medication.

Piecemeal necrosis. Necrosis or destruction of groups of hepatocytes within the limiting plate. Today the term interface hepatitis is preferred to prevent confusion with focal necrosis deeper within the lobule. Piecemeal necrosis is seen in chronic hepatitis.

Platelets. Blood components essential for clotting. Platelets are separated from the whole blood drawn from blood donors and available as units for transfusion.

Polyarteritis nodosa. Inflammatory process affecting the layers of the small and medium sized arteries associated with hepatitis manifested by various symptoms including febrile reactions.

Polyethylene glycol (PEG). Chemical substance added to interferon used in the treatment of hepatitis.

Polymerase chain reaction (PCR). Laboratory procedure used to amplify deoxyribonucleic acid and identify specific organisms, such as viruses. PCR can detect minute traces of HCV in any given medium. PCR blood tests for viral DNA can detect viruses as early as three days after infection.

Portal hypertension. High blood pressure occurring in the liver and its blood vessels commonly seen in cirrhosis.

Portal vein. One of the veins that carries blood to the liver.

Post transfusion hepatitis. Hepatitis that occurs following a transfusion of blood products.

Prevalence. The number of cases of disease in the community at any one time, usually expressed as a percentage of the population.

Protein. An assembly of amino acids with characteristic properties and functions, for instance, enzymes.

Prothrombin (Factor II). Protein produced by the liver essential for blood clotting.

Prothrombin time (PT test). Blood test that measures prothrombin levels by determining the time it takes for blood to clot when added to other clotting factors. The PT test is used as a measure of blood clotting and it increases as the liver fails to function.

Pruritis. Itching of the skin.

PT test. *See* Prothrombin time.

Purpura. Reddish or purple discolorations resembling small bruises found on the skin surface related to abnormal bleeding tendencies and ruptured blood vessels.

Raynaud's phenomenon. Condition of episodic constriction of small arteries of the extremities (usually fingers and toes) induced by cold temperatures or emotional stress; symptoms include a pale appearance (blanching) and numbness followed by redness and tingling associated with swelling or pain; Raynaud's phenomenon may also be seen in a syndrome frequently associated with various autoimmune disorders.

RBC. *See* Red blood cell.

Recombinant immunoblot assay (RIBA). Type of laboratory method used to confirm the presence of viral markers found by other screening methods.

Red blood cell (RBC). Cell of the reticuloendothelial system containing hemoglobin that transports oxygen to the body's tissues. RBCs are constantly produced in the body and constantly broken down. Each RBC survives for about 120 days at which time it is broken down into bilirubin.

Relapse. Recurrence of disease after a period of recovery.

Remission. Partial or complete disappearance of disease symptoms.

Reye's syndrome. Condition of acute encephalopathy in combination with fatty degeneration of the liver first described in Australia in 1963 primarily occurring in children with viral infections treated with analgesics, especially aspirin.

Rhabdomyolysis. Potentially fatal condition marked by destruction or degeneration of skeletal muscle tissue often associated with high levels of myoglobin in the urine.

RIBA. *See* Recombinant immunoblot assay.

Ribavirin. Antiviral compound shown to have activity against hepatitis C when used in combination with interferon.

Ribonucleic acid (RNA). A component of chromosomes that carries genetic identifying information used as a messenger for the production of new DNA; particles of RNA from specific infectious materials, such as viruses and bacteria, can be detected in blood tests used to confirm specific diseases.

RNA. See Ribonucleic acid.

RNA viruses. Viruses that contain the enzyme reverse transcriptase which allows them to replicate by producing new strands of RNA.

Sampling error. Possibility that inadequate or insufficient biopsy samples are taken, causing misleading results.

Sclera. The white part of the eye globe.

Scleral icterus. Yellow discoloration of the sclera commonly seen in liver disease.

S/Co Ratios. *See* Signal cutoff ratios.

Serology. Laboratory study of immunological markers of disease, including antigens and antibodies.

Serum. Liquid portion of blood separated from red blood cells.

Serum hepatitis. Former name for HBV infection, the disease caused by the hepatitis B virus.

Signal cutoff ratios (S/Co). Antibody tests for HCV use a cutoff value, which is compared to test results. Typically, results with signals higher than 1.0 are considered positive. Because false positives occasionally occur in these tests, laboratories report positive tests by including the exact signal/cutoff ratio. These results are accompanied by an interpretation for that method. For instance, with a cutoff of 1.0, S/Co ratios higher than 4.0 correlate with a 94.1 percent likelihood that this is a true positive. Results with signals close to the cutoff are interpreted as inconclusive, repeat analysis in one-two weeks recommended.

Smooth muscle antibody (SMA). Autoantibody that targets the smooth muscle tissue of the liver found in patients with autoimmune hepatitis.

Spider angiomatas. Enlarged, burst, spider-like blood vessels found on the chest, back, arms and face of patients with liver disease.

Spleen. Immune system organ situated opposite of the liver beneath the ribcage in the left upper abdominal quadrant that stores platelets and assists in the destruction of mature red blood cells.

Splenomegaly. Condition of enlarged spleen.

Steatohepatitis. Condition of liver inflammation accompanied by fatty liver.

Steatorrhea. Condition of loose, pale stool with excess fat, causing it to float to the top of the toilet bowl that occurs when the body is unable to properly digest dietary fat.

Steatosis. Condition of fatty liver in which triglycerides accumulate in liver tissue.

Superinfection. Condition of a second viral infection occurring and exacerbating symptoms in a patient who already has a viral infection.

Sustained response. A response to therapy that persists for a long period. In viral hepatitis, patients who continue to remain free of virus 6 months after stopping treatment are said to have a sustained response or sustained viral response.

Transaminases. Group of enzymes that aid in the liver's metabolic processes. See alanine aminotransferase and aspartate aminotransferase.

Transferrin. Protein produced by the liver that helps transport iron through the body.

Transplantation. Implanting tissue or organs taken from one patient into another.

Triglyceride. Fatty substance stored in the liver that accumulates in fatty liver disease.

Ursodeoxycholic acid (UCDA). Medication that reduces bile acids used for the treatment of cholestatic liver disease; UCDA decreases cholesterol saturation in the liver, reduces symptoms of itching, and prevents the formation of gallstones.

Varices. Enlarged and tortuous veins which can occur throughout the gastrointestinal tract, esophagus and stomach that occur in severe liver disease, especially portal hypertension. Bleeding varices are one of the leading causes of mortality in patients with cirrhosis.

Vascular. Having a rich supply of blood vessels.

Vasculitis. Inflammation of blood vessels.

Vertical transmission. Transmission of infectious agents during pregnancy.

Viral load. The amount of specific viral RNA or DNA viral particles present in blood usually expressed in international units (IU) per milliliter of blood. The viral load test is primarily used to confirm disease and monitor treatment response.

Virus. Very small parasitic microorganism capable of causing disease and reproducing in its host. The Nobel Prize winner Peter Medawar described viruses as "pieces of bad news wrapped in protein."

Vitiligo. Autoimmune condition characterized by patches of unpigmented skin often seen in association with thyroid conditions and viral disorders.

Western blot test. Test used to identify specific protein constituents used in the identification of antibodies and viral material.

Wilson's disease. Genetic disease causing excessive accumulations of copper in the liver which can cause liver damage progressing to hepatitis and cirrhosis.

Zones. The liver is divided into three functional zones, each containing a different mix of cells, endoplasmic reticulum, lysosomes and mitochondria. Certain types of liver disease may predominantly affect one or more of these zones.

Resources

Books

Armstrong, Donald and Jonathan Cohen. *Infectious Diseases*. London: Mosby. 1999.

Balch, James, and Mark Stengler. *Prescription for Natural Cures*. Danvers, MA: Balch Enterprises, 2004.

Blumberg, Baruch S. *Hepatitis B, The Hunt for a Killer Virus*. Princeton, New Jersey: Princeton University Press, 2002.

Blumenthal, Mark, Ed. *The Complete German Commission E Monographs Therapeutic Guides to Herbal Medicine*. Boston: The American Botanical Council/Integrative Medicine Communications, 1998.

Bruce, Cara, and Lisa Montanarelli. *The First Year — Hepatitis C: An Essential Guide for the Newly Diagnosed*. New York: Marlowe, 2002.

Buhner, Stephen Harrod. *Herbs for Hepatitis C and the Liver*. North Adams, MA: Storey Books, 2000.

Cohen, Jay. *Over Dose: The Case Against The Drug Companies. Prescription Drugs, Side Effects, and Your Health*. New York: Tarcher/Putnam, 2001.

Cohen, Misha, and Robert Gish. *The Hepatitis C Help Book*. New York: St. Martin's Griffin, 2000.

Chopra, Sanjiv. *Dr. Sanjiv Chopra's Liver Book: A Comprehensive Guide to Diagnosis, Treatment and Recovery*. New York: Simon and Schuster, 2001.

Goodman, Louis, and Alfred Gilman. *The Pharmacological Basis of Therapeutics*, second edition. New York: Macmillan, 1955.

Henry, John Bernard. *Clinical Diagnosis and Management by Laboratory Methods*. 17th edition. Philadelphia: W.B. Saunders, 1984.

Holmes, King K. *Sexually Transmitted Diseases. third edition*. New York: McGraw-Hill, 1999.

Life Extension Foundation. *Disease Prevention and Treatment*, expanded fourth edition. Hollywood, FL: Life Extension Media, 2003.

Mondoa, Emil, and Mindy Kitei. *Sugars That Heal*. New York: Ballantine, 2001.

Palmer, Melissa *Dr. Melissa Palmer's Guide to Hepatitis and Liver Disease*, revised Edition. New York: Penguin Group, 2004.

PDR for Herbal Medicine. Montvale, NJ: Medical Economics Company, 1997.

Sherlock, Sheila, and James Dooley. *Diseases of the Liver and Biliary System*, ninth edition, Oxford, London: Blackwell, 1993.

Zevin, Igor Vilevcich *A Russian Herbal, Traditional Remedies for Health and Healing*. Rochester, NY: Healing Arts Press, 1997.

317

Journals

Advance for Medical Laboratory Professionals
2900 Horizon Drive
King of Prussia, PA 19406
www.advanceweb.com

British Medical Journal
www.bmj.bmjjournals.com
Clinical Care Options in Hepatitis
http://clinicaloptions.com/hep/

Hepatitis Magazine
P.O. Box 16564
Sugarland, TX 77496
(800) 310-7047
www.hepatitismag.com

Hepatology Journal
W.B. Saunders Company
P.O. Box 628239
Orlando, FL 3286-8239
(800) 654-2452
Outside the U.S. (407) 345-4000
http://www.hepatologyjournal.org/

Journal of the National Academy of Acupuncture and Oriental Medicine
P.O. Box 62, Tarrytown, NY 10591-0062
(914) 332-4576
http://www.naaom.org

LabMedicine
Publication of the American Society for Clinical Pathology
21000 W Harrison Street
Chicago, IL 0612-3798

Life Extension
Publication of the Life Extension Foundation
1100 West Commercial Boulevard
Ft. Lauderdale, FL 33309
www.lef.org

Medical Laboratory Observer
2500 Tamiami Trail North
Nokomis, FK 34275
www.mlo-online.com

Natural Health
http://naturalhealthmag.com

New England Journal of Medicine
http://www.nejm.org

Transfusion
The Journal of the American Association of Blood Banks
350 Main Street
Malden, MA 02148
http://www.transfusion.org

Medical Journal Access and Search Engines

Computer Retrieval of Information on Scientific Projects (CRISP)
http://crisp.cit.nih.gov/
    Searchable database of federally-funded biomedical research projects conducted at universities, hospitals, and other research institutions.

Freereality Medical Search Engine
http://www.freeality.com/medicalt.htm

Hardin Library for the Health Sciences
University of Iowa
http://www.lib.uiowa.edu/hardin/

Health A to Z
http://www.healthatoz.com/

Medical World Search
http://www.mwsearch.com/

Medline Plus Health Topics
http://www.nlm.nih.gov/medlineplus/
    healthtopics.html

Medscape
http://www.medscape.com
    Medscape provides free online access to journal articles, reports and educational programs for registered users. Hepatitis is included under the Infectious Diseases topic

Medsite
http://www.medsite.com/

PubMed
National Library of Medicine's search service
http://www.ncbi.nlm.nih.gov/PubMed/

PubMed Central search engine
http://www.pubmedcentral.nih.gov/index.
    html

Virtual Med Online
http://www.virtualmedonline.com/
  journalcentral/

Webmedlit
http://www.webmedlit.com
  This site provides access to 22 medical journals including the *New England
Journal of Medicine* and the *British Medical Journal.*

Government Agencies

The following government agencies
provide current information on hepatitis,
including recent studies, clinical trials,
risk factors, prevention, vaccines and
treatment; some agencies provide fact
sheets, articles, and publications which
can be downloaded or requested to be
mailed at no charge.

Centers for Disease Control and
  Prevention (CDC)
Hepatitis Branch, Mailstop G37
Division of Viral and Rickettsial
  Diseases
National Center for Infectious Diseases
Centers for Disease Control and
  Prevention
Atlanta, GA 30333
(800) 311–3435; (888) 4HEPCDC
  (443–7232)
www.cdc.gov/hepatitis
www.cdc.gov/ncidod/diseases/hepatitis

CDC STD 2002 Treatment Guidelines for
  Hepatitis
http://www.cdc.gov/STD/treatment/
  7–2002TG.htm
  This site contains the current treatment
guidelines for STDs, including viral hepatitis, established by the CDC along with
information on symptoms and diagnosis.

CDC National Immunization Program
http://www.cdc.gov/nip/webutil/about/
  default.htm

Centers for Medicare and Medicaid Services
7500 Security Boulevard
Baltimore, MD 21244–1850

(877) 2267–2323
http://www.medicare.gov/
http://www.cms.hhs.gov/

Department of Veteran's Affairs
http://www.va.gov/hepatitisc
  Excellent resource with information on
hepatitis C and resources for veterans.

Environmental Health Services Branch
http://www.cdc.gov/nceh/emergency/
  default.htm

Food and Drug Administration (FDA)
Office of Consumer Affairs
HFE 88
5600 Fishers Lane
Rockville, MD 20857
(800) 523–4440
http://www.fda.gov

Food and Drug Administration
Center for Drug Evaluation and Research
  (CDER)
http://www.fda.gov/cder

HRSA National Vaccine Injury Compen-
  sation Program (VICP)
http://www.hrsa.gov/osp/vicp/index.htm

Indian Health Service
The Reyes Building
801 Thompson Avenue, Suite 400
Rockville, MD 20852–1627
(301) 443–1083
http://www.ihs.gov/

Institute of Medicine
http://www.iom.edu
  Nonprofit agency that works for the
interests of public health and evaluates
the efforts of the federal government.

National Center for Complementary and
  Alternative Medicine (NCCAM)
National Institutes of Health
http://nccam.nih.gov/
  This branch of the NIH investigates
complementary therapies used in clinical
trials in various locations throughout the
country.

National Council on Alcoholism and
  Drug Dependence (NCADD)
12 West 21st Street 7th Floor

New York, NY 10010
(212) 206–6770l (800) 622–2255
http://www.ncadd.org

National Institute on Alcohol Abuse and
  Alcoholism (NIAAA)
Suite 409, Willco Building
6000 Executive Boulevard
MSC 7003
Bethesda, MD 20892
(301) 443–3860
http://www.niaaa.nih.gov/

National Institute of Allergy and Infectious Diseases (NIAID)
NIAID Office of Communications
Building 31, Room 7A-50
31 Center Drive MSC 2520
Bethesda, MD 20982
(301) 496–5717
http://www.niaid.nih.gov

National Institute of Diabetes & Digestive & Kidney Diseases (NIDDK)
2 Information Way
Bethesda, MD 20892
(301) 654–3810
http://www.niddk.nih.gov
email: nddic@aerie.com

The National Institutes for Health (NIH)
Virology Section of the National Cancer
  Institute
31 Center Drive MSC 2580
Bethesda, MD 20892
(800) 4-CANCER (422–6237)
http://www.nih.gov

National Institutes of Health, Office of
  Dietary Supplements
http://www.dietary-supplements.info.
  nih.gov/

U.S. Department of Health and Human
  Services (USDHHS)
200 Independence Avenue, S.W.
Washington, D.C. 20201
(877) 696–6775
http://www.hhs.gov/

USDHSS Agency for Healthcare Research
  and Quality
540 Gaither Road
Rockville, MD 20850
(302) 427–1364
http://www.ahrq.gov/

World Health Organization
http://www.who.int/

CDC Publications

*Guidelines for Laboratory Testing and
Result Reporting of Antibody to Hepatitis C Virus.* CDC Morbidity and Mortality Weekly Report, Feb. 7, 2003, vol.
52/No. RR-3.

*Prevention and Control of Infections with
Hepatitis Viruses in Correctional Set-
tings.* CDC Morbididty and Mortality
Weekly Report, Jan. 24, 2003, vol. 52/
No. RR-1.

*Prevention of Hepatitis A Through Active
or Passive Immunization: Recommen-
dations of the Advisory Committee on
Immunization Practices (ACIP).* CDC
Morbidity and Mortality Weekly Report,
Oct. 1, 1999, vol. 48/No. RR-12.

*Recommendations for Prevention and Con-
trol of Hepatitis C Virus (HCV) Infection and HCV-Related Chronic Disease.*
CDC Morbidity and Mortality Weekly
Report, Oct. 16, 1998, vol. 47/No. RR-
19.

*Recommendations for Preventing Trans-
mission of Infections Among Chronic
Hemodialysis Patients.* CDC Morbidity
and Mortality Weekly Report, Apr. 27,
2002, vol. 50/No.RR-5.

Hotlines

American Liver Foundation Hotlines
(800) GO LIVER (465–4837)
  Help for patients and their families.

CDC Viral Hepatitis Hotline
(888) 4HEPCDC (443–7232)
  Hotline provides recorded information, fact sheets by fax, and an option to
speak to a counselor about viral hepatitis
issues.

Hep-C-Alert
Hepatitis C Hotline
(877) HELP-4-HEP
  Assistance and information for people
infected with hepatitis C.

HIV/AIDS/Hepatitis C Nightline
(800) 273-AIDS or (415) 434-AIDS (from
5P.M.–5A.M. Pacific time)
Spanish language hotline (800) 303-
SIDA or (415) 989–5212.

National Center for Nutrition and Diet-
ics Consumer Nutrition Hotline
(800) 366–1655

Educational Hepatitis Resources Online

Note: additional resources for Hepatitis C are listed after Hepatitis Organizations and foundations.

American Medical Association
http://www.ama-assn.org

British Liver Trust
http://www.britishlivertrust.org.uk

Diseases of the Liver
Columbia Presbyterian Hospital
http://www.cumc.columbia.edu/dept/gi/
disliv.html

EMedicine
Internet resource with comprehensive
articles on various medical conditions
and symptoms written by physicians from
various specialties including emergency
medicine with comprehensive information on hepatitis.
http://www.emedicine.com

Frontline Hepatitis Awareness
http://www.frontline-hepatitis-awareness.
com

Health on the Net Foundation
http://www.hon.ch/
Maintained by a non-profit Swiss
organization dedicated to accurate
healthcare information; websites are
inspected regularly and must meet certain regulations for documentation of
sources.

HepatitisActivist
http://www.hepatitistactivist.org
Hepatitis Central
http://www.hepatitis-central.com
Information on herbal medicine and

resources for hepatitis B and C; email
support list

Hepatitis Education Project
4603 Aurora Ave. N.
Seattle, WA 98103
(206) 732–0311
http://www.scn.org/health/hepatitis/
Non-profit organization which provides educational materials, a free newsletter, and support groups for hepatitis
patients and their families online and
through local chapters in the Pacific
Northwest region.

Hepatitis Information Network
http://www.hepnet.com
Excellent resource providing updates
on patient care issues, the latest research,
reports from guest speakers, news releases.

Hepatitis Neighborhood
Resource of the Priority Healthcare Corporation
http://www.hepatitisneighborhood.com
Excellent resource providing email alerts
announcing guest speakers and inservices;
regularly updated with current information, links to journal articles and more.

Hepatitis Online (Heponline)
http://www.heponline.net

Hepatitis Place
http://www.hepplace.com
Privately funded medical information
resource center for health professionals
and hepatitis patients.

Hepatitis Zone
http://www.hep-help.com
Provides facts and informative articles
on hepatitis and the liver.

Infectious Diseases Society of America
http://www.idsociety.org
Information on hepatitis, emerging
infectious diseases, with links to journal
articles and conference information.

Liver-Related World Wide Websites
University of California, San Francisco
http://hepar-sfgh.ucsf.edu/

Medicine.Net Liver Disease
http://www.medicinenet.com/liver/

Hepatitis Organizations and Foundations

These organizations and foundations provide educational and support resources.

American Association for the Study of Liver Diseases
1729 Kings Street Suite 1000
Alexandria, VA 22134
(703) 299–9766

The American Gastroenterological Association
http://www.gasro.org

The American Liver Foundation
75 Maiden Lane, Suite 603
New York, NY 10038
(800) Go Liver (465–4837); 888 4-HEP-ABC (443–7222)
http://www.liverfoundation.org
email: info@liverfoundation.org

Digestive Disorders Associates
Anne Arundel Medical Center
Sajak Building Conference Room
Annapolis, MD
(410) 224–4887, ext 432
Northeast Region support group with meetings first Monday of each month from 6:30–8:30 P.M.

Family Health International
P.O. Box 13950
Research Triangle Park, NC 27709
(919) 544–7040
http://www.fhi.org

Hepatitis B Foundation
700 East Butler Avenue
Doylestown, PA 18901–2697
(215) 489–4900
http://www.hepb.org
The Hepatitis B Foundation is a national non-profit organization solely dedicated to the global problem of hepatitis B; it provides educational resources for patients, healthcare professionals, families and researchers.

Hepatitis Foundation International
30 Sunrise Terrace
Cedar Grove, NJ 07009–1423
(800) 891–0707
http://www.hepfi.org

Infectious Diseases Society of America (IDSA)
IDSA provides information on STDs and emerging infectious diseases; links to journal articles and conference information.
http://www.idsociety.org

International Hepatitis Society
1804 Fifth Street
Berkeley, CA 94710
(510) 540–0920

Hepatitis C Organizations and Internet Resources

Alternative Hope for Hepatitis C
http://www.alternativehopeforhepc.com/
Provides information on diet and nutritional supplements including the antioxidant microhydrin.

American College of Gastroenterology (ACG)
P.O. Box 3099
Arlington, VA 22302
http://www.acg.gi.org/

Hamilton Hepatitis C Network
http://www.hamiltonhepc.net

HCV Advocate
http://www.HCVadvocate.org
Web site founded by activist Alan Franciscus offers comprehensive information on medical, social and political aspects of HCV, and alternative and Eastern therapies; includes a printed newsletter.

HCV Anonymous
http://www.hcvanonymous.com
This comprehensive website contains links, a chat group, bulletin board, current information, information on government resources, article links, free HCV e-books, FAQs, and personal stories.

Hep C Alert
(877) HELP-4-HEP
Hep-C Alert is a non-profit organization dedication to raising public awareness

and providing resources for individuals infected with HCV and other hepatitis viruses; offers a toll-free hotline for hepatitis C counseling and media support.
http://www.hep-c-alert.org

Hepatitis C:An Epidemic for Anyone
http://www.epidemic.org/index2.html

Hepatitis C Association
1351 Cooper Road
Scotch Plains, NJ 07076–4377
(866) 437–4377
http://www.hepcassoc.org/

The Hep C Connection
http://www.hepc-connection.org
email hepc-connection@worldnet.att.net

Hepatitis C Council of Victoria Inc, Australia
http://home.vicnet.net.au/~hepcvic/infof.htm

Hepatitis C Educational and Prevention Society
http://www.hepcbc.org/

Hepatitis C Info
http://www.hcop.org
Includes resources, FAQ, prevention information, articles

Janis & Friends Hepatitis C /Support
http://janis7hepc.com
Excellent resource with current information, resources and links

Hepatitis and HIV (AIDS Virus) Co-Infection Resources

CDC's FAQ about HIV and HCV co-infection
http://faq/HIV-HCV_coinfection.htm

Community Prescription Service
P.O. Box 1937, Old Chelsea Station
New York, NY 10113
(800) 842–0502
http://www.prescript.com
Publishes a free booklet, *Double Jeopardy*, with valuable information about co-infection with hepatitis C and HIV,

that can be downloaded or ordered by calling.

Hepatitis C Advocacy and Action Coalition (HAAC)
530 Divisadero Street #162
San Francisco, CA 94117
San Francisco email: haac_sf@hotmail.com
New York email: James_Learned@prodigy.net

HIV and Hepatitis Support
www.hivandhepatitis.com
An excellent resource regularly updated with information on HIV, HBV and HCV and co-infections with HIV and hepatitis, including information from 2005 3rd annual International Hepatitis Society Conference.

National AIDS Treatment Advocacy Project (NATP)
www.natap.org
This very informative site provides the latest information on HIV and co-infection with HIV and hepatitis.

National alliance of State and Territorial AIDS Directors (NASTAD)
NASTAD Viral Hepatitis Program
http://www.nastad.org/pro_viral_hepatitis.asp?menu=pro

The Body, An AIDS and HIV Information Resource
http://www.thebody.com

Drug and Alcohol Abuse and Toxins Resources

Advocates for the Integration of Recovery & Methadone
http://www.afirmfwc.org

Agency for Toxic Substances and Disease Registry
1600 Clifton Road NE, Building 16
Atlanta, GA 30333
(888) 422–8737
http://www.atsdr.cdc.gov/DRO/DRO-home.html

Alcoholics Anonymous (AA) World Services, Inc.

475 Riverside Drive, 11th Floor
New York, NY 10115
(212) 870–3400
http://www.aa.org/

Annie Appleseed Project
Excellent resource for drug and herb toxicity.
http://www.annieappleseedproject.org/

Center for Drug Evaluation and Research (CDER)
Food and Drug Administration
http://www.fda.gov/cder/

Curezone Toxins Resource
http://curezone.com/diseases/toxins

Drug-Induced Liver Injury: A National and Global Problem
Conference Proceedings of the CDER, February 2001
http://www.fda.gov/cder/livertox/stateArt.htm

MEDWATCH
Food and Drug Administration
5600 Fisher's Lane
Rockville, MD 20852
(800) 332–1088
http://www.fda.gov

Narcotics Anonymous World Service Office
PO Box 9999
Van Nuys, CA 91409
(818) 773–9999
http://www.na.org/

National Acupuncture Detoxification Association (NADA) Clearinghouse
3220 N Street N.W. Suite 275
Washington, D.C. 20007
(503) 222–1362
http://www.acupuncture.com
Excellent resource with information on herbal medicine and toxins.

National Association of Addiction Treatment Providers
313 W. Liberty Street, Suite 129
Lancaster, PA 17603–2748
(717) 392–8480
http://www.naatp.org/home.php

National Council on Alcoholism and Drug Dependence, Inc. (NCADD)
20 Exchange Place, Suite 2902
New York, NY 10005
(212) 269–7797
http://www.ncadd.org/

National Institute on Alcohol Abuse and Alcoholism (NIAAA)
5635 Fishers Lane, MSC 9304
Bethesda, MD 20892–9304
http://www.niaaa.nih.gov/
Links to publications, databases, clinical trials, and conferences.

National Institute on Drug Abuse (NIDA)
6001 Executive Boulevard, Room 5213
Bethesda, MD 20892–9561
(301) 443–1124
http://www.nida.nih.gov/
Information on all specific drugs of abuse and testing; drug information resources for health professionals, students, and parents.

Substance Abuse and Mental Health Services Administration (SAMHSA)
National Mental Health Information Center
PO Box 42557
Washington, D.C. 20015
(800) 789–2647
http://www.mentalhealth.org
http://www.samhsa.gov/index.aspx
SAMHSA Substance Abuse Treatment Facility Locator Service
http://findtreatment.samhsa.gov/facility-locatordoc.htm

Autoimmune Hepatitis Resources

American Association Autoimmune and Related Diseases Association
www.http://www.aarda.org
This site provides educational resources and publishes a monthly newsletter, *InFocus*, with information on research news, clinical trials, support and resources.

Autoimmune Diseases On-Line
http://www.autoimmune-disease.com/

Colleen's Autoimmune Hepatitis
http://members.tripod.com/~ddterry/col
leen/story.html

Emedicine on Autoimmune Hepatitis
http://www.emedicine.com/med/topic366.
htm

Hepatitis Central Resources
http://hepatitis-central.com/HCV/
autoimmune/toc.html

Metabolic Hepatitis Resources

The Alpha 1 Foundation
http://www.alphaone.org
This site provides information on Alpha
1 antitrypsin deficiency

American Hemochromatosis Society, Inc.
http://www.americanhs.org
Fatty Liver: NAFLD and NASH
MedicineNet.com
http://www.medicine.net.com/fatty.liver/
index.htm/

Galactosemia Page
http://www.galactosemia.org/galactosemia.
htm

Galactosemia Resources and Information
http://www.galactosemia.com/
Excellent resource with food lists, support group links

Hemochromatosis Foundation
P.O. Box 8569
Albany, NY 12208

Hemochromatosis, WebMD
http://mywebmd.com/hw/blood_
disorders/shc29hem.asp

Hereditary Fructose Laboratory at Boston
University
http://www.bu.edu/aldolase/HFI/diagnosis
/index.html

Iron Disorders Institute
http://www.irondisorders.org

Iron Overload Disease Association Inc.
(Hemochromatosis)
http://www.ironoverload.org

National Institute of Digestive Diseases
Information on Hemochromatosis
http://www.niddk.nih.gov/health/hematol/
pubs/hemoch/hemoc.htm

Wilson's Disease Association
4 Navaho Drive
Brookfield, CT 06804
(800) 39900266; (203) 775–9666
http://www.wilsonsdisease.org

Wilson's Disease Association International
http://wilsonsdisease.org

Wilson's Disease Information
National Digestive Diseases Information
Clearinghouse
http://digestive.niddk.nih.gov/ddiseases/
pubs/wilson

Pediatric Hepatitis Support Resources

Advocates for Youths
1025 Vermont Avenue NW, Suite 200
Washington, D.C. 20005
(202) 347–5700
http://www.advocatesforyouth.org

American Social Health Association Teen
Information
http://www.iwannaknow.org

Children's Liver Alliance
http://www.liverkids.org.au/

Australian resource dedicated to education on liver diseases and transplants.
Children's Liver Disease Foundation
http://www.childliverdisease.org
UK site with information on children's
liver diseases

Go Ask Alice
http://www.goaskalice.columbia.edu
Internet and bulletin board from
Columbia University's Health Education
Programs, providing health information
for teens on various health topics from
health educators, physicians, and researchers.

Parents of Kids with Infectious Diseases
http://www.pkids.org/

Excellent resource with information on hepatitis, AIDS, vaccines, and research.

Pediatric Viral Hepatitis Treatment
http://www.hepatitis.org/hepaetenfant_angl.htm

Viral Hepatitis Pediatric Advisor
http://www.medinformation.com/ac/crsa.nsf/file/crs-pa-hhg.hepatitis

Mental Health Resources

American Psychiatric Association (APA)
1000 Wilson Boulevard, Suite 825
Arlington, VA 22209–3901
(703) 907–733
http://www.psych.org/index.cfm

Center for Mental Health Services
Rm 12–105 Parklawn Building
5600 Fishers Lane
Rockville, MD 20857
(301) 443–8956
http://www.mentalhealth.samhsa.gov/

Freedom from Fear
308 Seaview Avenue
Staten Island, NY 10305
(718) 351–1717
http://www.freedomfromfear.com
    Excellent resource for teens and adults coping with stress related to disease.

National Institute of Mental Health
6001 Executive Boulevard, Room 8184, MSC 9663
Bethesda, MD 20892–9663
(866) 615–6464 (TollFree)
http://www.nimh.nih.gov

Clinical Trial Information

American Cancer Society, Diabetes Association and Heart Association
http://www.patientINFORM.org
    Information about trials involving cancer, heart disease, and diabetes.

Hepatitis B Foundation
Clinical Trials
http://www.hepb.org

Cancer Information Service (virology studies)
http://cancer.gov/clinical_trials

Centerwatch Clinical Trials: Hepatitis
http://www.centerwatch.com/studies/cat79.htm

Clinical Trials Database
http://www.emergingMed.com/

Clinical Trials, National Library of Medicine
Service of the U.S. National Institutes of Health
Linking Patients to Medical Research
http://www.clinicaltrials.gov

Columbia University
Research and Clinical Trials in Liver Disease
http://hora.cpmc.columbia.edu/dept/liverMD/researchtrials2.html

CRISP Computer Retrieval of Information
National Institutes of Health Scientific Projects
http://crisp.cit.nih.gov/CRISP

Medical Science Monitor
International Medical Journal for Experimental and Clinical Research
http://www.medscimonit.com/

Memorial Sloan-Kettering Cancer Center
1275 York Avenue
New York, NY 10021
(212) 639–2000
    Currently evaluating Japanese/Herbal Medicine for hepatitis C

National Center for Complementary and Alternative Medicine (NCCAM)
National Institutes of Health
http://nccam.nih.gov/
    NIH branch that investigates complementary and alternative medicine in clinical trials.

National Institutes of Health Clinical Research Studies Protocol Database
http://clinicalstudies.info.NIH.gov

University of Washington Virology Research Clinic
http://wwww.depts.washington.edu/

Veritas Medicine
Clinical Trials
http://www.veritasmedicine.com/HepatitisC

Drug Treatment Financial Assistance

Amgen (Manufacturer of Infergen)
Reimbursement Services
(888) 508–8088

Cancer Care Resource for Financial Assistance
http://www.cancercare.org/financialneeds/
financialneedslist.cfm?c=387
Links to many financial assistance medical assistance.

Directory of Prescription Drug Patient Assistance Programs
Pharmaceutical Research and Manufacturers of America
(800) 762–4636

Drug Company Patient Contacts
http://www.aegis.com/pubs/cria/2004/
cro41010.html

Epivir Patient Assistance, GlaxoWellcome
GlaxoSmithKline
(800) 722–9294
http://www.thebody.com/updates/2004–06
–16.html
Financial Assistance for People with HIV and Hepatitis

Free Medicine Foundation
http://www.freemedicinefoundation.com/
(573)-996–3333
Established by volunteers, this foundations helps patients eliminate or substantially reduce their prescription drug bills.

Gilead Patient Assistance Programs for Antivirals, Hep B meds
(800) 226–2056

Medical Needs Program
340 Kingland Street
Nutley, NJ 07110
(888) 300-PATH; (800) 285–4484
Hepsera for HBV made by Hoffman La Roche (Manufacturer of Roferon-A Interferon)

Infergen Assistance
InterMune Company
(888) 696–803

Medicare Replacement Drugs Demonstration
http://www.cms.hhs.gov/researchers/demos
/drugcoveragedemo.asp

Needy Meds
http://www.NeedyMeds.com

Ontario HepC Assistance Plan
http://www.health.gov/on.ca/english/
public/project/hepc/hepc.html

Partnership for Prescription Assistance
(888) 477–2669
http://www.pparx.org
Founded in 2005, this coalition of biopharmaceutical research companies, doctors, other health care providers, patient advocacy organizations, and community groups have joined forces to help qualifying patients who lack prescription coverage obtain needed medicines.

Pegasys/Copegus Assist
Roche Pegassist
(877) 734–2797

Roferon A Assistance
Roche
(877) 757–6243, option 4

RX Assist
http://www.rxassist.org

Schering-Plough Corporation (Manufactures Intron A, Peg-Intron, Rebetrol, and Rebetron)
Kenilworth, New Jersey
Schering's Commitment to Care Program
(800) 521–7157 (ext 147 for financial assistance)
http://www.hep-help.com

The Medicine Program
http://www.themedicineprogram.com

Antiviral Drug Resources

CDC consensus statement on viral load
http://www.cdc.gov/ncidod/diseases/
hepatitis
http://www.aasid.org/pdffiles/chronic
hepatolendorse.pdf

U.S. Food and Drug Administration (FDA)
http://www.fda.gov
(800) 593–2214

Ribavirin in Pregnancy
http://www.ribavirininpregnancy
registry.com

Roche Drug Safety Department
(800) 526–6367

Laboratory Test Interpretation

The Blood Book
http://www.bloodbook.com
This site has information about laboratory tests and blood products.

Common Lab Tests for Liver Disease
http://cpmcnet.columbia.edu/dept/gi/lab
tests.html

Home Access Laboratory Testing for HCV
(888) 888-HEPC
http://www.homeaccess.com

Laboratory Tests Online
http://www.labtestsonline.org
Free service with description of laboratory tests and interpretive values provided by the American Society of Clinical Pathologists.

Medical Tests
HealthEast Care System
http://yourhealth.healtheast.org/Library/
HealthGuide/MedicalTests/Default.htm
Free service providing information about laboratory and imaging tests.

Normal Lab Values & Explanations.
http://www.askemilyss.com/Livrtest.htm

National Center for Biotechnology Information
http://www.ncbi.nlm.nih.gov
This office of the NIH has information on laboratory tests and reference ranges.

The Virtual Hospital
http://www.vh.org
Numerous educational resources including laboratory test information.

Biopsy and Pathology Information

Dr. Greenson's Gastrointestinal and Liver
Pathology Page

http://www.pathology.med.umich.edu/
greensonlab/

Grading & Staging of Liver Biopsy
http://tpis.upmc.edu/tpis/schema/mHAI.
html

Hepatology Links of Interest
http://www.il-st-acad-sci.org/health/
liver.html

Liver and Biliary Disease by the Pathguy
(Dr. Ed Friedlander)
http://www.pathguyy.com/lectures/liver.
htm

Transplant Information

Children's Organ Transplant Association
http://www.cota.org

The James Redford Institute for Transplant Awareness
http://www.jrifilms.org/myths.html

National Foundation for Transplants
http://www.transplants.org

National Transplant Assistance Fund
http://www.transplantfund.org

Organ Procurement and Transplantation Network
http://www.optn.org/

The Tiger Fund
Helping Needy Organ Donor & Transplant Families
http://www.tigerfund.org/

Transplant Rejection
http://www.1uphealth.com/health/
transplant_rejection_info.html

Transweb
http://www.transweb.org/
Information, FAQs on organ transplants and donation

United Network for Organ Sharing Transplants (UNOS)
http://www.unos.org

Blood Products and Transfusions

American Association of Blood Banks
http://www.aabb.org

Premier organization established in 1947 to promote excellence in transfusion medicine. Inspects and certifies hospital blood banks and provides educational resources.

College of American Pathologists
http://www.cap.org
Organization that regulates laboratory medicine, including transfusion medicine, comprised of members of the American Society of Clinical Pathologists. Provides guidelines and criteria for transfusion medicine, inspects and certifies blood banks and provides numerous educational resources.

The American Red Cross (ARC)
http://www.arc.org
ARC is the largest single blood supplier in the United States. The ARC has a consent agreement with the FDA in which the two organizations work together to ensure the safety of the blood products manufactured by the ARC.

Food and Drug Administration Regulations for Blood Banks
http://www.fda.gov/cber

Joint Commission Accreditation Agency for Hospitals
http://www.jcaho.org

Prison Support

Morbidity and Mortality Weekly Report Centers for Disease Control and Prevention
Prevention and Control of Infections with Hepatitis Viruses in Correctional Settings
January 24, 2003 Bulletin 52, RR-1
Electronic copy available at http://www.cdc.gov/mmwr

National HCV Prison Coalition
http://www.hcvinprison.org
This organization, which is funded by the Robert Wood Johnson Foundation, was formed for the advocacy and support of prisoners with hepatitis and HIV/HCV co-infection.

Disability Information

Social Security Disability and Benefits Law
http://www.severe.net/

Social Security
www.ssa.gov/disability

Alternative Medicine Resources

Alternative Medicine Information Sauce
http://www.alternative-medicine-info.com

American Association of Oriental Medicine (AAOM)
433 Front Street
Catasauqpa, PA 18032–2506
(610) 266–1433
http://www.aaom.org
Provides a listing of practitioners

Food and Healing
The website of Annemarie Colbin, Ph.D.
http://www.foodandhealing.com
Information on nutrition and healing, holistic healing philosophies, links to articles.

Healingpeople.com
http://www.healingpeople.com
This Web site contains a listing of acupuncturists and naturopaths in the United States; provides information on all aspects of Chinese medicine for practitioners and consumers; includes links and excerpts from *The Chinese Way to Healing:Many Paths to Wholeness* and from *The HIV Wellness Sourcebook.*

Health Central
http://www.healthcentral.com
Dr. Dean Edell's Web site contains sections on alternative and complementary therapies, including a Hepatitis Conditions Center with numerous resources.

Herbal Medicine Resource
http://www.herbalremedies.com

Institute for Traditional Medicine
2017 S.E. Hawthorne Boulevard

Portland, OR 97214
(503) 233–4907
http://www.itmonline.org
   Includes a listing of traditional medicine practitioners and resources and information on herbal medicine.

Integrative Medical Arts Group
P.O. Box 308
Beaverton, OR 97075
http://www.HealthWWWeb.com
   Provides resources and information for integrative health care and educational services for patients and healthcare providers; inlcudeing Interactive Body/Mind Information System information and software.

M.D. Anderson Cancer Center
http://www.mdanderson.org/departments/
   CIMER

Memorial Sloan-Kettering Cancer Center's About Herbs Database
http://www.mskcc.org/mskcc/html/11571.
   cfm?RecdID=441&tab=HC

National Acupuncture and Oriental Medicine Alliance (NAOMA)
14637 Starr Road S.E.
Olalla, WA 98359
(253) 851–6896
   Professional membership organization of acupuncturists, Asian medicine providers and acupuncture-related organizations.

National Association for Alternative Medicine
158 Lafayette Street
Colusa, CA 95932
http://naam-liver.1le.org/

National Center for Complementary and Alternative Medicine (NCCAM)
National Institutes of Health
http://nccam.nih.gov/

National Institutes of Health, Office of Dietary Supplements
http:///wwww.dietary-supplements.info.
   nih.gov/

Alternative and Integrationist Clinics

Integrationists are physicians who use a combination of Eastern and Western medicine.

Body Health
20351 Irvine Ave Suite C-2
Santa Ana Heights, CA 92707
Email: energyscan@sbcglobal.net
   Exclusively, alternative therapies L.I.F.E. advanced biofeedback, colon hydrotherapy, custom mineral blends, lymph drainage, massage.

Center for Complementary Healing and Wellness
2265 Livernois Suite 500
Troy, MI 48083
http://www.cchw-troy.com
   Exclusively alternative therapies

City Clinic
356 Seventh Street
San Francisco, CA
(415) 487–5500
   Provides education and counseling services, hepatitis A and B vaccinations, women's health; STD testing; services are private and either free or low cost.

The Continuum Center for Health & Healing
Dr. Woodson Merrell
http://www.healthandhealingNY.org

DocMisha, Author of the Hepatitis C Help Book
Chicken Soup Chinese Medicine
3128 16th Street
San Francisco, CA 94103–3328
(415) 864–7234
Hep C workshop information email:
   TCMPaths@aol.com
Consultations, appointments email:
   CHINMEDSF@aol.com
http://www.docmisha.com
   Misha Cohen's Web site contains information on the treatment of hepatitis and HIV with acupuncture, herbs, Chinese medicine; includes question and answer forum.

Fenway Community Health Center
7 Haviland Street
Boston, MA 02115
(617) 267–0900
   Outpatient clinic with primary care services, massage and acupuncture for detox and chemical addiction.

Millenium Healthcare
4370 Georgetown Square
Atlanta, GA 30338
http://www.millenium-healthcare.com
   Holistic medicine and surgery, traditional Chinese medicine, Chelation, NAET, Reiki, Holistic family practice.

Olive Leaf Wholeness Center
145 E. 23rd Street
(212) 477–0405
http://www.oliveleafwholenesscenter.com
   Independent holistic and integrative healing modalities; clinical services and a diversified group of practitioners in both conventional and alternative medicine.

Pathways to Wellness
110 Main St. Lower Level #4
East Greenwich, RI 02818
(401) 884–0366
Email: pathways@helloworld.com
   Alternative therapies only, naturopathic doctor consults, nutritional consultations, herbal pharmacy.

Wei de Ren Clinic
Dr. Wei de Ren, M.D.
Treatment for Hepatitis and Cirrhosis Infection
Traditional Chinese Herbal Medicine
99 University Place, Room #201
New York, NY 10003
http://www.dr-ren.com

Zhang's Clinic
420 Lexington Avenue, #631
New York, NY 10170–0632
(212) 573–9584
www.dr-zhang.com
   Featured in articles by Dr. Andrew Weil on self-healing, Dr. Zhang specializes in the treatment of hepatitis C using alternative medicine.

Herbal and Alternative Product Resources

American Herbal Products Association
P.O. Box 2410
Austin, TX 78768
(512) 320–8555
http://www.ahpa.org
   This association provides a list of Eastern and Western herb suppliers.

Bob's Red Mill
(800) 552–2258
http://www.bobsredmill.com
   Natural food and grains.

Earthrise Nutritionals
http://www.earthrise.com
   Spirulina and other immune modulating products.

Enzymatic Therapy (for Thymuplex and Liquid Liver Extract with ginseng)
825 Challenger Drive
Green Bay, WI 54311
(800) 783–2286
http://www.enzy.com

Himalaya USA (for Liv.52/Livercare)
6950 Portwest Drive, Suite 170
Houston, TX 77024
(800) 869–4640
http://www.himalayausa.com

Kenshin Trading
1815 W. 213 Street, Suite 180
Torrance CA 90501
(800) 766–1313
Supplier of reishi mushrooms and other alternative products

Life Extension Foundation
1100 West Commercial Boulevard
Ft. Lauderdale, FK 33309
(800) 678–8989; (800) 644–4440
http://www.lef.org
   This company provides references to scientific abstracts and cutting-edge alternative medical information; supplier of vitamins, minerals, herbal and glandular products

Marilyn Neutraceuticals (for Hep-Forte)
14851 North Scottsdale Road
Scottsdale, AZ 85254

(800) 899–4499
http://www.naturallyvitamins.com

Mayway China Native Herbs and Produce
1338 Mandela Parkway
Oakland, CA 94607
(510) 208–3113
http://www.mayway.com
　One of the largest and most reputable
supplies of Chinese herbal medicines.

Neem America Incorporated
http://www.neemamerica.org

Neem Tree Farms
http://www.neemtreefarms.com

Tao of Herbs
3340 S. Wallace Street
Chicago, IL 60616
(312) 881–0078
(888) 828–8228
http://www.taoofherbs.com

References

1. Appold, Karen. "Overcoming hepatitis testing hurdles." *Advance for Medical Laboratory Professionals.* 16(9), May 3, 2004: 20–22.

2. Armstrong, Donald, and Jonathan Cohen. *Infectious Diseases.* Philadelphia: Mosby, 1999: 350–375.

3. Banks, Malcom, Richard Bendall, Sylvia Grierson, Graham Hath, and Jonathan Mitchell. "Human and Porcine Hepatitis E Virus Strains, United Kingdom." *Emerging Infectious Diseases* 10(5), May 204: 953–955.

4. Bianchi, L., and F. Gudat. "Chronic hepatitis." Chapter 9 in *Pathology of the Liver.* 3rd ed. Edited by Roderick Mac-Sween. London: Churchill Livingstone, 1994: 349–362.

5. Birnkrant, Arthur. "Cutaneous Manifestations of Hepatitis C." Available on-line at eMedicine.com. www.emedicine. com/derm/topic850.htm. Accessed 2004.

6. Blumberg, Baruch. S. *Hepatitis B, The Hunt for a Killer Virus.* Princeton, New Jersey: Princeton University Press, 2002: 84–118.

7. Brechot, Christian, and Bertrand Nalpas. Interactions between alcohol and hepatitis viruses in the liver." Chapter 2 in *Clinics in Laboratory Medicine, Hepatitis and Chronic Liver Disease.* Edited by Mark Feitelson and Mark Zern. Philadelphia: W. B. Saunders, 273–282.

8. Buggs, Adrienne. "Hepatitis. Available online at eMedicine.com. www. e.medicine.com/EMERG/topic244.htm. Accessed August. 2004.

9. Buhner, Stephen. *Herbs for Hepatitis C and the Liver.* North Adams, Massachusetts: Storey Books, 2000: 14–53.

10. Burt, a.d., and O. F. James. "Pathophysiology of the liver." Chapter 3 in *Pathology of the Liver.* 3rd ed. Edited by Roderick MacSween. London: Churchill Livingstone, 1994: 51–57.

11. Carman, William. "Molecular variants of hepatitis B virus." Chapter 10 in *Clinics in Laboratory Medicine, Hepatitis and Chronic Liver Disease.* Edited by Mark Feitelson and Mark Zern. Philadelphia: W.B. Saunders, 1996: 407–428.

12. Casey, John. "Hepatitis delta virus," Chapter 12 in *Clinics in Laboratory Medicine, Hepatitis and Chronic Liver Disease.* Edited by Mark Feitelson and Mark Zern. Philadelphia: W.B. Saunders, 1996: 451–462.

13. Centers for Disease Control and Prevention. Guidelines for laboratory testing and result reporting of antibody to hepatitis C virus. MMWR 2003, 52 (No. RR-3): 1–6.

14. Centers for Disease Control and Prevention, National Center for HIV, STD and TB Prevention. A comprehensive approach: Preventing blood-borne

infections among injection drug users, 2002. Online at www.cdc.gov/idu/Pubs/ca/chapter1.htm.

15. Centers for Disease Control and Prevention, National Center for Infectious Diseases, Guidelines for viral hepatitis surveillance and case management, 2004. Online at www.cdc.gov/ncidod/diseases/hepatitis/resource/surveillance.htm.

16. Centers for Disease Control and Prevention. Prevention and control of infections with hepatitis viruses in correctional settings. MMWR 2003; 52 (No. RR-1):13–20.

17. Centers for Disease Control and Prevention. Prevention of hepatitis A through active or passive immunization: recommendations of the Advisory Committee on Immunization Practices (ACIP). MMWR 1999; 48 (No. RR-12): 3–14.

18. Centers for Disease Control and Prevention. Recommendations for preventing transmission of infections among chronic hemodialysis patients. MMWR 2001; 50 (No. RR-5): 1–12.

19. Centers for Disease Control and Prevention. Recommendations for prevention and control of hepatitis C virus (HCV) infection and HCV-related chronic disease. MMWR 1998; 47 (No. RR-19): 18–33.

20. Centers for Disease Control and Prevention, Special Pathogens Branch. Questions and Answers about Marburg Hemorrhagic Fever, March 30, 2005. Online at www.cdc.gov/ncidod/dvrd/apb/mnpages/dispages/marburg/qa.htm.

21. Centers for Disease Control and Prevention. Updated U.S. Public Health Service guidelines for the management of occupational exposures to HBV, HCV, and HIV and recommendations for postexposure prophylaxis. MMWR 2001, 50 (No. RR-11): 2–9.

22. Chopra, Sanjiv. *Dr. Sanjiv Chopra's Liver Book: A Comprehensive Guide to Diagnosis, Treatment and Recovery.* New York: Simon and Schuster, 2001: 235–268.

23. Cohen, Misha, and Robert Gish. *The Hepatitis C Help Book.* New York: St. Martin's Press, 2000: 220–262.

24. Cook, Janine and Nancy Hooper. "Managing the immune response in transplantation." *Advance for Medical Laboratory Professionals,* 15(18) Aug 25, 2003:13–15.

25. Cuthbert, Jennifer. "Hepatitis A: Old and New." *Clinical Microbiology Review* (14)1, 2001: 39–58.

26. The Doctor's Prescription for Healthy Living. *Healing Hepatitis Naturally.* Topanga, California: Freedom Press, 2004: 11–50.

27. Dodd, R.Y., et.al. "Current prevalence and incidence of infectious disease markers and estimated window-period risk in the American Red Cross blood donor population." *Transfusion* 42, August 2002: 975–979.

28. Dufour, Robert. "Laboratory approach to acute and chronic hepatitis." *Medical Laboratory Observer* 35(9), Sept. 2003: 10–16.

29. Farber, Emmanuel. "Alcohol and other chemicals in the development of hepatocellular carcinoma." Chapter 8 in *Clinics in Laboratory Medicine, Hepatitis and Chronic Liver Disease.* Edited by Mark Feitelson and Mark Zern. Philadelphia: W.B. Saunders, 1996: 377–391.

30. Feitelson, Mark. "Hepatocellular injury in hepatitis B and C virus infections." Chapter 4 in *Clinics in Laboratory Medicine, Hepatitis and Chronic Liver Disease* Edited by Mark Feitelson and Mark Zern. Philadelphia: W.B. Saunders, 1996: 307–319.

31. French, Samuel. "Ethanol and hepatocellular injury." Chapter 3 in *Clinics in Laboratory Medicine, Hepatitis and Chronic Liver Disease.* Edited by Mark Feitelson and Mark Zern. Philadelphia: W. B. Saunders, 1996: 289–301.

32. Grimm, Ian, and Nicholas Shaheen. "Treatment of chronic viral hepatitis." Chapter 67 in *Sexually Transmitted Diseases.* 3rd ed. Edited by King Holmes. New York: McGraw-Hill, 1999: 913–920.

33. Harris, Helen, Mary Ramsay, Nick Andrews and Keith Eldridge. "Clinical course of hepatitis C virus during the first decade of infection: cohort study." *British Medical Journal* (324), Feb. 23, 2002: 1–6.

34. Kao, Jia-Horng, Pei-Jer Chen, Ming-Yang Lai, and Ding-Shinn Chen. "Occult hepatitis B virus infection and clinical outcomes of patients with chronic hepatitis C." *Journal of Clinical Microbiology*, 40(11), Nov. 2002: 4068–4071.

35. Kew, Michael. "Hepatitis B and C viruses and hepatocellular carcinoma." Chapter 9 in *Clinics in Laboratory Medicine, Hepatitis and Chronic Liver Disease.* Edited by Mark Feitelson and Mark Zern. Philadelphia: W.B. Saunders, 1996: 395–403.

36. Larke, Bryce. et. al. "Acute nocosomial HCV infection detected by NAT of a regular blood donor." *Transfusion* 42, June 2002: 759–766.

37. Lee, William M. "Drug-Induced Hepatotoxicity." *The New England Journal of Medicine* 333(17), Oct. 26, 1995: 1118–1127.

38. Lemon, Stanley and Miriam Alter. "Viral hepatitis." Chapter 26 in *Sexually Transmitted Diseases.* 3rd ed. Edited by King Holmes. New York: McGraw-Hill, 1999: 362–384.

39. Lokere, Jillian. "Gradual weight loss improves liver biochemistry and histopathology in NAFLD." *Clinical Care Options for Hepatitis,* April 17, 2005.

40. Thomas W., London, and Alison Evans." The epidemiology of hepatitis viruses B, C, and D. Chapter 1 in *Clinics in Laboratory Medicine, Hepatitis and Chronic Liver Disease.* Edited by Mark Feitelson and Mark Zern. Philadelphia: W.B. Saunders, 1996: 251–267.

41. Macedo de Oliveeira, Alexandre, Kathryn White, Dennis Leschinsky, Brady Beecham, Tara Vot, Ronald Moolenaar, Joseph Perz, and Thomas Safranek. "An Outbreak of Hepatitis C Virus Infections Among Outpatients at a Hematology/Oncology Clinic." *Annals of Internal Medicine,* 11(42), 2005: 892–902.

42. Marrone, Aldo, and Richard Sallie. "Genetic heterogeneity of hepatitis C virus. "Chapter 11 in *Clinics in Laboratory Medicine, Hepatitis and Chronic Liver Disease.* Edited by Mark Feitelson and Mark Zern Philadelphia: W.B. Saunders, 1996: 429–446.

43. Mendler, Michel. "Fatty Liver: Nonalcoholic Fatty Liver Disease (NAFLD) and Nonalcoholic Steatohepatitis (NASH)." Online at MedicineNet.com, www.medicinenet.com/script/main/art.asp?articlekey=1909&pf=3. Accessed November 2002.

44. *The Merck Manual of Diagnosis and Therapy* 10th ed. Edited by Charles Lyght. New York: Merck, Sharpe and Dome Research Laboratories, 1962: 948–966.

45. Mondoa, Emil, and Mindy Kitel. *Sugars That Heal, The New Healing Science of Glyconutrients.* New York: Ballantine, 2001:150–162.

46. Palmer, Melissa. *Dr. Melissa Palmer's Guide to Hepatitis & Liver Disease.* Rev. ed. New York: Avery Penguin, 2004: 311–356.

47. Perricone, Nicholas. *The Perricone Promise.* New York: Times Warner Books, 2004: 18–28.

48. Peter, James. *Use and Interpretation of Tests in Infectious Disease.* 4th ed. Santa Monica, California: Specialty Laboratories, 1996: 127–139.

49. Polish, Louis. Margaret Gallagher, Howard Fields and Stephen Hadler. "Delta hepatitis: molecular biology and clinical and epidemiological features." *Clinical Microbiology Reviews.* July 1993: 211–229.

50. Pratt, Daniel. *55th Annual Meeting of the American Association for the Study of Liver Diseases, Viral Liver Disease, Developments in the Management of Hepatitis B.* Medscape CME Course, Dec. 2004. Available online at www.medscape.com/viewprogram/3672_pnt.

51. Roseff, Susan. "Regulatory and quality initiatives—trends in transfusion medicine." *LabMedicine* 36(2), Feb. 2005: 108–114.

52. Rothstein, Kenneth, and Santiago Munoz. "Interferon and other therapies for hepatitis B and hepatitis C infections." Chapter 13 in *Clinics in Laboratory Medicine, Hepatitis and Chronic Liver Disease.* Edited by Mark Feitelson and Mark Zern. Philadelphia: W.B. Saunders, 1996: 466–485.

53. Ryder, Stephen. "Hepatitis." Chap-

ter 39 *Infectious Diseases*, Volume I. New York: Mosby, 1999: 1–13.

54. Scheuer, Peter. *Liver Biopsy Interpretation*. 4th ed. London: Bailliére Tindall, 1988: 67–78.

55. Seeff, Leonard. "Why is there such difficulty in defining the natural history of hepatitis C?" *Transfusion* (40), Oct. 2000:1162–1163.

56. Sherlock, Sheila, and James Dooley. *Diseases of the Liver and Biliary System*. 9th ed. Cambridge, MA:Blackwell Scientific Publications, 1993: 260–335.

57. Simmonds, Peter. "The origin and evolution of hepatitis viruses in humans." *Journal of General Virology* (82), 2001: 693–712.

58. Snowbeck, Christopher "Hepatitis outbreak claims first fatality." *Pittsburgh Post-Gazette* online. Available at www. postgazette.com/neigh_west/20031108hepatitis1108pl.asp. Accessed Nov. 8, 2003.

59. Steinmann, Daniel J., Heidi Barth, Bettina Gissler, et. al. "Inhibition of hepatitis C virus-like particle binding to target cells by antiviral antibodies in acute and chronic hepatitis C." *Journal of Virology* (78) 17, Sept. 2004: 9030–9040.

60. Stroh, Michael. "Hepatitis C Fatality in Baltimore Shrouded in Mystery." *The Baltimore Sun*, Jan. 4, 2005.

61. Sulkowski, MS, SH Mehat, M Torbenson, et. al. "Hepatic steatosis and antiretroviral drug use among adults coinfected with HIV and hepatitis C virus." *AIDS* 19(6), April 2005: 585–592.

62. Tolman, Keith, and Robert Rej. "Liver Function." Chapter 33 in *Tietz Textbook of Clinical Chemistry* 3rd ed. edited by Carl Burtis and Edward Ashwoood. Philadelphia: W. B. Saunders Company, 1999: 1125–1158.

63. U.S. Preventive Services Task Force Press Release. "Screening for Hepatitis C in Adults." March 2004. Available online at www.ahrq.gov/clinic/uspstf/uspshepc.htm.

64. Vento, Sandro. "Fulminant Hepatitis Associated with Hepatitis A Virus Superinfection in Patients with Chronic Hepatitis C." *The New England Journal of Medicine* 338(5), Jan 29, 1998: 286–290.

65. "Viral Hepatitis Among Injection Drug Users." Fact sheet published by Injection Drug Use/HIV Prevention Division of the National Institutes of Health.

66. Wright, Lloyd. *Triumph Over Hepatitis C*. Malibu, California: Lloyd Wright Publishing, 2000: 214–224.

67. Wright, Lloyd. *Hepatitis C Free*. Malibu, CA Lloyd Wright Publishing, 2002:214–224: 109–141.

68. Zachou, Kalliopi. Eirini Rigopoulou, and George Datekos. "Autoantibodies and autoantigens in autoimmune hepatitis: important tools in clinical practice and to study pathogenesis of the disease." *Journal of Autoimmune Diseases* 1(2); 2004: Available online at http://www.jautoimdis.com/content/1/1/2.

69. Zein, Nizar. "Clinical significance of hepatitis C virus genotypes." *Clinical Microbiology Reviews*. April, 2000: 223–235.

70. Zimmerman, H. J., and K. Ishak. "Hepatic injury due to drugs and toxins." Chapter 15 in *Pathology of the Liver*. 3rd ed. Edited by Roderick MacSween London: Churchill Livingstone, 1994: 563–629.

71. Zuckerman, Jane, and Arie Zuckerman. "Hepatitis Viruses." Chapter 4 in *Infectious Diseases*. Vol II. Edited by Donald Armstrong and Jonathan Cohen. New York: Mosby, 1999: 1–14.

72. Zuger, A. "Caution: That Dose May Be Too High." *New York Times*, Sept. 17, 2002.

Index